ESSENTIAL EMERGENCY PROCEDURES

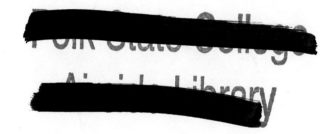

ESSENTIAL EMERGENCY PROCEDURES

Editor-in-Chief

Kaushal Shah, MD

Emergency Department Director of Trauma Services
St.Luke's-Roosevelt Hospital Center
University Hospital of Columbia University College of Physicians
and Surgeons
New York, New York

Associate Editor

Chilembwe Mason, MD

Attending
Department of Emergency Medicine
Bronx-Lebanon Hospital Center
Bronx, New York

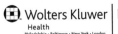 Wolters Kluwer | Lippincott Williams & Wilkins
Health
Philadelphia · Baltimore · New York · London
Buenos Aires · Hong Kong · Sydney · Tokyo

Acquisitions Editor: Frances DeStefano
Managing Editor: Nicole T. Dernoski
Project Manager: Alicia Jackson
Senior Manufacturing Manager: Benjamin Rivera
Marketing Manager: Angela Panetta
Creative Director: Doug Smock
Cover Designer: Shawn Girsberger
Production Service: Laserwords Private Limited, Chennai, India

Library of Congress Cataloging-in-Publication Data
Essential emergency procedures / [edited by] Kaushal Shah, Chilembwe Mason.
   p. ; cm.
  Includes bibliographical references and index.
  ISBN 978-0-7817-7490-1
  1. Emergency medicine–Handbooks, manuals, etc. I. Shah, Kaushal. II. Mason, Chilembwe.
  [DNLM: 1. Emergencies–Handbooks. 2. Emergency Medicine–methods–Handbooks. WB 39 E769 2008]
  RC86.8.E75 2008
  616.02'5–dc22

                                                                                    2007026925

Care has been taken to confirm the accuracy of the information presented and to describe generally accepted practices. However, the authors, editors, and publisher are not responsible for errors or omissions or for any consequences from application of the information in this book and make no warranty, expressed or implied, with respect to the currency, completeness, or accuracy of the contents of the publication. Application of the information in a particular situation remains the professional responsibility of the practitioner.

The authors, editors, and publisher have exerted every effort to ensure that drug selection and dosage set forth in this text are in accordance with current recommendations and practice at the time of publication. However, in view of ongoing research, changes in government regulations, and the constant flow of information relating to drug therapy and drug reactions, the reader is urged to check the package insert for each drug for any change in indications and dosage and for added warnings and precautions. This is particularly important when the recommended agent is a new or infrequently employed drug.

Some drugs and medical devices presented in the publication have Food and Drug Administration (FDA) clearance for limited use in restricted research settings. It is the responsibility of the health care provider to ascertain the FDA status of each drug or device planned for use in their clinical practice.

To purchase additional copies of this book, call our customer service department at (800) 638-3030 or fax orders to (301) 223-2320. International customers should call (301) 223-2300.

Visit Lippincott Williams & Wilkins on the Internet: at LWW.com. Lippincott Williams & Wilkins customer service representatives are available from 8:30 am to 6 pm, EST.

10 9 8 7 6 5

Dedication (Kaushal Shah)

I'd like to dedicate this book to all the attendings in my residency training program (Harvard Affiliated Emergency Medicine Residency at Beth Israel Deaconess Medical Center) and, specifically to my mentor, Jonathan Edlow. I will be forever indebted to them for making a significant impact on my world view. Because of them, I believed I could create a book such as this one.

I would also like to thank my wife, Vanisha Gilja Shah, who tolerated me through the making of this book and who is always supportive of my academic (in other words, nonlucrative) interests.

Dedication (Chilembwe Mason)

This is dedicated to the attendings from the University of Maryland School of Medicine, specifically Drs. Scalia, Brown, Cooper, and Bulter, who guided me as a student into the field of Emergency Medicine. Also, tremendous thanks to the entire residency program at St. Luke's-Roosevelt Hospital Center.

Contributors

Mitchell Adelstein, MD
Attending
Department of Emergency Medicine
St. Luke's-Roosevelt Hospital Center
New York, New York

Annie Akkara
Resident
Department of Emergency Medicine
St. Luke's-Roosevelt Hospital Center
New York, New York

Mara S. Aloi, MD
Assistant Professor
Department of Emergency Medicine
Drexel University School of Medicine
Philadelphia, Pennsylvania;
Residency Program Director
Department of Emeregncy Medicine
Allegheny General Hospital
Pittsburgh, Pennsylvania

Matthew R. Babineau, MD
Resident
Department of Emergency Medicine
Beth-Israel Deaconess Medical Center
Boston, Massachusetts

William Bagley
Chief Resident
Department of Emergency Medicine
St. Luke's-Roosevelt Hospital Center
New York, New York

Satchit Balsari, MBBS, MPH
Resident
Division of Emergency Medicine
New York-Presbyterian Hospital
New York, New York

Kevin M. Ban, MD
Instructor in Medicine
Division of Emergency Medicine
Harvard Medical School;
Attending Physician
Department of Emergency Medicine
Beth Israel Deaconess Medical Center
Boston, Massachusetts

David Barlas, MD
Assistant Professor
Department of Emergency Medicine
Weill College of Medicine
Cornell University;
Associate Residency Director
Department of Emergency Medicine
New York Hospital Medical Center
of Queens
Flushing, New York

Nelsson H. Becerra, MD
Emergency Ultrasound Fellow
and Attending Physician
Department of Emergency Medicine
St. Luke's-Roosevelt Hospital Center
Columbia University College of Physicians
and Surgeons
New York, New York

Anthony Berger, MD
Resident
Department of Emergency Medicine
New York Hospital Medical Center
of Queens
Queens, New York

David J. Berkoff, MD
Assistant Clinical Professor
Department of Surgery
Division of Emergency Medicine
and Sports Medicine
Duke University
Durham, North Carolina

Mitchell Bernstein, MD
Surgery Attending
Department of Surgery
St. Luke's-Roosevelt Hospital Center
Columbia University College of Physicians
and Surgeons
New York, New York

Elad Bicer, MD
Resident
Department of Emergency Medicine
St. Luke's-Roosevelt Hospital Center
New York, New York

Peter A. Binkley, MD
Resident
Department of Emergency Medicine
New York Hospital-Queens
Queens, New York

Evan Bloom, MD
Clinical Fellow in Medicine
Department of Emergency Medicine
Harvard University;
Resident
Department of Emergency Medicine
Beth Israel Deaconess Medical Center
Boston, Massachusetts

Elizabeth M. Borock, MD
Assistant Professor
Department of Emergency Medicine
New York University School of Medicine;
Attending Physician
Department of Emergency Medicine
New York University Hospital
Bellevue Hospital Center
New York, New York

David W. Callaway, MD
Resident
Department of Emergency Medicine
Harvard Medical School;
Beth Israel Deaconess Medical Center
Boston, Massachusetts

Wallace A. Carter, MD
Associate Professor of Emergency Medicine
Weill Medical College of Cornell University;
Associate Professor of Clinical Medicine
College of Physicians and Surgeons of
Columbia University;
Program Director
Emergency Medicine Residency
New York-Presbyterian Hospital
New York, New York

Andrew Chang, MD, MS
Assistant Professor
Department of Emergency Medicine
Albert Einstein College of Medicine;
Attending Physician
Montefiore Medical Center
Bronx, New York

Dan Chavira
Chief Resident
Department of Emergency Medicine
Harbor-UCLA Medical Center
Torrance, California

Jericca L. Chen, MD, RDHS
Assistant Clinical Professor
New York University School of Medicine;
Attending Physician
Department of Emergency Medicine
North Shore University Hospital
Manhasset, New York

Penelope Chun
Attending
Department of Emergency Medicine
North Shore University Hospital
Manhasset, New York

Brian Chung, MD
Resident
Emergency Medicine Residency
New York Hospital Queens
Flushing, New York

Wendy Coates
Attending
Department of Emergency Medicine
Harbor-UCLA Medical Center
Torrance, California

Clinton J. Coil, MD, MPH
Clinical Instructor
Division of Emergency Medicine
David Geffen School of Medicine
at UCLA
Los Angeles, California;
Quality and Process Improvement Fellow
Department of Emergency Medicine
LA County/Harbor-UCLA Medical Center
Torrance, California

Manuel A. Colón, MD, RDMS
Assistant Professor and Emergency Ultrasound
Director
Department of Emergency Medicine
University of Puerto Rico Hospital
Carolina, Puerto Rico

Mark Clark
Attending
Department of Emergency Medicine
St. Luke's-Roosevelt Hospital Center
New York, New York

Jason D'Amore, MD
Assistant Research Director
Department of Emergency Medicine
North Shore University Hospital;
Assistant Professor
Department of Emergency Medicine
New York University School of Medicine
New York, New York

Amir Darvish, MD
Department of Emergency Medicine
St. Luke's-Roosevelt Hospital Center
Columbia University College of Physicians
and Surgeons
New York, New York

Ami Kirit Dave, MD
Assistant Professor
Department of Emergency Medicine
New York University
Bellevue Hospital Center
New York, New York

Moira Davenport, MD
Assistant Professor
Department of Emergency Medicine
and Orthopaedic Surgery
New York University School of Medicine;
Attending Physician
Allegheny General Hospital
Department of Emergency Medicine
and Orthopedic Surgery
Pittsburgh, Pennsylvania

Erik P. Deede, MD
Attending Physician
Department of Emergency Medicine
Metrowest Medical Center
Framingham, Massachusetts

Marina Del Rios Rivera, MD
Fellow
Clinical Epidemiology and Health Services
Research
Department of General Medicine
Joan and Sanford I. Weill Medical College
and Graduate School of Medical
Sciences-Cornell University;
Fellow
Emergency Ultrasonography
Assistant Attending
Department of Emergency Medicine
New York Methodist Hospital
Brooklyn, New York

Joshua S. Easter, MD
Resident
Department of Emergency Medicine
Beth Israel Deaconess Medical Center
Boston, Massachusetts

Jonathan A. Edlow, MD
Associate Professor
Department of Medicine
Harvard Medical School;
Vice-chair
Department of Emergency Medicine
Beth Israel Deaconess Medical Center
Boston, Massachusetts

Robert P. Favelukes, MD
Resident
Department of Emergency Medicine
St. Luke's-Roosevelt Hospital Center
New York, New York

David Feller-Kopman, MD
Assistant Professor
Department of Medicine
Harvard Medical School;
Director
Medical Procedure Service
Interventional Pulmonology
Beth Israel Deaconess Medical Center
Boston, Massachusetts

Jenice Forde-Baker, MD
Resident
Department of Emergency Medicine
New York-Presbyterian Hospital;
The University Hospital of Columbia and Cornell
New York, New York

Ryan P. Friedberg, MD
Clinical Instructor
Departments of Medicine and Orthopedics
Harvard Medical School;
Director
Musculoskeletal Education
Department of Emergency Medicine
Beth Israel Deaconess Medical Center
Boston, Massachusetts

Maureen Gang, MD
Assistant Professor
Department of Emergency Medicine
New York University School of Medicine;
Chairperson
Tisch Education Quality Assurance Commission
Department of Emergency Medicine
Tisch Hospital
New York, New York

Jeffrey Green
Attending Physician
New York Hospital Queens
Flushing, New York

Sanjey Gupta, MD
Department of Emergency Medicine
Weill Medical College
Cornell University
New York Hospital-Queens
Flushing, New York

Cassandra Jo Haddox, DO
Resident
Department of Emergency Medicine
Allegheny General Hospital
Pittsburgh, Pennsylvania

Keeli A. Hanzelka, MD
Resident
Department of Emergency Medicine
St. Luke's-Roosevelt Hospital Center
New York, New York

Alberto Hazan, MD
Chief Resident
Department of Emergency Medicine
St. Luke's-Roosevelt Hospital Center
New York, New York

Timothy Horeczko, MD
Resident
Department of Emergency Medicine
Harbor-UCLA Medical Center
Torrance, California

Catherine H. Horwitz, MD
Department of Emergency Medicine
Beth Israel Deaconess Medical Center
Harvard Affiliated Emergency Medicine
Residency
Boston, Massachusetts

James Hsiao, MD
Resident
Department of Emergency Medicine
New York-Presbyterian Hospital
New York, New York

Heather Huffman-Dracht
Resident
Department of Emergency Medicine
Harbor-UCLA Medical Center
Torrance, California

Amy S. Hurwitz, MD
Clinical Fellow
Department of Emergency Medicine
Harvard Medical School;
Resident
Department of Emergency Medicine
Beth Israel Deaconess Medical Center
Boston, Massachusetts

Jason Imperato, MD, MBA
Instructor
Department of Emergency Medicine
Harvard Medical School;
Staff Physician
Department of Emergency Medicine
Mount Auburn Hospital
Cambridge, Massachusetts

Gregory S. Johnston, MD
Assistant Professor
Department of Emergency Medicine
New York University School of Medicine;
Attending Physician
Department of Emergency Medicine
Bellevue Hospital Center and New York
University Medical Center
New York, New York

Amy H. Kaji, MD, MPH
Assistant Clinical Professor
Department of Emergency Medicine
David Geffen School of Medicine
at UCLA
Los Angeles, California;
Emergency Physician
Department of Emergency Medicine
Harbor-UCLA Medical Center
Torrance, California

Taylor J. Kallas, MD
Division of Emergency Medicine
Duke University
Durham, North Carolina

Julie K.A. Kasarjian, MD, PhD
Resident
Department of Emergency Medicine
Harbor-UCLA Medical Center
Torrance, California

Jennifer Kaufman, MD
Fellow
Gastroenterology and Nutrition
Memorial Sloane Kettering
Cancer Center
New York, New York

Barbara Kilian, MD
Attending Physician
Department of Emergency Medicine
Columbia University
St. Luke's-Roosevelt Hospital Center
New York, New York

Shadi Kiraiki
Resident
Department of Emergency Medicine
North Shore University Hospital
Manhasset, New York

Ted Korszun
Attending
Department of Emergency Medicine
North Shore University Hospital
Manhasset, New York

Lara Kulchycki, MD
Attending Physician
Department of Emergency Medicine
Beth Israel Deaconess Medical Center
Boston, Massachusetts

Andreana Kwon, MD
Resident
Department of Emergency Medicine
St. Luke's-Roosevelt Hospital Center
New York, New York

Brian Kwong
Chief Resident
Department of Emergency Medicine
St. Luke's-Roosevelt Hospital Center
New York, New York

Heidi E. Ladner, MD
Clinical Instructor Pending
Weill Medical College of Cornell University;
Director of Emergency Ultrasound
Department of Emergency Medicine
New York Hospital Queens
Flushing, New York

Alden Matthew Landry, MD
Resident
Department of Emergency Medicine
Harvard Medical School;
Beth Israel Deaconess Medical Center
Boston, Massachusetts

Richard Lanoix, MD
Residency Director
Department of Emergency Medicine
St. Luke's-Roosevelt Hospital Center
Columbia University College of
Physicians and Surgeons
New York, New York

Faye Maryann Lee, MD
Resident
Department of Emergency Medicine
New York University Bellevue Hospital
New York, New York

Jay Lemery
Director of Wilderness Medicine
Department of Emergency Medicine
New York Presbyterian Hospital
Weill Cornell Medical College
New York, New York

Resa Lewiss
Attending
Department of Emergency Medicine
St. Luke's-Roosevelt Hospital Center
New York, New York

Ari M. Lipsky, MD
Assistant Clinical Professor
Department of Medicine
David Geffen School of Medicine at UCLA
Los Angeles, California;
Faculty
Department of Emergency Medicine
Harbor-UCLA Medical Center
Torrance, California

Brenda L. Liu, MD
Attending Physician
Department of Emergency Medicine
New York Hospital of Queens
Flushing, New York

Timothy C. Loftus, MD
Resident
Department of Emergency Medicine
New York-Presbyterian Hospital;
The University Hospital of Columbia and Cornell
New York, New York

Gregory J. Lopez, MD
Resident
Department of Emergency Medicine
New York University-Bellevue Hospital
New York, New York

Veda Maany, MD
Department of Emergency Medicine
St. Luke's-Roosevelt Hospital Center
New York, New York

William C. Manson, MD
Resident
Department of Emergency Medicine
New York Hospital Queens
Flushing, New York

Tania V. Mariani, MD
Resident
Department of Emergency Medicine
New York University-Bellevue Hospital Center
New York, New York

Adrian Martinez, MD
Resident
Department of Emergency Medicine
St. Luke's-Roosevelt Hospital Center
New York, New York

Chilembwe Mason, MD
Attending
Department of Emergency Medicine
Bronx-Lebanon Hospital Center
Bronx, New York

Todd A. Mastrovitch, MD
Director, Pediatric Education
Emergency Medicine Residency
New York Hospital Queens
Flushing, New York

Daniel C. McGillicuddy,
Clinical Instructor
Department of Emergency Medicine
Harvard Medical School;
Assistant Program Director
Department of Emergency Medicine
Beth Israel Deaconess Medical Center
Boston, Massachusetts

Daniel Mūnoz-Acabá, MD
Chief Resident
Emergency Medical Department
University of Puerto Rico Hospital
Carolina, Puerto Rico

Richard G. Newell, MD, MPH
Department of Emergency Medicine
Harbor/UCLA Medical Center
Torrance, California;
Administrative Fellow
California Emergency Physicians
Sutter Roseville Medical Center
Roseville, California

David H. Newman, MD
Assistant Professor of Clinical Medicine
Department of Emergency Medicine
Columbia University;
Director of Clinical Research
Department of Emergency Medicine
St. Luke's-Roosevelt Hospital Center
New York, New York

Emilola Ogunbameru, MD
Director, Child Abuse Services
Department of Emergency Medicine
St. Luke's-Roosevelt Hospital Center
Columbia University College of
Physicians and Surgeons
New York, New York

Jessica Paisley, MD
Resident
Department of Emergency Medicine
Columbia University;
St. Luke's-Roosevelt Hospital Center
New York, New York

Neil Patel, MD
Resident
Department of Emergency Medicine
Harbor-UCLA Medical Center
Torrance, California

Audrey Paul
Assistant Professor of Emergency Medicine
Mount Sinai Hospital
New York, New York

Jayson R. Pereira, MD
Chief Resident
Department of Emergency Medicine
Harvard University
Beth Israel Deaconess Medical Center
Boston, Massachusetts

Eric Perez
Attending
Department of Emergency Medicine
St. Luke's-Roosevelt Hospital Center
New York, New York

Jennifer V. Pope, MD
Clinical Fellow
Department of Medicine
Harvard University;
Resident
Department of Emergency Medicine
Beth Israel Deaconess Medical Center
Boston, Massachusetts

Armin Perham Poordabbagh
Resident
Department of Emergency Medicine
North Shore University Hospital
Manhasset, New York

Robert J. Preston, MD
Division of Emergency Medicine
Duke University
Durham, North Carolina

Joshua Quaas, MD
Director of Medical Student Education
Department of Emergency Medicine
St. Luke's-Roosevelt Hospital Center
Columbia University College of
Physicians and Surgeons
New York, New York

Oscar Rago, MD, MBA
Resident
Department of Emergency Medicine
St. Luke's-Roosevelt Hospital Center
New York, New York

Rama B. Rao, MD
Assistant Clinical Professor
Department of Emergency Medicine
New York University School of Medicine
Bellevue Hospital Center
New York, New York

Kimberly Reagans, MD
Resident
Department of Emergency Medicine
St. Luke's-Roosevelt Hospital Center
New York, New York

Kathleen G. Reichard, DO
Senior Attending Physician
Department of Pediatric Emergency Medicine
St. Luke's-Roosevelt Hospital Center
New York, New York

David C. Riley, MD, MS, RDMS
Assistant Clinical Professor
Department of Medicine
Columbia University College of
Physicians and Surgeons;
Director
Ultrasound Fellowship-Education
Department of Emergency Medicine
St. Luke's-Roosevelt Hospital Center
New York, New York

Marina Del Rios
Attending
Department of Emergency Medicine
St. Luke's-Roosevelt Hospital Center
New York, New York

Melissa Rockefeller
Resident
Department of Emergency Medicine
St. Luke's-Roosevelt Hospital Center
New York, New York

James E. Rodriguez, MD
Resident
Department of Emergency Medicine
New York University Medical Center
Bellevue Hospital Center
New York, New York

Leon D. Sanchez, MD, MPH
Assistant Professor
Division of Emergency Medicine
Harvard Medical School;
Attending
Department of Emergency Medicine
Beth Israel Deaconess Medical Center
Boston, Massachusetts

Turandot Saul, MD
Resident
Department of Emergency Medicine
New York University;
Bellevue Hospital-New York University
Medical Center
New York, New York

Kari Scantlebury
Resident
Department of Emergency Medicine
St. Luke's-Roosevelt Hospital Center
New York, New York

Todd A. Seigel, MD
Clinical Fellow
Department of Medicine
Harvard University;
Resident
Department of Emergency Medicine
Beth Israel Deaconess Medical Center
Boston, Massachusetts

Kaushal Shah, MD
Emergency Department Director of Trauma
Services
St.Luke's-Roosevelt Hospital Center
University Hospital of Columbia University
College of Physicians and Surgeons
New York, New York

Lekha Ajit Shah, MD
Fellow in Emergency Ultrasound
Department of Emergency Medicine
Columbia University;
Attending Physician
Department of Emergency Medicine
St. Luke's-Roosevelt Hospital Center
New York, New York

Hiral H. Shah, MD, JD
Resident
Department of Emergency Medicine
North Shore University Hospital
Manhasset, New York

Ashley Shreves, MD
Director of Medical Student Education
Department of Emergency Medicine
St. Luke's-Roosevelt Hospital Center
Columbia University College of Physicians
and Surgeons
New York, New York

Steven Shuchat, MD
Attending
Department of Emergency Medicine
New York Hospital Medical Center of Queens
Flushing, New York

Jay Smith, MD
Resident
Department of Emergency Medicine
Beth Israel Deaconess Medical Center
Boston, Massachusetts

Peter B. Smulowitz, MD
Instructor in Medicine
Department of Emergency Medicine
Beth Israel Deaconess Medical Center
Boston, Massachusetts

Dean Jared Straff, MD
Resident
Department of Emergency Medicine
New York-Presbyterian Hospital
The University Hospital of Columbia and Cornell
New York, New York

Jennifer Stratton
Attending
Department of Emergency Medicine
St. Luke's-Roosevelt Hospital Center
New York, New York

Alison E. Suarez, MD, MS
Resident
Department of Emergency Medicine
Weill Medical College
Cornell University
New York Hospital-Queens
Flushing, New York

Ramona S. Sunderwith, MD, MPH
Attending
Pediatric Emergency Medicine
Department of Emergency Medicine
St. Luke's-Roosevelt Hospital Center
New York, New York

Anand K. Swaminathan, MD, MPH
Resident
Department of Emergency Medicine
New York University-Bellevue Hospital Center
New York, New York

Angela M. Tangredi, MD
Director
Pediatric Emergency Services
St. Luke's-Roosevelt Hospital Center
New York, New York

Jennifer Teng, MD
Resident
Department of Emergency Medicine
Columbia University
St. Luke's-Roosevelt Hospital Center
New York, New York

Jason A. Tracy, MD
Clinical Instructor
Department of Emergency Medicine
Harvard University;
Director of Operations
Department of Emergency Medicine
Beth Israel Deaconess Medical Center
Boston, Massachusetts

Joseph P. Underwood, MD
Instructor of Clinical Medicine
Columbia University
College of Physicians and Surgeons
Columbia University Medical Center
New York, New York

Diana Valcich, MD
Resident
Department of Emergency Medicine
New York Methodist Hospital
Brooklyn, New York

Maria Vasilyadis, MD
Resident
Department of Emergency Medicine
New York University-Bellevue Hospital
New York, New York

Ann Vorhaben, MD
Resident
Department of Emergency Medicine
St. Luke's-Roosevelt Hospital Center
New York, New York

Raymond V. Wedderburn, MD, FACS
Chief, Trauma and Critical Care
Associate Director, Surgical Residency
Program
St. Luke's-Roosevelt Hospital Center
New York, New York

Scott G. Weiner, MD, MPH
Assistant Professor
Department of Emergency Medicine
Tufts University;
Attending Physician
Department of Emergency Medicine
Tufts-New England Medical Center
Boston, Massachusetts

Lucy Willis, MD
Resident
Department of Emergency Medicine
St. Luke's-Roosevelt Hospital Center
New York, New York

Laura T.G. Withers, MD
Department of Surgery
Columbia University;
Chief Resident
Department of Surgery
St. Lukes-Roosevelt Hospital Center
New York, New York

Michael M. Woodruff, MD
Instructor
Department of Medicine
Harvard Medical School;
Attending Physician
Department of Emergency Medicine
Beth Israel Deaconess Medical Center
Boston, Massachusetts

Tina Wu, MD
Staff Physician
Department of Emergency Medicine
New York University School of Medicine
Bellevue Hospital Center
New York, New York

Julie A. Zeller, MD
Resident
Department of Emergency Medicine
Beth Israel Deaconess Medical Center
Boston, Massachusetts

Preface

Procedures in the emergency department (and the hospital in general) are frequent and varied. They range from simple suturing to complicated thoracotomies. Procedures that are performed for the first few times or infrequently are the ones that cause the most anxiety. The ability to review the procedure quickly from a reliable source is clearly invaluable to a physician (and the patient).

This procedure handbook is designed primarily for any physician, resident, or medical student who will be doing emergency procedures. The aim of the book is to have a bedside refresher of the key components of a procedure. This creates accuracy, confidence, and likely fewer complications. There will be times when you want to read an entire chapter to fully grasp every detail and there will be times when you want just the critical information. This book was designed to meet both needs.

The highlights of this book are the "Landmarks" and "Pearls" sections. The "Landmarks" section contains the key anatomical locations for quick reference and the "Pearls" section contains the pertinent clinical information relevant to the procedure (e.g., "place the subclavian central line on the same side as the chest wound or pneumothorax" and guidelines on how to interpret the cerebrospinal fluid or the diagnostic peritoneal lavage).

Key chapters that are worth reviewing and very unlikely to be found in other procedure books are: Induced Therapeutic Hypothermia, Epley Maneuver and Hallpike Test for positional vertigo, Occipital Nerve Block, Open Joint Evaluation/Methylene Blue Injection, and six different goal-directed ultrasound procedures.

There is no doubt that increased comfort with medical procedures translates to increased comfort as a physician. Enjoy the read.

Acknowledgments

We are extremely grateful to all the Section Editors who really used their vision and expertise (with only a very general framework provided by us) to make the chapters shine. We will never know the innumerable hours that were likely invested but their efforts are tremendously appreciated. Thank you to Leon, Newman, Erik, Josh, Ari, Jerrica, Jonathan, Ami, Wally, Moira, Sanjey ("Jay"), Jay, Jason, Angela, and Riley.

Acknowledgements

Contents

Section Editor: Leon D. Sanchez

1   Intubation: Tracheal and Nasotracheal

Todd A. Seigel and Leon D. Sanchez

General

In emergent management of the airway, the likelihood that a patient has fasted before intubation is very small. These patients are at risk for aspiration of gastric contents, and for this reason, rapid sequence intubation (RSI) is the preferred method of airway management in the emergency department. The following discussion of orotracheal intubation refers to the appropriate procedures of RSI. Nasotracheal intubation is also discussed.

Indications

- Failure to protect the airway
- Failure to maintain the airway
- Failure of ventilation
- Failure of oxygenation
- Other therapeutic indications such as need for paralysis or hyperventilation

Contraindications

- **Orotracheal and Nasotracheal Intubation**
  - Total upper airway obstruction
  - Total loss of facial landmarks
- **Nasotracheal Intubation**
  - Apnea
  - Basilar skull or facial fracture
  - Neck trauma or cervical spine injury
  - Head injury with suspected increased intracranial pressure (ICP)
  - Nasal or nasopharyngeal obstruction
  - Combative patients or patients *in extremis*
  - Patients with coagulopathy
  - Pediatric patients

Landmarks

- Viewing the oropharynx from above, the tongue will be the most anterior structure.
- The pouchlike vallecula separates the tongue from the epiglottis, which sits above the airway. The larynx sits anterior to the esophagus.
- The vocal cords sit as an inverted "V" within the larynx.

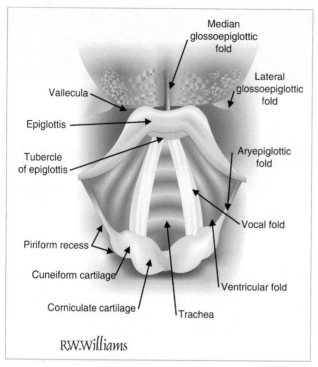

FIGURE 1.1: Larynx visualized from the oropharynx. Note the median glossoepiglottic fold. It is pressure on this structure by the tip of a curved blade that flips the epiglottis forward, exposing the glottis during laryngoscopy. Note the valleculae and the pyriform recesses are different structures, a fact often confused in the anesthesia literature. The cuneiform and corniculate cartilages are called the arytenoid cartilages. The ridge between them posteriorly is called the posterior commissure. (Reused with permission from Redden RJ. Anatomic considerations in anesthesia. In: Hagberg CA, ed. *Handbook of difficult airway management.* Philadelphia: Churchill Livingstone; 2000:9.)

Technique for Orotracheal Intubation

The approach to the technique for RSI can be summarized in seven discrete steps, each beginning with the letter P.

- **Preparation**
  - Assess airway: Use LEMON mnemonic to predict difficulty of airway.
    - **L**ook externally: If you sense that an airway appears difficult, it likely is.
    - **E**valuate anatomy: The 3-3-2 Rule
      - Thyromental distance: A distance less than three of the patient's finger widths is predictive of difficult airway.
      - Mouth opening: If the patient's open mouth can fit less than three of the patient's own fingers, it is predictive of a difficult airway.
      - Hyomental distance: A distance of less than two of the patient's finger widths is predictive of a difficult airway.
    - **M**allampati Score: Roughly correlates the view of internal oropharyngeal structures with successful intubation attempts. Graded as class I to IV.
    - **O**bstruction: Any evidence of upper airway obstruction heralds a difficult airway.
    - **N**eck mobility: Neck mobility is crucial to obtaining the optimum view of the larynx. Hindrance to neck extension, including cervical spine immobilization, predicts difficulty in intubation.

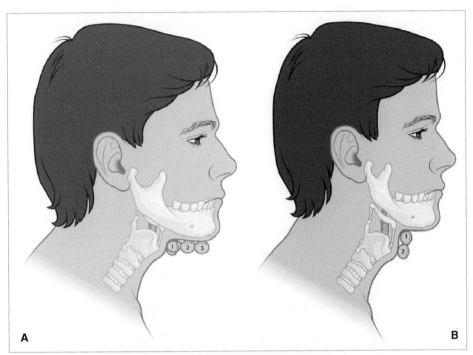

FIGURE 1.2: **A:** The second 3 of the 3-3-2 rule. **B:** The 2 of the 3-3-2 rule. (From Walls RM, Murphy MF, Luten RC, et al. *Manual of emergency airway management*. Philadelphia: Lippincott Williams & Wilkins; 2004:77, with permission.)

- Equipment
  - Endotracheal tubes: Prepare two endotracheal tubes, 7.5 or 8.0 AND 7.0. The larger tube is suitable for most adult men, the smaller for most adult women. If difficulty is encountered using a larger tube, the smaller tube is readily available. Check the integrity of the cuff before use. Place the stylet in the tube.
  - Laryngoscope and blades: Ensure the light source works in two laryngoscopes, and prepare blades (Macintosh 3 and 4, Miller 3 and 4). Use a blade you feel comfortable with.
- Prepare for likely surgical intervention.
- Ensure patient is monitored with a functional IV line.
- Position patient and adjust bed height.
- Have pharmacologic agents drawn and ready to push.
- Assign roles to the other members of the team in the room.

■ **Preoxygenation**
- Theoretically, deliver 100% oxygen for 3 minutes (in reality, nonrebreather mask delivers approximately 70%).
- This fills the functional residual capacity with oxygen, replacing nitrogen.
- When time is critical or patient is following commands, preoxygenation is achieved in eight vital capacity breaths.
- This allows approximately 8 minutes of apnea in a 70-kg adult; this time period varies based on patient body habitus, medical history, and present issue.

■ **Pretreatment**
This refers to the administration of medications to attenuate the potential adverse side effect of intubation. Not every patient requires pretreatment. Pretreatment is

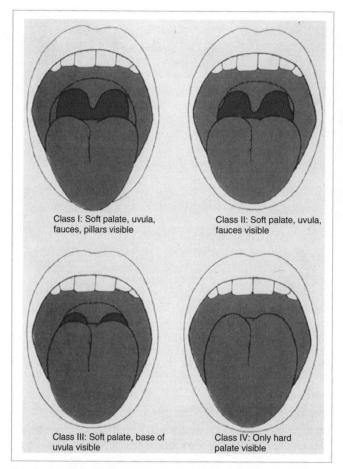

Class I: Soft palate, uvula, fauces, pillars visible

Class II: Soft palate, uvula, fauces visible

Class III: Soft palate, base of uvula visible

Class IV: Only hard palate visible

FIGURE 1.3: The Mallampati Scale. (From Walls RM, Murphy MF, Luten RC, et al. *Manual of emergency airway management*. Philadelphia: Lippincott Williams & Wilkins; 2004:78, with permission.)

considered most often in patients with increased ICP, in children, or to mitigate the sympathetic response to intubation.

- Increased ICP: The patient should be intubated with a standard ''five-drug cocktail.''
    - **Lidocaine** 1.5 mg/kg—mitigates physiologic response to laryngoscope blade insertion that may increase ICP.
    - **Vecuronium** 0.01 mg/kg—as a defasciculating agent before administration of succinylcholine because fasciculations can increase ICP.
    - **Fentanyl** 3 μg/kg—if the patient is hemodynamically stable.
    - **Succinylcholine** and **etomidate** as standard induction and paralytic agents. Ketamine raises ICP and should be avoided in patients with increased ICP.

Protection and Positioning

- Sellick maneuver: Firm pressure against cricoid cartilage to protect from aspiration.
- ''Sniffing'' position: Place a towel underneath the patient's head. This creates neck extension with slight flexion of lower cervical spine and optimally aligns the pharyngeal and laryngeal airway.

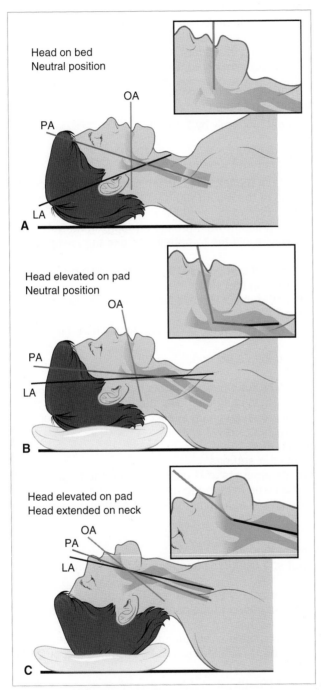

FIGURE 1.4: **A:** Anatomic neutral position. The oral axis (*OA*), pharyngeal axis (*PA*), and laryngeal axis (*LA*) are at greater angles to one another. **B:** Head, still in neutral position, has been lifted by a pillow flexing the lower cervical spine and aligning the *PA* and *LA* axes. **C:** The head has been extended on the cervical spine, aligning the *OA* with the *PA* and *LA* axes, creating the optimum sniffing position for intubation. (From Walls RM, Murphy MF, Luten RC, et al. *Manual of emergency airway management.* Philadelphia: Lippincott Williams & Wilkins; 2004:56, with permission.)

- **Paralysis and Induction**
  - The induction agent should be given first, as a bolus, in sufficient dose to produce immediate loss of consciousness. Common induction agents are propofol (1.5–3 mg/kg) and etomidate (0.3 mg/kg).
  - The paralytic agent should then be administered. Succinylcholine (1.5–2 mg/kg) is the paralytic of choice in RSI because of its rapid onset.
  - Fasciculations will occur approximately 20 to 30 seconds after the administration of succinylcholine.
  - Apnea will occur almost uniformly by 1 minute.
- **Placement of the Tube**
  - Open the patient's mouth.
  - Laryngoscopy
    - Holding the handle in the left hand, insert the blade of choice starting from the right side of the mouth with the goal of sweeping the tongue fully to the left.
    - Apply gentle upward and forward pressure (approximately 45 degrees) to visualize the airway; avoid the temptation to use the laryngoscope as a lever.
    - If cords are not immediately visible, try withdrawing laryngoscope slowly to allow the cords to drop into view.
    - Keep the cords under direct visualization; ask someone to hand you the endotracheal tube.
    - Pass the tube through the vocal cords and stop when the cuff is just past the cords.
    - Remove stylet and inflate balloon.
- **Proof of Tube Placement**
  - Direct visualization of the tube passing through the cords is paramount.
  - Auscultate over the stomach and then over the lungs to confirm placement.
  - Must confirm with color change on end-tidal carbon dioxide detector.
  - Obtain postintubation chest x-ray.
- **Postintubation Management**
  - Maintain proper ventilator settings.
  - Administer appropriate amounts of sedation to keep the patient comfortable.
  - Nasogastric tube should be inserted to decompress the stomach.
  - Obtain arterial blood gas to determine adequate oxygenation and ventilation.

Technique for Nasotracheal Intubation
The seven Ps are modified but still useful in nasotracheal intubation.
- **Preparation**
  - Obtain 6.0 to 7.5 endotracheal tube and test the cuff.
  - Inspect nares to assess ease of tube passage; right is the default if there is no clear preference.
  - Administer topical vasoconstrictor solution to help prevent bleeding.
  - If time permits, consider nasal anesthesia: 4% cocaine pack or 2% lidocaine jelly.
  - Lubricate the tube and nostril.
- **Preoxygenate**
- **Pretreatment and Paralysis do not have a role in nasotracheal intubation**
  - If elevated ICP is suspected, do not perform nasotracheal intubation!
- **Positioning**
  - The patient should be comfortable. Sitting helps keep the tongue anterior in the airway.

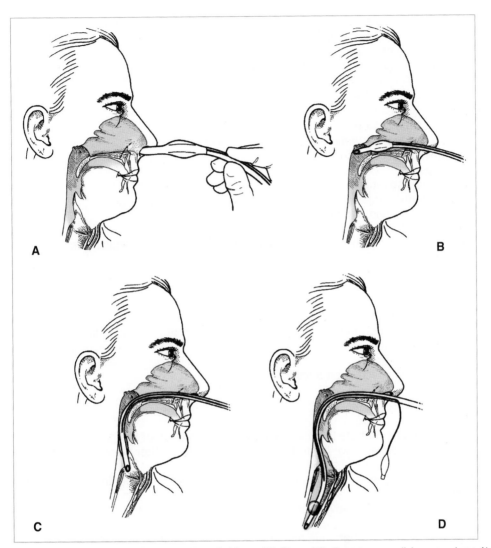

FIGURE 1.5: Nasotracheal intubation. (From Reichman EF, Simon RR. *Emergency medicine procedures*. New York: McGraw-Hill; 2004, with permission.)

- Maintain "sniffing" position: Head extended on the neck with slight flexion of the neck on the chest.
- **Placement and Proof**
  - Enter the nostril with the bevel of the tube facing laterally, aware of the vascular supply against the anterior septum.
  - Follow the floor of the nasal cavity directly back; nasal airway is located beneath the inferior nasal turbinate.
  - Once the turbinate is reached, direct the tube slightly caudad.
  - Slight resistance will occur in the posterior pharynx; rotate the tube such that the bevel is facing up.
  - Once the nasopharynx is entered, return the bevel to the lateral position and advance until breath sounds are heard through the tube; tube will be just above vocal cords.

* Place pressure against the larynx with the nondominant hand and ask the patient to take a deep breath. Cords abduct during inspiration and tube can be gently passed.
* Confirm tube placement as with orotracheal intubation.

Complications
* Incorrect tube placement
  * Esophageal intubation—remove endotracheal tube.
  * Mainstem intubation—pull back endotracheal tube to ventilate both lungs.
* Witnessed aspiration
* Broken teeth, excessive bleeding secondary to mucosal damage
* Pneumothorax and pneumediastinum
* Cardiac dysrhythmia
* Complications or side effects from pharmacologic therapy, including hypotension

Common Pitfalls
* Failure to confirm IV access and patency
* Not waiting for adequate sedation and paralysis before attempting intubation
* Failure to maintain visualization of cords when passing the endotracheal tube
* Using the laryngoscope as a lever

Pearls
* The decision to intubate is a clinical decision: the status of the gag reflex and arterial blood gases have limited utility in assessing whether a patient needs to be intubated.
* RSI is ultimately intended to place an endotracheal tube without interposed ventilation.
* Intubation is time sensitive, but in most patients you have more time than you think.
* If an esophageal intubation is detected, the tube should be removed and the patient should be ventilated.
* Stridor in a patient may be suggestive of obstruction and a difficult intubation.
* Nasotracheal intubation is relatively uncommon. It should be considered in the spontaneously breathing patient where paralytics may be contraindicated, if a short period of intubation is required, or if oral airway management is deemed difficult.

Suggested Readings
Vissers RJ. Advanced airway support. *Emergency medicine manual*. New York: McGraw-Hill; 2004.

Walls RM, Murphy MF, Luten RC, et al. *Manual of emergency airway management*, 2nd ed. Philadelphia: Lippincott Williams & Wilkins; 2004.

Wolfson AB, Reichman, EF. In: Wolfson AB, ed. Resuscitation. *Harwood Nuss' clinical practice of emergency medicine*. Philadelphia: Lippincott Williams & Wilkins; 2004.

2 Cricothyroidotomy—Standard and Needle

Alden Matthew Landry and Jason Imperato

Indications

- Cricothyroidotomy is used to provide emergent airway access if a safer, less invasive airway (oral or nasotracheal intubation) cannot be established or is contraindicated.
- For children younger than 12 years, needle cricothyroidotomy is the surgical airway of choice.

Contraindications

- **Absolute**
  - An oral or nasal airway can be established
  - Significant injury or fracture of the cricoid cartilage or larynx (tracheostomy is the procedure of choice)
  - Partial or complete transection of the airway
  - Patients younger than 12 years (needle cricothyroidotomy is the procedure of choice for this age-group)
- **Relative**
  - Neck mass, swelling, or cellulitis
  - Neck hematoma
  - Coagulopathy

Landmarks

The cricothyroid membrane is best identified by palpating the laryngeal prominence ("Adam's apple"), which is the palpable protuberance at the anterosuperior aspect of the larynx. Approximately one finger breadth inferior to the laryngeal prominence is a small depression which is the cricothyroid membrane and below it is the cricothyroid cartilage.

Technique—Standard Cricothyroidotomy

- **Identify the Landmarks** (see earlier "Landmarks" section)
- **Prepare the Neck**
  - If time permits, apply appropriate antiseptic solution.
  - If time permits and patient is conscious, infiltrate skin of anterior neck with 1% lidocaine solution.
- **Immobilize the Larynx**
  - This is done by placing the thumb and long finger on opposite sides of the superior laryngeal horns, allowing the physician to relocate and reidentify the cricothyroid membrane at any time during the procedure.
- **Incise the Skin**
  - Using a no. 11 blade, make a vertical midline incision approximately 2 cm in length.
  - Care should be taken to extend the incision down to but not through any of the deep structures of the neck.

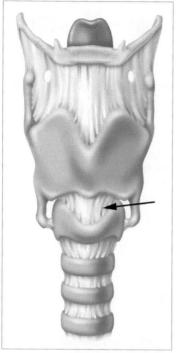

FIGURE 2.1: Anatomy of the larynx. The cricothyroid membrane (*arrow*) is bordered above by the thyroid cartilage and below by the cricoid cartilage. (From Walls RM, Murphy MF, Luten RC, et al. *Manual of emergency airway management,* 2nd ed. Philadelphia: Lippincott Williams & Wilkins; 2004:162, with permission.)

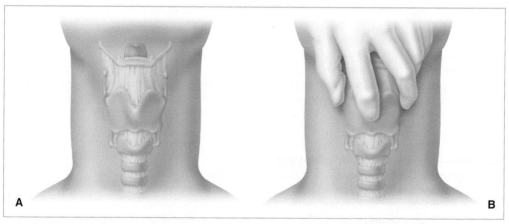

FIGURE 2.2: **A:** Surface anatomy of the airway. **B:** The thumb and long finger immobilize the superior cornua of the larynx; the index finger palpates the cricothyroid membrane. (From Walls RM, Murphy MF, Luten RC, et al. *Manual of emergency airway management,* 2nd ed. Philadelphia: Lippincott Williams & Wilkins; 2004:163, with permission.)

- **Reidentify the Membrane**
  - Use your index finger to palpate the anterior larynx, while maintaining immobilization of the larynx with your thumb and long finger.
  - Keep your index finger on the cricothyroid membrane.
- **Incise the Membrane**

- Remove index finger.
- Incise the cricothyroid membrane at least 1 cm in length in a horizontal direction.

Insert the Tracheal Hook
- Insert and turn the tracheal hook so it is oriented in a cephalad direction.
- Light upward and anterior traction is applied to bring the airway immediately out of the skin incision.

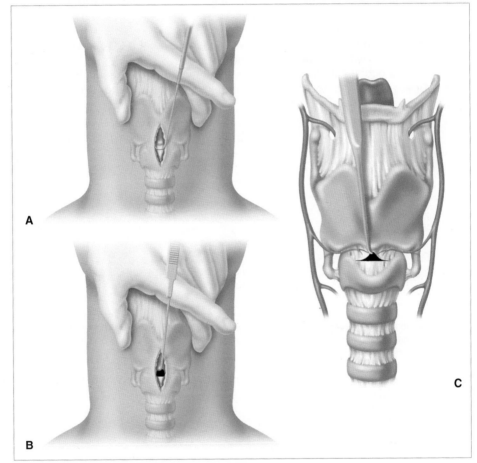

FIGURE 2.3: **A:** The tracheal hook is oriented transversely during insertion. **B** and **C:** After insertion, cephalad traction is applied to the inferior margin of the thyroid cartilage. (From Walls RM, Murphy MF, Luten RC, et al. *Manual of emergency airway management,* 2nd ed. Philadelphia: Lippincott Williams & Wilkins; 2004:166, with permission.)

Insert the Trousseau Dilator
- Insert minimally into the wound with the blades oriented superiorly and inferiorly, allowing the dilator to open and enlarge the wound vertically.

Insert the Tracheostomy Tube
- With its inner cannula in place, gently insert the tracheostomy tube through the incision between the blades of the Trousseau dilator.
- Rotate the Trousseau dilator to allow advancement of the tube.
- Remove the Trousseau dilator once the tube is firmly seated against the anterior neck.

■ **Inflate the Cuff and Confirm Tube Position**
  ○ Ventilate the patient and auscultate both lungs for equal breath sounds.
  ○ Confirm color change of carbon dioxide detector.

Technique—Needle Cricothyroidotomy

■ Find landmarks in the same way as for standard cricothyroidotomy.
■ Attach a large-bore needle (12- or 14-gauge) with a catheter to a 3-mL syringe.
■ Partially fill the syringe with saline.
■ Immobilize the trachea.
■ Insert the needle into the cricothyroid membrane at a 90-degree angle.
■ Attempt to withdraw air through the needle.
  ○ Air bubbles in the syringe is confirmation that the needle is in the trachea.
■ Change the angle to 45 degrees and advance the catheter over the needle into the trachea (see Fig. 2.4).

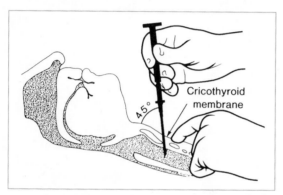

FIGURE 2.4: Percutaneous transtracheal catheter ventilation. Insert the needle into the cricothyroid membrane at a 45-degree angle, directed inferiorly. (From Simon RR, Brenner BE. *Emergency procedures and techniques,* 4th ed. Philadelphia: Lippincott Williams & Wilkins; 2002:100, with permission.)

■ Withdraw the needle and syringe and attach an endotracheal tube connector to the catheter.
■ Stabilize the tube.
■ Ventilate the patient and check for proper placement of tube.

Complications

■ Hemorrhage
■ Subcutaneous emphysema
■ Pneumomediastinum
■ Infection
■ Voice change
■ Subglottic stenosis
■ Laryngeal/tracheal injury

Common Pitfalls

■ Malposition of the needle, including creation of a false lumen
■ Poor identification of anatomic landmarks
■ Failure to stabilize trachea

Pearls

- Numerous commercial cricothyroidotomy devices are available. Be familiar with the one at your institution. Several use a modified Seldinger technique which is similar to the method used for placement of central venous catheters.
- Cricothyroidotomy is the surgical airway of choice in an emergency.
- In addition to the standard cricothyroidotomy technique, there is a rapid four-step technique that entails: (a) palpation, (b) stab incision, (c) inferior traction, and (d) tube insertion.

Suggested Readings
Brofeldt BT, Panacek EA, Richards JR. An easy cricothyrotomy approach: The rapid four-step technique. *Acad Emerg Med*. 1996;3:1060–1063.

Vissers RJ. Advanced airway support. *Emergency medicine manual*. New York: McGraw-Hill; 2004.

Walls RM, Murphy MF, Luten RC, et al. *Manual of emergency airway management*, 2nd ed. Philadelphia: Lippincott Williams & Wilkins; 2004.

Wolfson AB, Reichman, EF. Resuscitation. In: Wolfson AB, ed. *Harwood Nuss' clinical practice of emergency medicine*. Philadelphia: Lippincott Williams & Wilkins, 2004.

3 Laryngeal Mask Airway

Evan Bloom and Lara Kulchycki

Indications
- Require airway management but cannot be intubated by direct laryngoscopy.
- For patients who cannot be intubated or ventilated by bag valve mask (BVM), laryngeal mask airway (LMA) insertion should be accompanied by simultaneous preparation for a surgical airway in the unlikely event of LMA failure.

Contraindications
- Absolute (when used as an airway rescue device): Able to establish a definitive airway with endotracheal intubation
- **Relative Contraindications**
  - Trismus
  - High risk of aspiration
    - ▶ Vomiting
    - ▶ Brisk upper gastrointestinal bleeding
    - ▶ Massive hemoptysis
  - Laryngeal injuries/tracheal disruption
  - Recent head and neck radiation
  - Significant upper airway infection, such as epiglottitis
  - Foreign body in upper airway
  - Conditions requiring high ventilation pressures

Risks/Consent Issues
- During an emergent airway, consent is implied unless the patient has a valid "Do not resuscitate" order.
- The most serious risks of the procedure are ventilation failure and aspiration.

Anatomy/Landmarks
The device is blindly inserted into the oropharynx and advanced until the mask rests over the glottic opening.

Technique—Standard Laryngeal Mask Airway
- **Preparation**
  - Confirm all monitoring equipment is in place and functional, including the oxygen saturation probe and cardiac telemetry.
  - Prepare BVM ventilation and confirm oxygen supply.
  - Draw up any necessary medications, such as sedatives.
  - Select the appropriate LMA based on estimated patient weight (see Table 3.1).
  - Inflate the cuff to assess for air leaks.

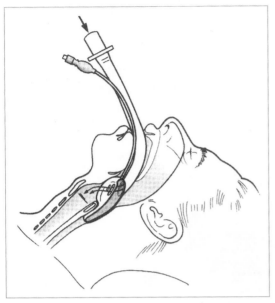

FIGURE 3.1: The laryngeal mask airway (LMA) mask rests in the hypopharynx over the glottic opening. (From Reichman EF, Simon RR. *Emergency medicine procedures.* New York: McGraw-Hill; 2004, with permission)

  ▷ Inject the amount of air appropriate to the selected LMA (Table 3.1).
  ▷ Deflate while pressing the cuff against a flat surface to provide a smooth leading edge for insertion.
  ◦ Apply water-soluble lubricant to the cuff surface.
- **Preoxygenation**
  ◦ Deliver 100% oxygen via a nonrebreather mask (for spontaneously breathing patients) or BVM ventilation (for apneic patients) until the surgeon is ready to insert the device.
  ◦ Administer medications, such as sedation, if needed.
- **Position**
  ◦ Sniffing position is optimal for nonintubating LMAs.

TABLE 3.1: Guidelines for laryngeal mask airway selection and mask inflation

LMA size	Weight (kg)	Volume of air inflation (mL)	Maximum ETT size (mm)
1	Neonates/infants <5	4	3.5
1.5	Infants 5–10	7	4.0
2	Infants/children 10–20	10	4.5
2.5	Children 20–30	14	5
3	Children 30–50	20	6.0 cuffed
4	Adults 50–70	30	6.0 cuffed
5	Adults 70–100	40	7.0 cuffed
6	Adults >100	50	7.0 cuffed

LMA, laryngeal mask airway; ETT, endotracheal tube.

- If neutral head position is necessary for cervical spine immobilization, LMA success rates are still high.
- **Placement**
  - LMA insertion
    - ▸ Hold the LMA in a pencil grip manner with the dominant hand.
    - ▸ Insert the device into the oropharynx with the aperture facing the tongue.

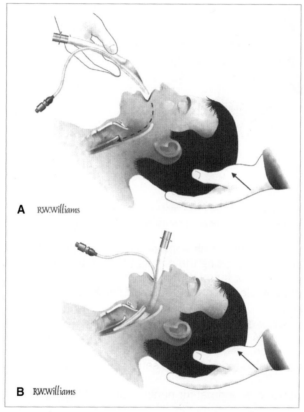

A   R.W.Williams

B   R.W.Williams

FIGURE 3.2: Laryngeal mask airway (LMA) insertion. **A:** Starting insertion position for the LMA Classic and Unique. **B:** Insert the LMA to the limit of your finger length. (From Walls RM, Murphy MF, Luten RC, et al. *Manual of emergency airway management,* 2nd ed. Philadelphia: Lippincott Williams & Wilkins; 2004:105)

  - ▸ Advance the LMA along the contour of the palate past the posterior border of the tongue.
  - ▸ Resistance to further movement will be noted when the mask rests in the hypopharynx over the glottic opening.
  - ▸ Inflate the collar with the appropriate amount of air (Table 3.1) or until there is no audible air leak with ventilation.
  - ▸ Confirm successful ventilation with auscultation and use of an end-tidal carbon dioxide (CO_2) detector.
  - ▸ If unable to advance the LMA past the tongue, invert the device so the aperture is facing the palate and rotate the mask into position once the LMA has reached the posterior oropharynx.
- **Protection**
  - Secure the LMA in the midline with tape or a tube-securing device.
  - Place a bite block to prevent tube occlusion.

Technique—Intubating Laryngeal Mask Airway
- Inflate the intubating laryngeal mask airway (I-LMA) mask collar and the endotracheal tube (ETT) cuff to ensure integrity (then deflate both).
- Apply water-soluble lubricant to both devices.
- Hold the I-LMA by the metal handle and insert along the contour of the palate until the device rests in the hypopharynx and resists further movement.

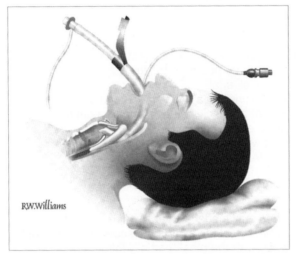

FIGURE 3.3: Intubating laryngeal mask airway (I-LMA) insertion. (From Walls RM, Murphy MF, Luten RC, et al. *Manual of emergency airway management,* 2nd ed. Philadelphia: Lippincott Williams & Wilkins; 2004:101)

- Inflate the I-LMA mask collar.
- Connect to BVM and confirm ventilation of the patient.
- Pass the ETT through the I-LMA lumen with the black vertical line on the tube facing the surgeon (this line indicates correct bevel orientation).
- At the 15-cm marker, the ETT is about to emerge from the mask.
- Lift the handle of the I-LMA as the ETT is advanced into the trachea to improve intubation success (Verghese maneuver).
- Inflate the ETT cuff and confirm tube placement.
- Deflate the I-LMA mask collar.
- To remove the I-LMA.
  - Disconnect the I-LMA from the BVM.
  - Hold the ETT firmly in place with one hand while gently withdrawing the I-LMA.
  - When the proximal I-LMA has reached the surgeon's hand that is stabilizing the ETT, insert the stabilizer rod into the lumen to prevent dislodgement of the tube as the I-LMA is removed from the oropharynx.
  - Reconnect the ETT with a BVM to continue ventilation.
- If the surgeon is unfamiliar with I-LMA removal and is concerned about dislodging the ETT with this maneuver, the I-LMA can be left in place.

Complications
- **Aspiration**
  - The main limitation of the LMA as an emergency airway rescue device is that it cannot protect against aspiration.
  - Gastric inflation from air leak may cause reflux of stomach contents.

- **Inadequate Ventilation**
  - Malpositioned device
  - Inappropriate LMA size
- **Laryngospasm**
- **Pulmonary Edema**
  - Reports exist of patients developing negative pressure pulmonary edema after biting the LMA and then inhaling against an occluded tube.

Common Pitfalls
- Poor estimation of patient weight leading to incorrect LMA size selection
- Failure to pass the LMA beyond the posterior tongue
- Inability to obtain adequate mask seal
- Aggressive BVM ventilation leading to gastric inflation and aspiration
- Failure to transition the patient as quickly as possible to a definitive airway
- Tube occlusion from failure to employ a bite block
- Accidental ETT dislodgement with I-LMA removal
- Inadequate sedation after LMA insertion

Pearls
- Avoid cricoid pressure as this may hinder proper LMA placement.
- If the leading edge of the LMA is kinking as it is advanced into the oropharynx, the surgeon can insert the device with the mask partially inflated.
- If the patient desaturates during I-LMA placement, bag ventilate to restore normal oxygenation before attempting tracheal intubation.
- Never force passage of the ETT.
- If an I-LMA is not available, a standard LMA can also be used to facilitate blind endotracheal intubation by inserting a gum elastic bougie through the lumen, removing the deflated LMA, and then passing a ETT over the bougie into the trachea (success rates are lower than with an I-LMA).

Suggested Readings
Brain AI, Verghese C, Addy EV, et al. The intubating laryngeal mask: II. A preliminary clinical report of a new means of intubating the trachea. *Br J Anaesth.* 1997; 79(6):704–709.

Murphy FM. Laryngeal mask airways. In: Walls RM, ed. *Manual of emergency airway management*, 4th ed. Philadelphia: Lippincott Williams & Wilkins; 2004:97–109.

Reichman E. Airway procedures. In: Wolfson AB, ed. *Harwood-Nuss' clinical practice of emergency medicine*, 2nd ed. Philadelphia: Lippincott Williams & Wilkins; 2005: 12–27.

Rosenblatt WH, Murphy M. The intubating laryngeal mask: Use of a new ventilating-intubating device in the emergency department. *Ann Emerg Med.* 1999;33(2): 234–238.

4

Thoracentesis

David W. Callaway, David Feller-Kopman,

and Daniel C. McGillicuddy

Indications

- Diagnostic: Acquisition of pleural fluid for diagnostic analysis
- Therapeutic: Relief of respiratory distress caused by the accumulation of fluid in the pleural space

Contraindications

- **Absolute**
  - Traumatic hemo- or pneumothorax (tube thoracostomy more appropriate)
- **Relative**
  - Platelet count <50,000
  - Prothrombin time (PT)/partial thromboplastin time (PTT) greater than twice normal
  - Cutaneous infection (e.g., herpes zoster)
  - Mechanical ventilation (can convert small pneumothorax into tension pneumothorax)
  - Uncooperative or agitated patient
  - An effusion that is contralateral to a prior pneumonectomy side

Risks

Thoracentesis is generally an elective procedure. Informed consent is required.

- The needle may cause injury to the lung (tube thoracostomy may be required if a pneumothorax develops).
- The potential for infection exists (sterile technique will be utilized).
- Rarely, other organs such as the spleen or liver may be injured.
- The procedure can cause mild pain (local anesthesia will be given).
- The needle puncture can cause localized bleeding; if this happens, a pressure dressing will be applied.

Landmarks

- The posterior approach is most common.
  - Identify the midscapular line and mark the thoracentesis site one to two rib spaces below the superior portion of the effusion.
  - The intercostal neurovascular bundle runs along the inferior portion of the rib. Therefore, the needle should be inserted superiorly (see Fig. 4.1).
- The hemidiaphragm changes level with respiration. You should not proceed with thoracentesis below the eighth intercostal space, given the risk for splenic or hepatic injury.

Technique

- **Preparation**
  - Place patient on supplemental oxygen.

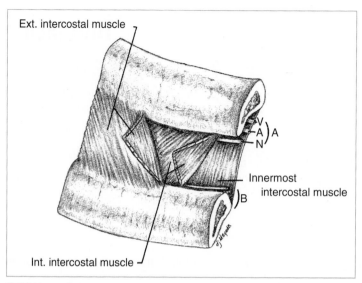

Ext. intercostal muscle

V
A } A
N

Innermost intercostal muscle

B

Int. intercostal muscle

FIGURE 4.1: Relations of structures within an intercostal space **A**. Intercostal vessels and nerves are shown in **B**. Collateral vessels are shown. A, artery; V, vein; N, nerve.

- Place the patient in upright (most common), lateral decubitus, or supine position.
- Arrange your material on a sterile towel atop a Mayo stand (or equivalent) (see Fig. 4.2).

Identify the Thoracentesis Site

- On physical examination, dullness to percussion, decreased breath sounds, and decreased tactile fremitus identify the superior margin of the effusion.
- Ultrasound localization is more accurate than physical examination for identifying effusions.
- Mark needle insertion site one to two rib spaces below the superior margin of the effusion.

Sterilize and Anesthetize the Area

- Sterilize a wide area surrounding the designated insertion site.
- Drape the area with sterile towels.
- Observe sterile technique from this point forward.
- Analgesia: Achieve local anesthesia using lidocaine with epinephrine (1% lidocaine is 10 mg/mL of solution). Typically, only 5 to 10 mL are required.
- Inject the subcutaneous tissue with a small-bore (25-gauge) needle and raise a wheal at the superior margin of the selected rib in the midscapular or posterior axillary line.
- Alternating between aspiration and injection, advance to the superior portion of the posterior rib and anesthetize the periosteum.
- Gently advance the needle over the superior portion of the rib while infiltrating with lidocaine.
- Slowly advance the needle until pleural fluid is aspirated. Withdraw the needle 1 to 2 mm and inject 2 to 4 mL of lidocaine to anesthetize the parietal pleura. Though the visceral pleura are not innervated with pain fibers, the parietal pleura are quite sensitive.
- Mark the depth of the chest wall by grasping the needle at the level of the skin with either your thumb and index finger or a Kelly clamp and withdraw the needle.

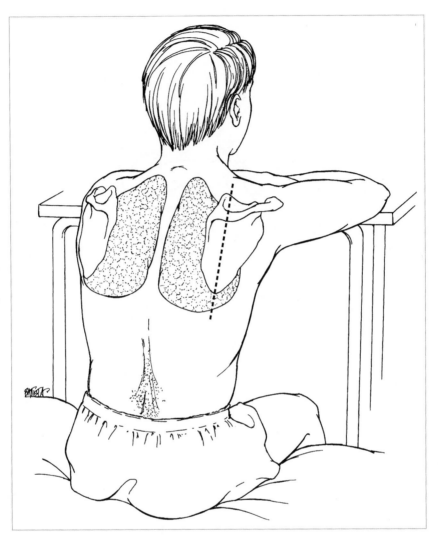

FIGURE 4.2: Landmarks for the posterior approach.

■ **Needle Insertion**
   ● Make a stab incision parallel to the rib at the marked site for easier insertion of the thoracentesis needle.
   ● Attach a 60-mL syringe to the catheter-clad needle. Insert the thoracentesis needle, bevel directed inferiorly, through the skin over the selected rib while maintaining negative pressure.
   ● Advance the needle over the superior portion of the posterior rib, applying constant steady pressure and aspirating until pleural fluid is encountered.
   ● As the catheter enters the pleural space, angle the needle caudally and push the catheter off the needle into the pleural space.
   ● Occlude the lumen of the catheter (see Fig. 4.3).
■ **Drain Pleural Fluid**
   ● Attach the three-way stopcock to the catheter hub. Set the stopcock valve to occlude the catheter port.
   ● Attach the 60-mL syringe to one port of the three-way stopcock.

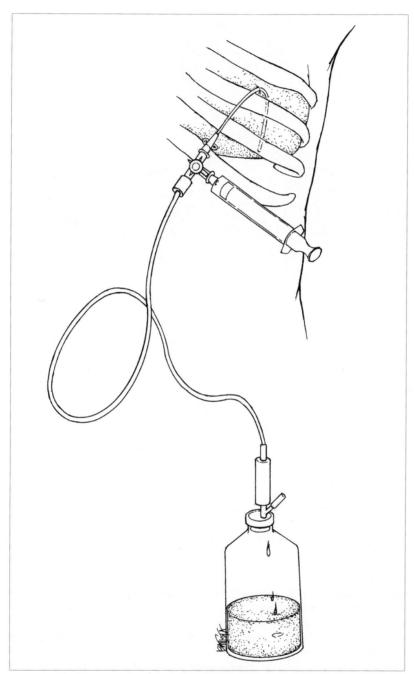

FIGURE 4.3: Needle insertion.

- Turn the stopcock valve to connect the syringe with the catheter and withdraw fluid from the pleural space. Turn the stopcock to connect the syringe to the intravenous tubing and empty the syringe into the collection bag or bottle.

Postprocedure

- When no further fluid can be withdrawn, ask the patient to hum/exhale while the catheter is withdrawn.

- Cover the insertion site with a sterile dressing or plastic adhesive bandage(Band-Aid).
- Send a Red-top specimen tube (for Gram stain and culture) and a Purple-top specimen tube (for cell count) to the laboratory.
- Indications for chest radiograph are:
  - Aspiration of air
  - Prior chest radiation therapy
  - Prior thoracentesis
  - Hemodynamic instability
  - Shortness of breath during the procedure
  - Multiple needle passes
  - To assess underlying lung parenchyma (i.e., to evaluate for pneumonia or malignancy).
- Hemodynamic and respiratory monitoring for 1 to 2 hours is recommended.

Complications
- Pneumothorax
- Lung laceration
- Hemopneumothorax
- Intra-abdominal injuries
- Diaphragmatic tear
- Hypotension from removal of massive amounts of fluid
- Chest wall bleeding from lacerated intercostal artery
- Re-expansion pulmonary edema
- Subsequent development of empyema

Fluid Analysis
The primary goal of fluid analysis is to identify the etiology of the effusion (see Table 4.1).
- **Light Criteria**
  - Presence of more than one of the following findings is 98% sensitive for exudates.
    - Pleural fluid to serum protein ratio >0.5

TABLE 4.1: Common etiologies of effusions

Transudate	Exudate
Congestive heart failure	Infection:
Cirrhosis with ascites	Bacterial pneumonia
Nephrotic syndrome	Lung abscess
Hypoalbuminemia	Tuberculosis
Myxedema	Neoplasm:
Peritoneal dialysis	Primary lung
Glomerulonephritides	Mesothelioma
Superior vena cava obstruction	Metastases
Pulmonary embolus	Lymphoma
	Connective tissue disease
	Miscellaneous
	Pulmonary infarct
	Uremia
	Chylothorax

> ▷ Pleural fluid to serum lactate dehydrogenase (LDH) ratio >0.6
> ▷ Pleural fluid LDH >200 or two thirds of upper limit of normal serum LDH
> • Meeting none of Light criteria is considered the standard for excluding an exudative effusion.

Common Pitfalls

- Failure to sit patient completely upright causing increase in risk of hepatic or splenic injury
- Failure to perform thoracentesis when effusion may be causing patient's respiratory distress
- Failure to maintain sterile technique resulting in postprocedure empyema

Pearls

- Therapeutic thoracentesis should not remove >1,000 to 1,500 mL to reduce likelihood of postexpansion pulmonary edema.
- If the clinical picture suggests a transudative effusion (e.g., history of congestive heart failure [CHF] with clear/light yellow fluid) but the pleural fluid is exudative according to Light's criteria, calculation of the serum:pleural fluid albumin gradient may assist in the diagnosis. Serum albumin >1.2 g/dL higher than the pleural fluid is consistent with a transudative effusion (sensitivity 92%).
- Ultrasound is very useful in detecting the proper needle insertion site, thereby reducing complications (see Fig. 4.4).

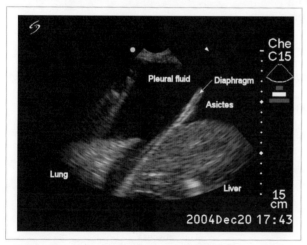

FIGURE 4.4: Ultrasound imaging of pleural effusion.

Suggested Readings

Ultrasound Guidance

Feller-Kopman D. Ultrasound- guided thoracentesis. *Chest.* 2006;129:1709–1714.

Jones PW, Moyers P, Rogers JT, et al. Ultrasound- guided thoracentesis- is it a safer method? *Chest.* 2003;123:418–423.

Tibbles CD, Porcaro W. Procedural applications of ultrasound. *Emerg Med Clin North Am.* 2004;22(3):797–815.

Post-thoracentesis Chest Radiography

Colt HG, Brewer N, Barbur E. Evaluation of patient- related and procedure- related factors contributing to pneumothorax following thoracentesis. *Chest*. 1999;116(1): 134–138.

Doyle JJ, Hnatiuk OW, Torrington KG, et al. Necessity of routine chest roentgenography after thoracentesis. *Ann Int Med*. 1996;124(9):816–820.

Petersen WG, Zimmerman R. Limited utility of chest radiograph after thoracentesis. *Chest*. 2000;117(4):1038–1042.

General

Collins TR, Sahn SA. Thoracentesis. Clinical value, complications, technical problems, and patient experience. *Chest*. 1987;91:817.

Villena V, López-Encuentra A, Pozo F, et al. Measurement of pleural pressure during therapeutic thoracentesis. *Am J Respir Crit Care Med*. 2000;162:1534.

Light Criteria

Light RW. Pleural effusion. *N Engl J Med*. 2002;346(25):1971–1977.

5 Tube Thoracostomy

Chilembwe Mason

Indications

"Chest tube" is used to evacuate abnormal collections of air or fluid from the pleural space in the following conditions:

- Pneumothorax
- Hemothorax
- Chylothorax
- Empyema
- Drainage of recurrent pleural effusion
- Prevention of hydrothorax after cardiothoracic surgery

Contraindications

- None for unstable injured patients
- **Relative Contraindications**
  - Anatomic abnormalities—pleural adhesions, emphysematous blebs, or scarring
  - Coagulopathy

Landmarks

- Chest tube placement preferred at the fourth or fifth intercostal space at the mid- to anterior axillary line but multiple sites are possible (see Fig. 5.1).
- Intercostal nerve and vessels are located along the inferior margin of each rib, therefore the tube should pass immediately over the superior surface of the lower rib.

Supplies

There exist several commercially packaged thoracostomy kits. However, the surgeon should be familiar with the required equipment should these kits not be available. Standard equipment includes:

- Antiseptic solution, drapes, and towel clips
- 1% Lidocaine, 20 mL
- 25-gauge needle, 22-gauge needle, 10-mL syringe
- No. 10 scalpel blade with handle, Kelly clamps (two), and forceps
- Thoracostomy tube selection
  - Trauma: No. 36–40 French
  - Nontraumatic: No. 24–32 French
  - Children: No. 20–24 French
  - Infants: No. 18 French
- Pleurivac (collection bottle, underwater seal, suction control)
- Connecting tubing

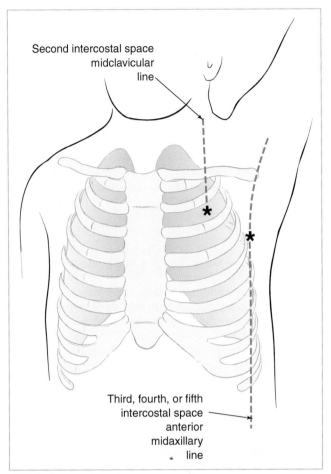

Second intercostal space
midclavicular
line

Third, fourth, or fifth
intercostal space
anterior
midaxillary
line

FIGURE 5.1: Possible sites for chest tube placement. (From Connors KM, Terndrup TE. Tube thoracostomy and needle decompression of the chest. In: Henretig FM, King C, eds. *Textbook of pediatric emergency procedures*. Philadelphia: Lippincott Williams & Wilkins; 1997:399.)

- Gauze pads, adhesive tape, 4 × 4-in. pads, Xeroform gauze dressing, antibiotic ointment
- 2, 1, or 0 suture (not 2–0 or 1–0), needle driver, and suture scissors

Technique
- **Preparation**
  - Nasal oxygen and continuous pulse oximetry monitoring should be arranged for.
  - If patient is stable, parenteral analgesics or conscious sedation should be used.
  - Elevate the head of the bed to 30 to 60 degrees.
  - Patient's arm on the affected side is placed over the patients head.
  - Sterilize the area where the tube will be inserted with povidone-iodine or chlorhexidine solution.
  - Drape the area with sterile towels.

- Assemble the suction-drain system according to manufacturer's recommendations; adjust the suction until a steady stream of bubbles is produced in the water column.

General Basic Steps

Analgesia
Incision
Blunt dissection
Verification
Insertion
Securing the tube
Confirmation

- **Analgesia**
  - Produce local anesthesia using up to 5 mg/kg of 1% lidocaine with epinephrine (1:100,000).
  - Inject the subcutaneous area with a small-bore (25-gauge) needle.
  - Generously infiltrate the muscle, periosteum, and parietal pleura in the area of the tube's eventual passage using a larger bore needle.
- **Incision**
  - Using a no. 10 scalpel blade make at least a 3 to 4 cm transverse incision through the skin and subcutaneous tissue.
  - One method is to make the incision at an intercostal space lower than the thoracic wall entry site, so the tube may be "tunneled" up over the next rib.
- **Blunt Dissection**
  - Use a large Kelly clamp or scissor (this often takes considerable force).
  - Track is created over the rib by pushing forward with the closed points and then spreading and pulling back with the points spread.
  - Push through the muscle and parietal pleural with the closed points of the clamp until the pleural cavity is entered.
  - A palpable pop is felt when the pleura is penetrated, and a rush of air or fluid should occur at this point.
- **Verification**
  - Once the pleura is penetrated, insert a gloved finger into the chest wall track to verify that the pleura has been entered and that no solid organs are present.
  - The finger can be left in place to serve as a guide for tube insertion.
- **Insertion**
  - It is recommended that the tube be held in a large curved clamp with the tip of the tube protruding from the jaws.
  - Pass the tube over, under, or beside the finger into the pleural space.
  - The tube is advanced superiorly, medially, and posteriorly until pain is felt or resistance is met; then pulled back 2 to 3 cm.
  - Ensure that all the holes in the chest tube are within the pleural space.
- **Securing the Tube** (numerous methods are acceptable)
  - Close the remainder of the incision using a large 0 or 1 silk or nylon suture keeping the ends long.
  - Suture ends are wrapped and tied repeatedly around the chest tube, then knotted securely. The sutures are tied tightly enough to indent the chest tube slightly to avoid slippage.

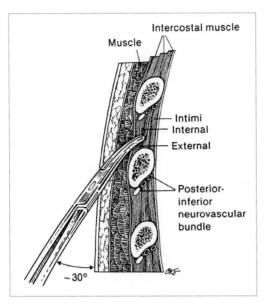

FIGURE 5.2: Perform blunt dissection through the subcutaneous tissues and intercostal muscles with a Kelly clamp. (From Feliciano DV. Tube thoracostomy. In: Benumof JL, ed. *Clinical procedures in anesthesia and intensive care*. Philadelphia: JB Lippincott Co; 1992, with permission.)

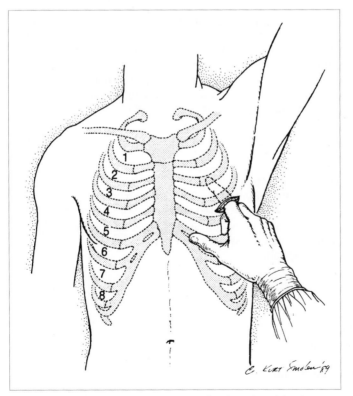

FIGURE 5.3: Perform finger thoracotomy before insertion of the thoracostomy tube. (From Feliciano DV. Tube thoracostomy. In: Benumof JL, ed. *Clinical procedures in anesthesia and intensive care*. Philadelphia: JB Lippincott Co; 1992, with permission.)

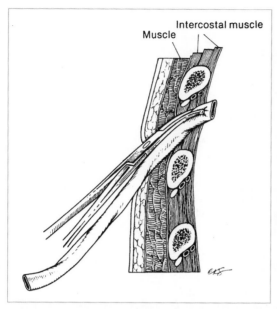

Muscle
Intercostal muscle

FIGURE 5.4: Direct the thoracostomy tube posteriorly and superiorly in patients with pleural effusions including hemothoraces. (From Feliciano DV. Tube thoracostomy. In: Benumof JL, ed. *Clinical procedures in anesthesia and intensive care*. Philadelphia: JB Lippincott Co; 1992, with permission.)

- A horizontal mattress (or Purse-string) suture is placed approximately 1 cm across the incision on either side of the tube, essentially encircling the tube. This suture helps secure the tube and eventually facilitates closing the incision when the chest tube is removed.
- Place occlusive dressing of petroleum-impregnated gauze where the tube enters the skin; then cover with two or more gauze pads.
- Wide cloth adhesive tape can be used to hold the tube more securely in place.

- **Confirmation**
  - Indicators for correct placement are as follows:
    - Condensation on the inside of the tube
    - Audible air movement with respirations
    - Free flow of blood or fluid
    - Ability to rotate the tube freely after insertion
  - Attach tube to previously assembled water seal or suction.
    - Observing bubbles in the water seal chamber when the patient coughs is a good way to check for system patency.
  - Obtain chest radiograph.

Complications
- Hemothorax
- Pulmonary edema
- Bronchopleural fistula
- Empyema
- Subcutaneous emphysema
- Infection
- Contralateral pneumothorax
- Subdiaphragmatic placement of the tube
- Localized hemorrhage

Common Pitfalls

- Use of inadequate local anesthesia
- Making the initial skin incision too small
- Failure to advance the chest tube far enough into the pleural space
- Directing the tube towards the mediastinum can cause a contralateral pneumothorax

Pearls

- For a pneumothorax, direct the tube superiorly and anteriorly. For a hemothorax, direct the tube posteriorly.
- Clamp both ends of the tube during insertion to avoid being contaminated by fluid.
- If there is no lung re-expansion after chest tube placement consider that the tube may not be in the pleural cavity, that the most proximal hole is outside the chest cavity, or that there is a large air leak from the tracheobronchial tree.
- Immediate drainage of more than 20 mL/Kg (approximately 1000–1500 mL in an adult) of blood from the pleural cavity or a continued output of at least 200 mL/hour for 4 hours is an indication for a thoracotomy.

Suggested Readings

Kirsch TD, Mulligan JP. Tube thoracostomy. In: Roberts JR, Hedges JR, eds. *Clinical procedures in emergency medicine*, 4th ed. Philadelphia: WB Saunders, 2004:187–209.

Simon RR, Brenner BE. *Emergency procedures and techniques*, 4th ed. Philadelphia: Lippincott Williams & Wilkens; 2002:172–179.

Section Editor: David H. Newman

6

Cardiac Pacing

Oscar Rago and Richard Lanoix

Indications
- **Hemodynamically Unstable or Symptomatic Bradycardia**
  - Hypotension
  - Pulmonary edema
  - Angina
  - Altered mental status
  - Other signs of significant end-organ hypoperfusion
- **Transvenous Pacing**
  - Failure or nontolerance of transcutaneous pacing
  - Need for extended duration of cardiac pacing without rapid access to consultants or facilities capable of providing transvenous or permanent pacemaker placement

Contraindications
- Absolute: None
- **Relative**
  - Severe hypothermia (due to propensity for induction of ventricular fibrillation)
  - Severe digoxin toxicity
    - ▶ Attempt infusion of digoxin immune Fab (Digibind)
    - ▶ Treat hyperkalemia with intravenous calcium

Transcutaneous Pacing Procedure
Landmarks
Pacer pads should be placed over the precordium anteriorly and in the intrascapular paraspinous region posteriorly.
Technique
- **Patient Preparation**
  - In conscious patients, reassurance and explanation of the procedure including expectations for discomfort are extremely important.
  - Continuous cardiac and pulse oximetry monitoring, intravenous access, and bedside capability for resuscitation including airway management, defibrillation, and arrhythmia treatment should be at the bedside *before initiation*.
- **Pacer/Electrode Placement**
  - Pads are placed as shown in Figure 6.1.

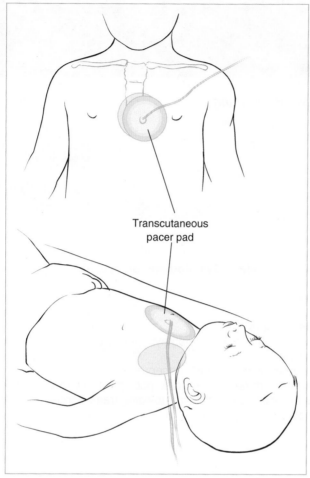

Transcutaneous
pacer pad

FIGURE 6.1: Proper placement of transcutaneous pacing electrodes. (From Kelly KP, Altieri MF. Cardiac pacing. In: Henretig FM, King C. *Textbook of pediatric emergency procedures.* Philadelphia: Williams & Wilkins; 1997:310, with permission.)

- Anterior chest pacing pad (negative charge electrode) is placed over the point of maximal impulse.
- If access to the posterior chest wall is limited or difficult, posterior pacer pad may also be placed in cardiac apex/base position (identical to electrical cardioversion placement).
- Electrocardiogram (ECG) electrodes should be placed in typical anterior chest wall positions.

- **Pacing**
  - Identify pacemaker mode on equipment and turn to ''on''.
  - Set heart rate to 70 bpm.
  - Place and maintain one hand in pulse-check position (radial, femoral, or carotid).
  - In bradyasystole and unconscious patients, set current to 150 to 200 mA and lower in 10-mA decrements; set current at the lowest level that will consistently achieve mechanical capture.
  - In stable and conscious patients, set current to 10 mA and raise in 10-mA increments until mechanical capture is achieved.

- Observe cardiac monitor for pacemaker spikes and electrical capture—"electrical capture" refers to narrow pacemaker spikes followed by typical, wide ventricular complexes.
- Monitor constantly for "mechanical capture"—*this is the goal of cardiac pacing* and refers to a palpable arterial pulse induced by pacemaker discharges.
- Titrate sedation/analgesia/anxiolysis to allow for tolerance of ongoing pacing.
- Failure to achieve mechanical capture should prompt immediate preparation for transvenous pacer placement.

Transvenous Pacing Procedure

Landmarks

- The **right internal jugular** and **left subclavian** approaches have the advantage of anatomic proximity and directional ease in accessing the superior vena cava.
- For specific venous access techniques and corresponding landmarks the reader is referred to the "Vascular" section in this book.

Equipment

- **Pacing Generator** (see Fig. 6.2) contains the following:

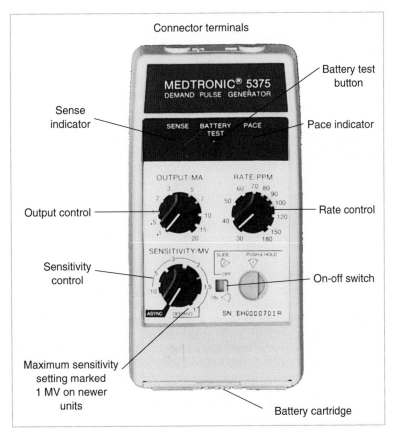

FIGURE 6.2: Medtronic cardiac pacer. (From Kelly KP, Altieri MF. Cardiac pacing. In: Henretig FM, King C. *Textbook of pediatric emergency procedures.* Philadelphia: Williams & Wilkins; 1997:303, with permission.)

- On/off switch
- Rate switch (numerical): Set at 70 bpm
- Demand versus Asynchronous switch (detection–sensitivity modes):
  - In "Demand" mode, the pacemaker will sense intrinsic cardiac impulses and pace only when the intrinsic rate falls below the set rate.
  - In "Asynchronous" mode the pacemaker will discharge at the set rate regardless of intrinsic activity. (Some generator units will have an additional numerical sensitivity setting, typically from 20 mV to 0.5 mV. **Higher** numerical settings cause **less sensitive** detection of intrinsic impulses while **lower** numerical settings cause **more sensitive** detection.)
- Output switch (numerical): Determines energy output (mA) per discharge.
- Sense indicator light: Flashes with each detected intrinsic impulse.
- **Flexible Pacing Catheter** (typically 3–5 French, ~100 cm in length) contains the following:
  - Negative and positive terminals at the proximal end
  - Distal balloon (test inflate with 1.5 mL normal saline)
  - Electrode at the distal tip (delivers the current stimulus)
- Central venous cannulation equipment—choose an "introducer" sheath **one size larger than the size of the pacing catheter**
- ECG monitoring
- If available, an ultrasound unit .

Technique
- **Patient Preparation**
  - Patient should be reassured and the procedure fully explained.
  - Physician should wear mask, sterile gown, and sterile gloves.
  - Sterile technique should be fully maintained throughout.
  - 100% O_2 via nonrebreather face mask should be administered.
  - Continuous cardiac and pulse oximetry monitoring should be placed.
  - Trendelenburg position is preferred for central venous dilation.
- **Pacemaker Catheter Insertion**
  - Obtain central venous access using the introducer sheath.
  - Set the pacemaker generator to demand mode, 70 bpm, 5 mA output.
  - Choose one of three common methods:
    - ECG monitor-assisted
    - Unassisted or blind catheter positioning
    - Ultrasound-guided

Electrocardiogram Monitor-Assisted
- Attach the negative terminal at the proximal end of the pacemaker catheter into the V_1 lead on the ECG monitor, if adaptable (displaces the monitor's V_1 wire).
- Inflate the balloon with 1.5 mL of air in a container of sterile saline to assess balloon integrity (the presence of bubbles in the saline indicates a balloon leak).
- Insert the catheter through the introducer sheath into the vein while noting depth.
- At 10 cm insertion depth inflate the balloon with 1.5 mL of sterile saline.
- While advancing the catheter, monitor P waves and QRS complexes to determine the location of the catheter tip.
- P wave and QRS morphology correlations with catheter position (see Fig. 6.3) as follows:
  - Subclavian/internal jugular vein: P wave and QRS are small, negative
  - Superior vena cava: Larger P wave, QRS unchanged
  - High right atrium: Very large P wave, QRS unchanged

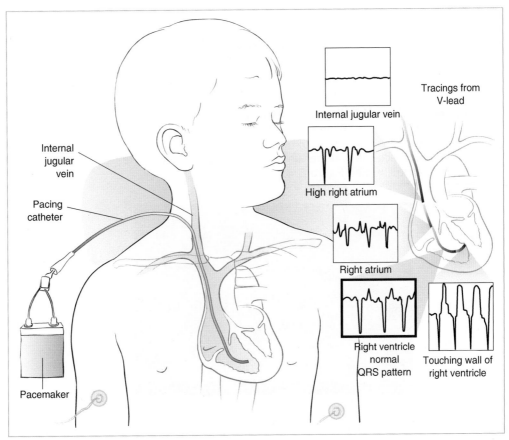

FIGURE 6.3: Transvenous pacemaker placement via the right internal jugular vein. (From Kelly KP, Altieri MF. Cardiac pacing. In: Henretig FM, King C. *Textbook of pediatric emergency procedures.* Philadelphia: Williams & Wilkins; 1997:304, with permission.)

- Low right atrium: Large positive P wave, larger negative QRS
- Right ventricle: Small positive P wave, large negative QRS
- Abutting the right ventricular wall: Injury pattern (ST elevation)
- Pulmonary artery: P wave negative, QRS becomes smaller
- Inferior vena cava: P wave positive, QRS negative, both smaller
- If the catheter is in the pulmonary circulation or inferior vena cava, withdraw 3 to 5 cm until typical right ventricular morphology appears, rotate catheter 90 degrees in either direction, advance again.

Unassisted or Blind Catheter Positioning
- Connect the pacemaker catheter to the generator by both electrodes and turn to "on."
- Set demand mode, rate of 100, output dial to 2 mA.
- If a balloon tipped pacemaker is used, test balloon integrity as above.
- Insert the catheter through the introducer sheath into the vein while noting depth.
- At 10 cm insertion depth, inflate the balloon with 1.5 mL of sterile saline.
- While advancing, the sensing indicator light will blink with each native beat until the catheter enters the right ventricle, when it will blink with every other beat. At this point stop advancing the catheter and deflate the balloon.

- Increase the output to 5 mA and slowly advance the catheter until mechanical ventricular capture occurs.
- If ventricular capture is not successful within 10 cm from the point where the sensing indicator began to blink with every other heartbeat, withdraw the catheter 10 cm, rotate it 90 degrees, and re-advance. Repeat until capture is successful.

Ultrasound-Guided Catheter Positioning
- As above in "Blind Catheter Positioning", plus the following:
- Visualize the heart utilizing the subxiphoid window
- Advance the catheter until it is visualized entering the right atrium and right ventricle. See Figure 6.4.

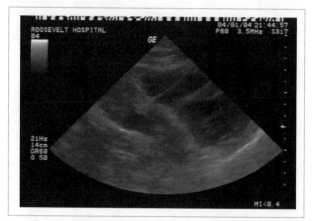

FIGURE 6.4: Subcostal view of the heart with the pacing wire in the right ventricle. (Picture courtesy of Amir Darvish, MD.)

- Once in the right ventricle, stop advancing the catheter and deflate the balloon.
- Slowly advance until ventricular capture is achieved.
- **Pacing**
  - If utilizing the ECG monitoring technique, disconnect the negative electrode (from the V_1 lead) and re-attach to the negative port in the generator.
  - Keep generator on.
  - Turn the pacer on (Demand mode, 70 bpm, 5 mA energy output).
  - Increase energy output dial until electrical capture (pacing spikes, wide QRS).
  - Check for mechanical capture (corresponding pulses with each electrical capture).
  - Once mechanical capture is achieved, decrease output until mechanical capture is lost ("threshold point"), and resume at 2 mA above this point.
- **Secure the Pacemaker**
  - Once mechanical capture is achieved withdraw the introducer sheath, suture the catheter to the chest wall with a 3-0 nylon and apply sterile dressing.
- **Confirmation**
  - A LBBB pattern should be seen on the 12-lead ECG during pacing.
  - Obtain a chest x-ray to confirm right ventricle placement.

Complications
- Identical to those related to central venous cannulation
- Ventricular dysrhythmias

- Left ventricular pacing from atrial septal defect (ASD) or ventricular septal defect (VSD)
- Right ventricular perforation with hemopericardium and tamponade
- Displacement or fracture of the electrode causing dysrhythmias

Common Pitfalls
- Forgetting to ensure mechanical capture after pacemaker placement
- Mistaking ventricular fibrillation or tachycardia for a paced rhythm
- Forgetting to inflate the balloon after the pacing catheter is placed in the vein

Pearls
- Electrical capture does not assure mechanical capture—CHECK FOR PULSES when confirming capture (not just pacemaker complexes on the ECG!).
- Transvenous pacers can be placed in less than 20 minutes in most patients.
- The right internal jugular or left subclavian are the most direct approaches.
- After pacemaker placement, a 12-lead ECG with RBBB pattern indicates septal perforation, VSD, or coronary sinus placement.
- Always check a chest x-ray after placing a pacemaker.
- Most common causes of failure to capture in transcutaneous pacers are improper electrode placement or large patient size.

Suggested Readings
Birkhahn R, Gaeta TJ, Tloczkowski J, et al. Emergency medicine-trained physicians are proficient in the insertion of transvenous pacemakers. *Ann Emerg Med.* 2004; 43:469–474.

Roberts J, Hedges J. *Clinical procedures in emergency medicine*, 4th ed. Philadelphia: WB Saunders; 2004.

7

Emergency Pericardiocentesis

Hiral H. Shah and Jason D'Amore

Indications
- Pericardial tamponade with hemodynamic decompensation
- Pulseless electrical activity with clinical suspicion of tamponade or with ultrasonographic evidence of pericardial effusion

Contraindications
- None for the unstable patient
- Coagulopathy is a relative contraindication

Risks/Consent
- In the emergent situation no consent is required.
- For risks see "Complications" section below.

Landmarks
- **Anatomic Approaches**
  - Subxiphoid
    - Needle is inserted between the xiphoid process and the left costal margin in a 30- to 45-degree angle to the skin.
    - Recommendations regarding needle aim vary widely including right shoulder, sternal notch, and left shoulder.
  - Parasternal approach (more common with bedside ultrasonography)
    - Needle is inserted perpendicular to the skin in the left fifth intercostal space immediately lateral to the sternum.
  - Ultrasound-guided approach
    - Place a 3.5- to 5.0-MHz probe in the subcostal position to directly visualize both the area of maximal effusion and location of vital structures.
    - Insert needle in left chest wall using a parasternal approach where the largest pocket of fluid is seen.

Technique
- **Patient Preparation**
  - A 100% oxygen via face mask should be administered if patient is conscious and nonintubated.
  - Ensure continuous cardiac and pulse oximetry monitoring.
  - Patient should be placed in the semiupright position (15–30 degrees) if possible to pool pericardial fluid dependently.
  - If patient is awake, local analgesia should be utilized.
  - Sterilize locally with chlorhexidine or povidone-iodine solution and use sterile gloves, if time permits.

Procedural Steps
- Attach an 18-gauge spinal needle to a 10- to 30-mL syringe.
- Attach an alligator clip to the base of the needle and the other end to the precordial (V) lead of the electrocardiogram (ECG) machine to monitor for ST elevations indicating penetration of the myocardium (see Figs. 7.1–7.3).

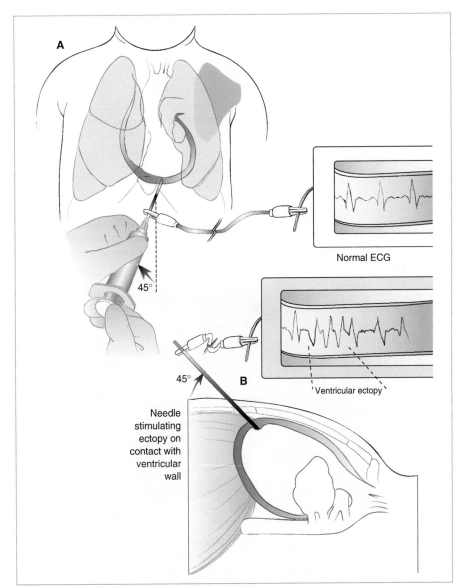

FIGURE 7.1: Pericardiocentesis in child using substernal approach. ECG, electrocardiogram. (From Reeves SD. Pericardiocentesis. In: Henretig FM, King C, eds. *Textbook of pediatric emergency procedures*. Philadelphia: Williams & Wilkins; 1997:780, with permission.)

- Using either a subxiphoid or parasternal approach (see "Landmarks" section above for details), insert and advance the spinal needle while gently aspirating the syringe, preferably with ultrasonographic assistance.

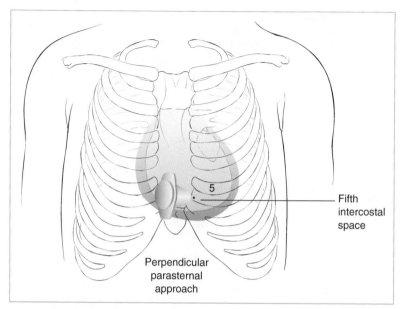

FIGURE 7.2: Pericardiocentesis in adolescent using parasternal approach. (From Reeves SD. Pericardiocentesis. In: Henretig FM, King C, eds. *Textbook of pediatric emergency procedures.* Philadelphia: Williams & Wilkins; 1997:780, with permission.)

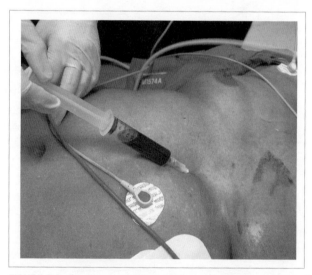

FIGURE 7.3: Emergency pericardiocentesis. (From Wiler J. Pericardiocentesis. In: Greenberg MI, Hendrickson RG, Silverberg M, et al. *Greenberg's text-atlas of emergency medicine.* Philadelphia: Lippincott Williams & Wilkins; 2005:29, with permission.)

- Pericardium should be reached at approximately 6 to 8 cm below the skin in adults.
- Stop advancing once fluid is aspirated.
- Remove as much fluid as possible.
- Remove the needle when done.
- If patient is successfully resuscitated, check for pneumothorax with portable (preferably upright) chest x-ray (CXR).

- **Confirmation**
  - Aspiration of blood may indicate cardiac puncture or hemorrhagic pericardial fluid
  - Clotting of blood does not confirm intracardiac aspirate (brisk bleeding can cause hemorrhagic pericardial fluid to clot)
  - Nonclotting blood confirms a pericardial source (defibrinated)
  - Nonbloody fluid confirms a pericardial source

Complications

- Dry tap (no fluid aspirated, more common without ultrasonography)
- Pneumothorax
- Myocardial or coronary vessel injury
- Hemopericardium
- Air embolism
- Dysrhythmias
- Cardiac arrest and/or death (rare)
- Liver injury

Common Pitfalls

- Inserting needle below xiphoid process as opposed to between the xiphoid process and the left costal margin

Pearls

- Whenever possible let ultrasonography dictate approach.
- Most complications occur in patients who have no pericardial effusion.
- Obtain chest radiography to rule out pneumothorax after the procedure.

Suggested Readings

Harper RJ. Pericardiocentesis. In: Roberts JR, Hedges JR, eds. *Clinical procedures in emergency medicine*, 4th ed. Chapter 16, WB Saunders; 2003.

Markovchick VJ. Pericardiocentesis. Rosen P, Chan T, Vilke G, et al. *Atlas of emergency procedures*, 5th ed. Mosby; 2001.

Tsang TS, Freeman WK, Sinak LJ, et al. Echocardiographically guided pericardiocentesis: Evolution and state-of-the-art technique. [Review]. *Mayo Clin Proc*. 1998;73(7): 647–652.

8

Emergency Department Thoracotomy

Oscar Rago and Barbara Kilian

Indications
- **Penetrating Chest Trauma**
  - Loss of pulses at any time with initial vital signs in the field
  - Systolic blood pressure <70 mm Hg after aggressive fluid resuscitation
- **Blunt Trauma**
  - Witnessed loss of pulses or systolic blood pressure <70 mm Hg after aggressive fluid resuscitation AND
    - ▷ Initial chest tube output >20 mL/kg of blood, OR
    - ▷ Confirmed or highly suspected pericardial effusion, OR
    - ▷ Confirmed or highly suspected ongoing intra-abdominal hemorrhage (controversial)
- **Goals**
  - Relief of cardiac tamponade
  - Support of cardiac function with open massage, aortic cross-clamping, and/or internal cardiac defibrillation
  - Control of cardiac, pulmonary, or great vessel hemorrhage

Contraindications
- Injuries with no witnessed vital signs
- Multisystem blunt trauma
- Severe head injury

Risks/Consent Issues
- This is an emergent procedure and does not require written consent.

Landmarks
- Left-sided supine anterolateral approach over the fifth rib, fourth intercostal space.
- In males incise below the nipple, in females below the inframammary fold.

Technique
- **Patient Preparation**
  - Patient should be intubated and a nasogastric tube should be placed.
  - Order IV fluids, epinephrine 1 mg IV, and stat blood.
  - Place towels under the left chest and the left arm above the head.
  - Sterilize the incision area with copious povidone-iodine solution.
  - In patients with signs of life, consider induction, sedation, and paralysis.
- **Incision and Dissection**
  - Using a no. 20 blade, incise from the sternal border to the posterior axillary line.

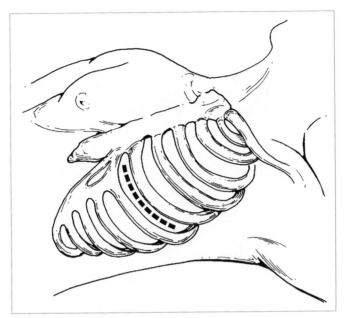

FIGURE 8.1: Thoracotomy landmark.

- Cut firmly through subcutaneous tissue to the intercostal muscle.
- Using scissors cut the intercostal muscles.
- Temporarily stop ventilations just before exposing the pleura to avoid lacerating the lung.
- Insert rib spreader (handle down) once the intercostal muscles are separated.
- Use a Gigli saw or trauma shears to cut the sternum for right-sided exposure.

- **Pericardiotomy**
  - Hold the pericardium with forceps, and use scissors to cut from the cardiac apex to the aortic root.
  - The incision should be made anterior and lateral, avoiding the left phrenic nerve.
  - Evacuate fresh blood and clots from the pericardial cavity.

- **Cardiac Massage**
  - Direct, two-handed cardiac massage should be started as soon as possible (see Fig. 8.3); the left hand is placed over the right ventricle while the right hand supports the surface of the left ventricle.
  - Avoid fingertip pressure and apply the compression force perpendicular to the septum.
  - Avoid direct pressure on coronary arteries and allow for relaxation in diastole.
  - To defibrillate, apply paddles perpendicular to the ventricles; use 20 to 60 J.

- **Control of Hemorrhagic Wounds**
  - Ventricular cardiac wounds
    - Initially, apply direct finger pressure.
    - Use staples to repair large ventricular wounds.
    - Nonabsorbable 2-0 silk sutures can also be used.
    - The use of Teflon pledgets may help prevent tearing of the myocardium (see Fig. 8.4).
  - For atrial wounds, use occlusion clamps (digital pressure may not work) or Foley catheter (see Fig. 8.5) for temporary control of bleeding.

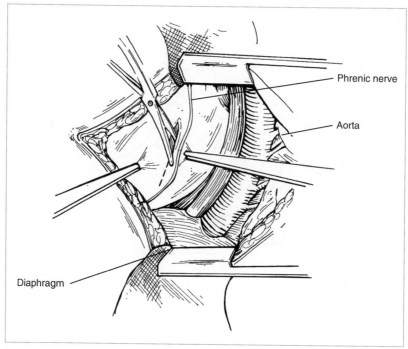

FIGURE 8.2: Pericardium.

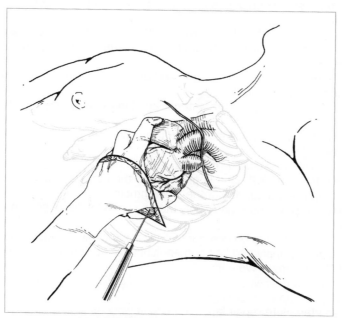

FIGURE 8.3: Internal cardiac massage.

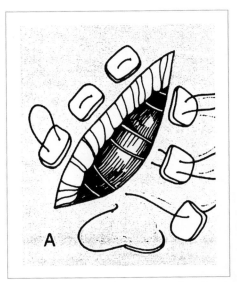

FIGURE 8.4: A ventricular septal defect resulting from a penetrating injury. Penetrating communications can often be closed by simple pledgeted mattress sutures. (From Simon RR, Brenner BE. *Emergency procedures and techniques,* 4th ed. Philadelphia: Lippincott Williams & Wilkins; 2002:166, with permission.)

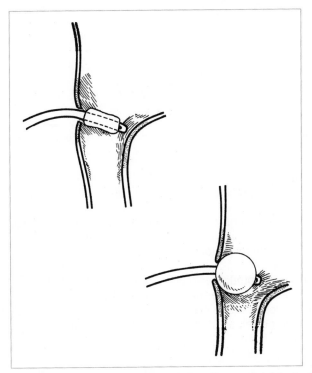

FIGURE 8.5: Place a Foley catheter tip into the wound. Inflate the balloon and pull back the catheter to control bleeding. Then proceed with more definitive repair. (From Simon RR, Brenner BE. *Emergency procedures and techniques,* 4th ed. Philadelphia: Lippincott Williams & Wilkins; 2002:167, with permission.)

- Great vessel wounds
  - ▶ Hemorrhage can generally be controlled using clamps or digital pressure (see Fig. 8.6).
  - ▶ Both subclavian arteries can be cross-clamped as needed.
  - ▶ Laparotomy pads can be used to tamponade hemorrhage.

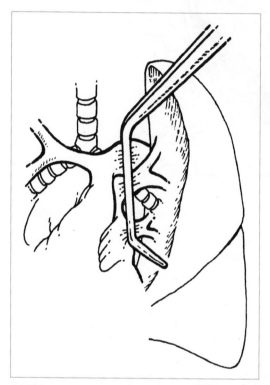

FIGURE 8.6: Occlusion of the pulmonary hilum with a Satinsky clamp. (From Simon RR, Brenner BE. *Emergency procedures and techniques*, 4th ed. Philadelphia: Lippincott Williams & Wilkins; 2002:170, with permission.)

Aortic Cross-Clamping
- Indicated if the systolic blood pressure cannot be maintained above 70 mm Hg.
- The aorta can be found posterior and lateral to the esophagus by running the fingers from the incision posteriorly towards the vertebral column, identifying the esophagus by palpation of the nasogastric tube, and dissecting away the anterior pleura.
- Once aorta is isolated, a vascular clamp is applied to the aorta by using the left index finger to secure the clamp (see Fig. 8.7).
- Check the brachial artery pressure and if it is greater than 120 mm Hg the clamp should be released and adjusted to maintain a blood pressure below 120 mm Hg.

Complications
- Aortic or esophageal injuries due to cross-clamping
- Myocardial injury secondary to open cardiac massage
- Phrenic nerve transaction

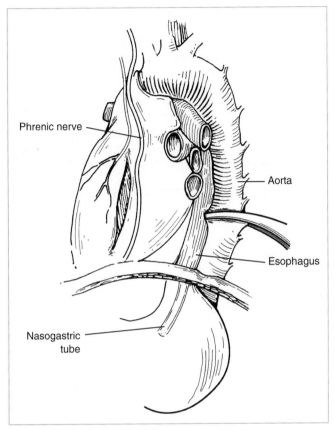

FIGURE 8.7: Aortic clamp.

- Fractured ribs
- Wound infection and/or sepsis (rare)

Common Pitfalls
- Incision too small: It is acceptable to incise past the posterior axillary line
- Rib spreader handle up: Does not allow for extension of incision to right chest
- Pericardium not opened: Myocardial injuries cannot be excluded without direct visualization
- Phrenic nerve injury: The nerve runs vertically on the anterior pericardial surface

Pearls
- The most important predictors of survival include injury mechanism (stab wounds carry the most favorable prognosis), injury location, and the presence of pulses.
- Always perform tube thoracotomy to identify potential right-sided injuries, if not extending the thoracotomy to the right side.
- A patient with an organized cardiac rhythm is a good candidate for a thoracotomy.
- Make the incision on top of the fifth rib to avoid the intercostal arteries.
- Start the incision 2 cm lateral to the sternal edge to avoid the internal mammary arteries.
- When cutting the pericardium diligently avoid myocardial laceration.

- Ribs may be broken while deploying the spreader, avoid getting cut by sharp bone edges.
- Health care needle-stick exposures have been reported at a high rate during emergency department (ED) thoracotomy. Be careful to take universal precautions and avoid needle injuries!

Suggested Readings

Cothren CC, Moore EE. Emergency department thoracotomy for the critically injured patient: Objectives, indications, and outcomes. *World J Emerg Surg*. 2006;1:4.

Roberts J, Hedges J. *Clinical procedures in emergency medicine*, 4th ed. Philadelphia: WB Saunders; 2004.

http://www.trauma.org/index.php/main/article/361/accessed june, 2007.

9 Induction of Therapeutic Hypothermia

Alberto Hazan and David H. Newman

Indications
- Comatose patients resuscitated from cardiac arrest with restoration of spontaneous circulation (see ''Pearls'' section)

Contraindications
- **Absolute Contraindications**
  - Patients without a pulse
  - Patients responsive to verbal commands
- **Relative Contraindications**
  - Delay in onset of cardiopulmonary resuscitation (CPR) of >10 minutes from cardiac arrest
  - Delay of >1 hour in restoration of spontaneous circulation
  - Pregnancy
  - Terminal illness

Risks/Consent Issues
- Procedure requires constant monitoring of body temperature by trained medical personnel to prevent severe iatrogenic hypothermia
- Eligible patients will not be able to consent to this procedure. (Given the brief time window that has been established for potential benefit and the degree of that benefit, risks of this procedure are considered few and mild enough that proxy consent is also unnecessary before initiation.)

Technique
- **Patient Preparation**
  - Sedation: Midazolam at 0.10 mg/kg/hour IV (alternate: propofol)
  - Analgesia: Fentanyl at 0.5 μg/kg/hour IV
  - Shivering prophylaxis: Vecuronium at 0.1 mg/kg IV, then 0.01 mg/kg IV every 30 minutes prn (alternate: any maintenance infusion paralytic agent)
  - Rectal temperature probe for continuous monitoring
- **Induction**
  - Place a commercial cooling blanket on top of the patient.
  - Keep temperature between 32°C and 34°C (90°F–93°F).
  - Use cold IV fluids or place ice packs on the axilla/groin to reach and maintain target temperature.
  - Target temperature should be reached within 2 to 4 hours from time of arrest.
- **Maintenance**
  - Continue to monitor and maintain body temperature between 32°C and 34°C (90°F–93°F) for a total of 12 to 24 hours.
  - Continue using cold IV fluids and ice packs if temperature exceeds 34°C (93°F).

- Remove cold packs or use IV fluids at room temperature if body temperature drops below 32°C (90°F).
- Continue medications as needed for sedation, analgesia, and shivering prophylaxis.
- Monitor electrolytes (check a basic metabolic panel every 6–8 hours).
- **Withdrawal**
  - After 24 hours of hypothermia, remove commercial cooling blanket and begin passive rewarming of the patient with warm blankets and IV fluids at room temperature to raise the body temperature back to normal.
  - Normal body temperature should be reached within 6 to 8 hours; use active external rewarming agents (e.g., warm humidified oxygen, warm IV fluids) to attain this target temperature.

Complications
- Severe iatrogenic hypothermia
- Adverse reactions to induction/maintenance medications

Pearls
- Although some authors have recommended induction of hypothermia only for those with ventricular fibrillation–associated cardiac arrests (based on trial enrollment criteria), we support a wider view of potential benefit: any comatose survivor of cardiac arrest regardless of rhythm subtype (presuming that hypoxic brain injury is present) may benefit from therapeutic hypothermia.

Suggested Readings
Bernard SA, Gray TW, Buist MD, et al. Treatment of comatose survivors of out-of-hospital cardiac arrest with induced hypothermia. *N Engl J Med*. 2002;346:557–563.

Holzer M, et al. The Hypothermia After Cardiac Arrest Study Group. Mild therapeutic hypothermia to improve the neurologic outcome after cardiac arrest. *N Engl J Med*. 2002;346:549–556.

Polderman KH, Rijnsburger ER, Peerdeman SM, et al. Induction of hypothermia in patients with various types of neurologic injury with use of large volumes of ice-cold intravenous fluid. *Crit Care Med*. 2005;33(12):2744–2751.

Section Editor: Erik P. Deede

10

Femoral Vein — Central Venous Access

Amir Darvish

Indications
- Emergency venous access for fluid resuscitation and drug infusion
- Infusions requiring central venous administration (vasopressors, calcium chloride, hyperosmolar solutions, hyperalimentation)
- Routine venous access due to inadequate peripheral IV sites; patients in respiratory distress who cannot be placed flat or in Trendelenburg position
- Introduction of transvenous pacemaker

Contraindications
- No absolute contraindications
- **Relative Contraindications**
  - Coagulopathic patients (if emergent need, femoral approach preferred over subclavian or internal jugular [IJ] because it is more compressible)
  - Overlying infection, burn or skin damage at puncture site
  - Trauma to ipsilateral groin or lower extremity
  - Suspected proximal vascular injury, particularly of inferior vena cava (IVC)

Risks/Consent Issues
- Pain (local anesthesia will be given)
- Local bleeding and hematoma
- Infection (sterile technique will be utilized)

Landmarks
Site of insertion is 2 to 3 cm inferior to the midpoint of inguinal ligament and 1 finger breadth medial to the femoral artery pulse. Anatomically, the structures underlying the inguinal ligament, from lateral to medial are recalled by mnemonic **NAVEL**

Femoral **N**erve
Femoral **A**rtery
Femoral **V**ein
Empty space
Lymphatics

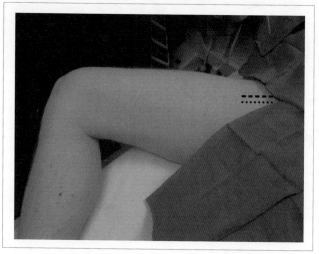

FIGURE 10.1: The *dashed line* represents the pulsatile femoral artery and the *dotted line* that is 1 finger breadth medial to it is the femoral vein.

Technique
- **Patient Preparation**
  - Ensure electrocardiogram (ECG) monitoring in case wire reaches the heart, causing dysrhythmia.
  - Externally rotate the leg and bend the knee to expose the groin.
  - Sterilize entire groin with povidone-iodine solution.
  - Drape with sterile sheets to cover from legs to head.

  Note: Unless immediate emergent access is warranted the surgeons attempting procedure must wear cap, eye shields, and mask with sterile gown and gloves.
- **Procedure**
  - Analgesia: Use 25- or 27-gauge needle to anesthetize skin and subcutaneous tissue with 1% lidocaine.
  - Vessel localization
    - If attempting to localize right femoral vein, use right hand to hold needle and syringe. With left hand palpate femoral artery to avoid arterial puncture while guiding needle insertion. If attempting to localize left femoral vein, reverse hands.
    - Insert introducer needle attached to a syringe at a 30- to 60-degree angle to skin using above landmarks.
    - Apply negative pressure to plunger while advancing needle 3 to 5 cm or until flash of blood seen in syringe.
    - If vessel is not identified, withdraw the needle while continuing to aspirate.
    - If redirecting needle, always retract needle to level of skin before advancing again.
    - Once needle punctures vessel, blood will flow freely into syringe.
    - Stabilize and hold introducer needle with free hand.
    - Remove syringe and ensure that venous blood continues to flow easily. Occlude needle hub with thumb to prevent air embolism.
  - Seldinger technique
    - Advance guide-wire through introducer needle. Wire should pass easily (Don't force it!).

▷ If resistance is met, withdraw the wire and rotate it, adjust angle of needle entry, or remove wire and reaspirate with syringe to ensure needle is still in vessel.

▷ Once most of the guide-wire is advanced through the needle, remove needle over wire. **Never let go of guide-wire!**

▷ Make a superficial skin incision with a scalpel to allow passage of the dilator, with sharp bevel of the scalpel angled away from the wire.

▷ Thread dilator over guide-wire. Advance dilator through skin and into vessel with a firm, twisting motion. Always hold onto wire.

▷ Remove dilator while keeping guide-wire in place.

▷ Thread catheter tip over guide-wire. Retract guide-wire until it emerges from the catheter's proximal end. **While holding the distal tip of the wire,** advance catheter over the guide-wire through the skin and into the vessel to the desired length.

▷ Withdraw guide-wire from proximal end of catheter while keeping catheter in place.

▷ Attach syringe to catheter hub and aspirate blood to confirm catheter is in the vein. Flush and heplock catheter.

○ Final steps

▷ If inserting multilumen central line, always aspirate, flush, and heplock all lumen.

▷ Suture catheter to skin using silk or nylon sutures.

▷ Cover skin insertion site with sterile dressing.

Complications

▪ Arterial puncture or cannulation
▪ Vessel laceration or dissection
▪ Retroperitoneal hemorrhage due to puncturing vessel above inguinal ligament
▪ Local hematoma
▪ Air embolism
▪ Catheter tip embolism
▪ Catheter malposition
▪ Lost guide-wire
▪ Venous thrombosis
▪ Insertion site cellulitis
▪ Line sepsis

Common Pitfalls

▪ Use of inadequate local anesthesia.
▪ Inadequate incision with scalpel will make passing of the dilator difficult.
▪ If location of vessel is in doubt, a ''finder'' 25-gauge needle attached to a 5-mL syringe can be used to note the depth and location of vein.
▪ During cardiac arrest, inadvertent cannulation of femoral artery may occur. Infusion of vasopressors through the artery may cause limb ischemia.

Pearls

▪ Never let go of the guide-wire. One end must always be held to prevent its embolism into the vessel.
▪ Never force the guide-wire or catheter. Applying excessive force on insertion and removal may cause vessel injury, breakage, or embolism.

▪ Always occlude open hub of needle to prevent air embolism.
▪ During chest compression, the only palpable pulse at the groin may be the retrograde blood flow from the vein. Attempt cannulation at the site of palpable "pulse."
▪ Use of ultrasonography in placing central catheters has shown to cause the following:
   ◦ Decrease in number of attempts, skin to blood flash time, and complications
   ◦ Increase in first attempts and success when traditional attempts have failed
▪ Technique (static or dynamic)
   ◦ Use high-frequency, 7- to 9-MHz linear probe.
   ◦ In a sterile manner, center the probe over vessel.

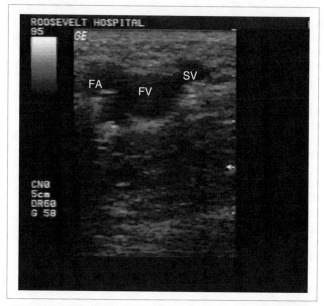

FIGURE 10.2: Appearance and orientation of femoral artery (FA), femoral vein (FV), and saphenous vein using a high-frequency, linear ultrasound probe.

   ◦ Identify femoral vein (FV), femoral artery (FA), and saphenous vein (SV).
      ▸ Blood vessels are *ANECHOIC* (appear black).
      ▸ Veins are *COMPRESSIBLE* (arteries are not).
      ▸ Veins *do not* have pulsatile flow (arteries do).
   ◦ The center of probe corresponds to center of the ultrasound screen where vessel is centered.
   ◦ Aim needle toward the femoral vein.
   ◦ As needle enters, the subcutaneous tissue distorts. Needle cannot be visualized on ultrasonography. Therefore, to identify needle location and direction, look for reverberation artifact of the needle and vessel wall tenting as described in Chapter 11.

Suggested Readings

Agee KR, Balk RA. Central venous catheterization in critically ill patient. *Critical Care Clin*. 1992;8(4):677–686.

Hind D, Calvert N, Mcwilliams R, et al. Ultrasonic locating devices for central venous cannulation: Meta-analysis. *Br Med J*. 2003;327(7411):361.

Miller AH, Roth BA, Mills TJ, et al. Ultrasound guidance versus the landmark technique for the placement of central venous catheters in the emergency department. *Acad Emerg Med*. 2002;9(8):800–805.

Reichman EF, Simon RR. *Emergency medicine procedures*. New York: McGraw-Hill; 2004:331–336.

11

Internal Jugular Vein — Central Venous Access

Amir Darvish

Indications

- Emergency venous access for fluid resuscitation and drug infusion
- Central venous pressure and O_2 monitoring
- Infusions requiring central venous administration (vasopressors, hyperosmolar solutions, hyperalimentation)
- Routine venous access due to inadequate peripheral IV sites
- Introduction of pulmonary artery catheter
- Introduction of transvenous pacing wire

Contraindications

- No absolute contraindications
- **Relative Contraindications**
  - Coagulopathic patients (femoral approach preferred)
  - Overlying infection, burn, or skin damage at puncture site
  - Combative or uncooperative patients
  - Distorted anatomy or trauma at the cannulation site
  - Penetrating trauma with suspected proximal vascular injury
  - Suspected cervical spine fracture

Risks/Consent Issues

- Pain (local anesthesia will be given)
- Local bleeding and hematoma
- Infection (sterile technique will be utilized)
- Pneumothorax or hemothorax and need for potential chest tube

Landmarks

Site of insertion is the apex of a triangle formed by the sternal and clavicular heads of the sternocleidomastoid muscle and the clavicle. This point is lateral to the carotid pulse. The needle is pointed toward the ipsilateral nipple (see Fig. 11.1).

Technique

- **Patient Preparation**
  - Administer supplemental oxygen.
  - Ensure continuous pulse oximetry, electrocardiogram (ECG), and blood pressure monitoring.
  - 15 degree Trendelenburg position to prevent air embolism.
  - Rotate the patient's head opposite to site of cannulation.
  - Prep neck with povidone-iodine solution, including clavicular area in case internal jugular (IJ) cannulation fails and subclavian vein access is necessary.
  - Drape with sterile sheets to cover from head to legs.

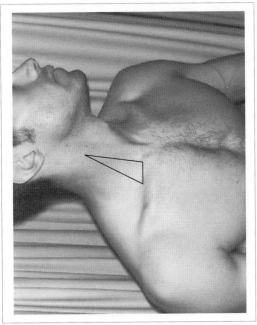

FIGURE 11.1: Identifying the triangle formed by the sternal and clavicular heads of the sternocleidomastoid and the clavicle. In the anterior approach to the jugular vein, the needle is inserted at the apex of the triangle toward the ipsilateral nipple.

Note: Unless immediate emergent access is warranted the surgeons attempting procedure must wear cap, eye shields, and mask with sterile gown and gloves.

- **Locate the Internal Jugular Vein (IJV)**
  - Stand at head level of patient.
  - Analgesia: Use 25- or 27-gauge needle to anesthetize skin and subcutaneous tissue with 1% lidocaine.
  - If attempting localization of right IJ, use right hand to hold syringe and introducer needle. With left hand, palpate carotid artery to avoid arterial puncture while guiding needle insertion. If attempting left IJ, reverse hands.
  - Using landmarks as described above, insert introducer needle attached to a syringe at 30 to 60 degrees to the skin. The point of insertion is at the apex of the triangle just lateral to the carotid pulse.
  - Apply negative pressure to plunger while advancing needle 3 to 5 cm or until flash of blood seen in syringe.
  - If vessel is not identified, withdraw the needle while continuing to aspirate.
  - If redirecting needle, always retract needle to level of skin before advancing again.
  - Once needle punctures vessel, blood will flow freely into syringe.
  - Stabilize and hold introducer needle with free hand.
  - Remove syringe and ensure that venous blood continues to flow easily. Occlude needle hub with thumb to prevent air embolism.
- **Seldinger Technique**
  - Advance wire through introducer needle.
  - Resistance to advancement may indicate that needle is no longer in vessel or against the vessel wall. Withdraw guide-wire, slightly rotate needle, or adjust angle of entry, then advance guide-wire again. Or reaspirate with the syringe to ensure needle is in the vessel.

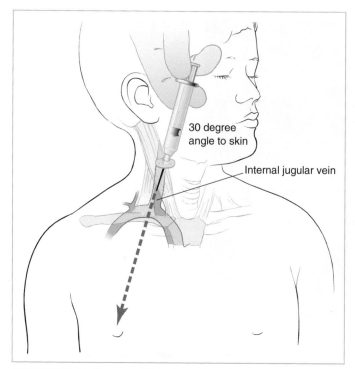

30 degree
angle to skin

Internal jugular vein

FIGURE 11.2: Median approach for internal jugular vein cannulation. (From Lavelle J, Costarino A Jr. Central venous access and central venous pressure monitoring. In: Henretig FM, King C, eds. *Textbook of pediatric emergency medicine procedures*. Philadelphia: Williams & Wilkins, 1997:271, with permission.)

- Once most of the guide-wire is advanced through needle, remove needle over the wire. **Never let go of the guide-wire!**
- Make a superficial skin incision with a scalpel to allow passage of the dilator, with sharp bevel of the scalpel angled away from the wire.
- Thread dilator over guide-wire. Advance dilator through skin and into vessel with a firm, twisting motion. Always hold onto wire.
- Remove dilator, while keeping guide-wire in place.
- Thread catheter tip over guide-wire. Retract guide-wire until it emerges from the catheter's proximal end. **While holding wire**, advance catheter over the guide-wire through the skin and into the vessel to the desired length.
- Withdraw guide-wire from proximal end of catheter while keeping catheter in place.
- Attach syringe to catheter hub and aspirate blood to confirm catheter is in the vein. Flush and heplock the catheter.

- **Final Steps**
  - If inserting multilumen central line, always aspirate, flush, and heplock all lumen.
  - Suture catheter to skin using silk or nylon sutures.
  - Cover skin insertion site with sterile dressing.
- **Confirmation**
  - Obtain chest radiograph to verify line placement and rule out complications. The catheter tip should be in the superior vena cava just proximal to the right atrium.

Complications
- Arterial puncture or cannulation
- Vessel laceration or dissection
- Pneumothorax or hemothorax
- Neck hematoma with tracheal compression
- Air embolism
- Catheter tip embolism
- Catheter malposition
- Dysrhythmias
- Lost guide-wire
- Tracheal puncture or endotracheal cuff perforation
- Venous thrombosis
- Insertion site cellulitis

Common Pitfalls
- Use of inadequate local anesthesia
- Inadequate incision with scalpel
- Advancing the guide-wire into the atrium and right ventricle can cause dysrhythmias, which can be corrected by retracting the guide-wire. Always have patient on cardiac monitor.

Pearls
- If unsuccessful, move to ipsilateral subclavian. Never attempt the opposite side without a chest x-ray first to avoid bilateral pneumothoraces.
- Never let go of guide-wire. One end must always be held to prevent its embolism into the vessel. Never force the guide-wire or catheter. Applying excessive force on insertion and removal may cause vessel injury, breakage, or embolism.
- Always occlude open hub of needle to prevent air embolism.
- Use of ultrasonography in placing central catheters has shown to cause the following:
  - Decrease in number of attempts, skin to blood flash time, and complications
  - Increase in first attempts and success when traditional attempts have failed
- Technique (static or dynamic)
  - Use high-frequency 7- to 9-MHz linear probe.
  - In a sterile manner, center the probe over the vessel.
  - Identify IJV and carotid artery (CA).
    - Blood vessels are *ANECHOIC* (appear black)
    - Veins are *COMPRESSIBLE* (arteries are not)
    - Veins *do not* have pulsatile flow (arteries do)
  - The center of probe corresponds to center of the ultrasound screen where vessel is centered.
  - Aim needle toward the IJV.
  - As needle enters, the subcutaneous tissue distorts.
  - Needle cannot be visualized on ultrasonography. Therefore, to identify needle location and direction, look for the following:
    - Reverberation artifact of the needle
    - Tenting of the vessel wall
  - Once vessel is entered, proceed with Seldinger technique explained earlier.

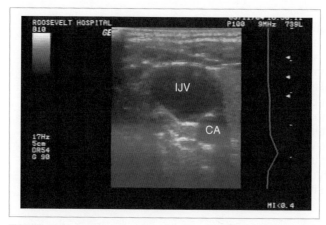

FIGURE 11.3: Appearance and orientation of internal jugular vein (IJV) and the carotid artery (CA) using a high-frequency, linear ultrasound probe.

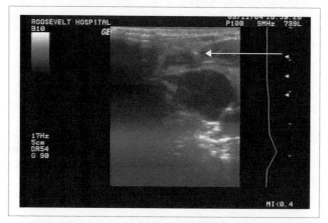

FIGURE 11.4: Reverberation artifact of the needle moving toward the internal jugular vein (IJV).

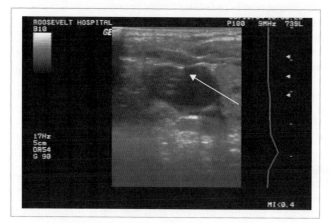

FIGURE 11.5: Tenting of the internal jugular vein (IJV) vessel wall as the needle enters the vein.

Suggested Readings

Daily PA, Scjwartz AJ, Greenhow DE, et al. Percutaneous internal jugular vein cannulation. *Arch Surg*. 1970;101:534.

Denys BG, Uretsky BF. Anatomical variations of internal jugular vein location: Impact on central venous access. *Crit Care Med*. 1991;19(12):1516–1519.

Hind D, Calvert N, McWilliams R, et al. Ultrasonic locating devices for central venous cannulation: Meta-analysis. *Br Med J*. 2003;327(7411):361.

Miller AH, Roth BA, Mills TJ, et al. Ultrasound guidance versus the landmark technique for the placement of central venous catheters in the emergency department. *Acad Emerg Med*. 2003;9(8):800–805.

Rosen P, Sternbach G, Chan T, et al. *Atlas of emergency medicine procedure*. Mosby; 2001:82–86.

12 Subclavian Vein—Central Venous Access

Lucy Willis

Indications
- Emergency venous access for fluid resuscitation and drug infusion
- Central venous pressure and O_2 monitoring
- Infusions requiring central venous administration (vasopressors, hyperosmolar solutions, hyperalimentation)
- Routine venous access due to inadequate peripheral IV sites
- Introduction of pulmonary artery catheter
- Introduction of transvenous pacing wire

Contraindications
- No absolute contraindications
- **Relative Contraindications**
  - Coagulopathic patients
  - Overlying infection, burn, or skin damage at puncture site
  - Distorted anatomy or trauma at the cannulation site
  - Combative or uncooperative patients
  - Penetrating trauma with suspected proximal vascular injury
  - Pneumothorax on contralateral side (risk of bilateral pneumothoraces)
  - Chronic obstructive pulmonary disease (COPD)

Risks/Consent Issues
- Pain (local anesthesia will be given)
- Local bleeding and hematoma
- Infection (sterile technique will be utilized)
- Pneumothorax or hemothorax, and need for potential chest tube

Landmarks
- The right side is often preferred because of the lower pleural dome on the right and also because the thoracic duct is on the left.
- **Infraclavicular Approach** (most commonly used)
  - Make needle entry at bisection of middle and medial thirds of the clavicle.
  - Aim toward suprasternal notch.
  - Orient bevel inferomedially to facilitate wire entry.
- **Supraclavicular Approach**
  - Make needle entry just above clavicle, 1 cm lateral to insertion of clavicular head of sternocleidomastoid (SCM).
  - Aim to bisect angle between SCM and clavicle (or towards contralateral nipple).
  - Orient bevel upward.

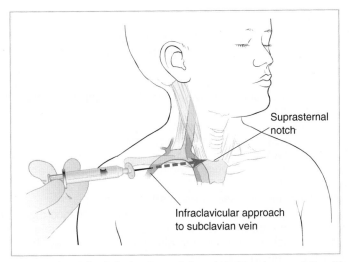

FIGURE 12.1: Infraclavicular approach for subclavian vein cannulation. (From Lavelle J, Costarino A Jr. Central venous access and central venous pressure monitoring. In: Henretig FM, King C, eds. *Textbook of pediatric emergency procedures.* Philadelphia: Williams & Wilkins; 1997:273, with permission.)

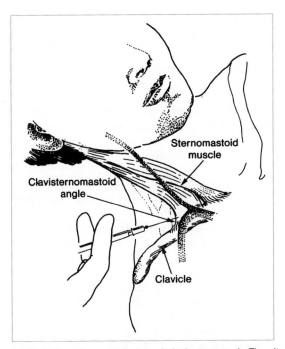

FIGURE 12.2: Supraclavicular subclavian approach. The site of entry is at the junction of the lateral aspect of the clavicular head of the sternocleidomastoid muscle with the superior border of the clavicle, called the clavisternomastoid angle. Direct the needle at a 5-degree angle from the coronal plane, at 50 degrees from the sagittal plane, and at 40 degrees from the transverse plane. (From Simon RR, Brenner BE. *Emergency procedures and techniques,* 4th ed. Philadelphia: Lippincott Williams & Wilkins; 2002:463, with permission.)

Technique
- **Patient Preparation**
  - Place patient in 15-degree Trendelenburg position.
  - Ensure continuous pulse oximetry, electrocardiogram (ECG), and blood pressure.
  - Prep the clavicular area with povidone-iodine solution, including the neck in case subclavian vein access fails and internal jugular vein access is necessary.
  - Apply sterile drapes.

  Note: Unless immediate emergent access is warranted the surgeons attempting procedure must wear cap, eye shields, and mask with sterile gown and gloves.

- **Locate the Subclavian Vein**
  - Analgesia: Use 25- or 27-gauge needle to anesthetize skin and subcutaneous tissue with 1% lidocaine.
  - Insert introducer needle (see ''Landmarks'' section).
    - Infraclavicular: At a shallow angle to the skin, advance the needle just posterior to the clavicle at the junction of medial and middle thirds. Apply posterior pressure on needle to direct it under the clavicle, aiming toward suprasternal notch.
    - Supraclavicular: Insert the needle 1 cm superior to clavicle and 1 cm lateral to SCM clavicular head. Direct the needle 10 to 15 degrees upward from the horizontal plane, just posterior to the clavicle aiming toward the contralateral nipple or bisection of angle between SCM and clavicle.
      - Aspirate continuously with the dominant hand while advancing the needle.
  - If redirecting needle, always withdraw to the level of skin first.
  - Once the vessel is located, free-flowing venous blood is aspirated.

- **Seldinger Technique**
  - Stabilize and hold needle in place with nondominant hand. Remove the syringe from the needle and cap the hub with your thumb to minimize risk of air embolism.
  - Advance guide-wire through introducer needle. The wire should pass easily and not be forced. **Never let go of the guide-wire!**
  - If resistance is met, withdraw the wire and rotate it, adjust location or angle of needle entry, or remove wire and reaspirate with syringe to ensure needle is still in vessel.
  - Remove the needle, always holding wire in place.
  - Make a superficial skin incision with the sharp scalpel bevel angled away from wire to allow easy passage of the dilator.
  - Pass the dilator over the guide-wire, always holding onto wire.
  - Advance the dilator through the skin and into the vessel with a slow, firm, twisting motion.
  - Remove dilator, leaving the guide-wire in place.
  - Pass the catheter over the wire until it emerges from the catheter's proximal end. **While holding the guide-wire,** advance catheter through the skin and into the vessel with a similar slow, firm, twisting motion.
  - Withdraw the guide-wire through the catheter.
  - Attach syringe to catheter hub and aspirate blood to confirm placement in the vein.
  - Flush and heplock catheter lumen.

- **Final Steps**
  - If inserting multilumen central line, always aspirate, flush, and heplock all lumen.

- Suture the catheter to the skin using silk or nylon sutures.
- Cover skin insertion site with sterile dressing.
- **Confirmation**
  - Obtain chest x-ray to verify correct line placement and to rule out complications. The line tip should be in the superior vena cava, just superior to the right atrium.

Complications

- Arterial puncture or cannulation
- Vessel laceration or dissection
- Pneumothorax or hemothorax
- Air embolism
- Catheter tip embolism
- Catheter malposition
- Dysrhythmias
- Lost guide-wire
- Tracheal puncture or endotracheal cuff perforation
- Venous thrombosis
- Insertion site cellulitis
- Line sepsis

Common Pitfalls

- Use of inadequate local anesthesia
- Inadequate incision with scalpel
- Advancing the guide-wire into the atrium and right ventricle can cause dysrhythmias, which can be corrected by retracting the guide-wire. Always have patient on cardiac monitor.

Pearls

- In cases of penetrating thoracic trauma, place subclavian line on the same side as the chest wound because of the risk of bilateral pneumothoraces, unless proximal vascular injury is suspected.
- If unsuccessful, move next to the ipsilateral internal jugular (IJ). Do not attempt the opposite side without a chest x-ray first (risk of bilateral pneumothoraces).
- Never let go of guide-wire. One end must always be held to prevent its embolism into the vessel.
- Never force the guide-wire or catheter. Applying excessive force on insertion and removal may cause vessel injury, breakage, or embolism.
- Always occlude open hub of needle to prevent air embolism.

Suggested Readings

Rosen P, Sternbach G, Chan T, et al. *Atlas of emergency medicine procedure*. Mosby; 2001:78–81.

Simon RR, Brenner BE. *Emergency procedures and techniques*. Philadelphia: Lippincott Williams & Wilkins;2002:452–469.

13 Intraosseous Vascular Access

Kimberly Reagans

Indications
- Used as emergent vascular access for fluid resuscitation and drug infusion when unable to obtain peripheral venous access.
- Primarily used in pediatric cardiac arrest—generally faster access than central line in infants or children.
- Used in adult resuscitation if other forms of vascular access cannot be established.

Contraindications
- **Absolute Contraindications**
  - Fracture at the insertion site
- **Relative Contraindications**
  - Previous attempt to place intraosseous (IO) needle on the same bone
  - Osteogenesis imperfecta
  - Osteoporosis
  - Overlying infection, burn, or skin damage at insertion site

Risks/Consent Issues
- Pain (local anesthesia can be given)
- Local bleeding and hematoma
- Growth plate injuries or fractures
- Extravasation of fluid or drugs through iatrogenic fracture/puncture site
- Osteomyelitis and cellulitis

Landmarks
- Standard placement of the IO line is 1 to 2 cm distal to the tibial tuberosity on the anteromedial aspect of the tibia (see Fig. 13.1)
- Alternate sites for placement
  - Medial aspect of the distal tibia approximately 1 to 2 cm proximal to the medial malleolus (see Fig. 13.2)
  - Anterior aspect of the distal femur just proximal to the junction of the femoral shaft and the lateral and medial condyles

Technique
- Sterilize the insertion site with povidone-iodine solution or alcohol.
- If the patient is awake, administer a local anesthetic to the skin and periosteum.
- Grasp the IO needle in the palm of the hand using the index finger and thumb to guide and stabilize the needle.
- Use nondominant hand to stabilize the leg.

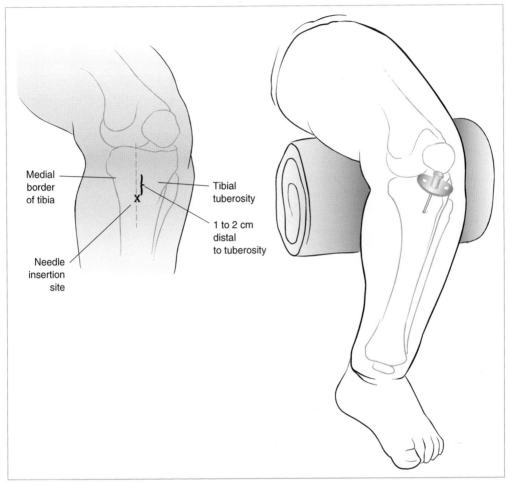

Medial
border
of tibia

Tibial
tuberosity

1 to 2 cm
distal
to tuberosity

Needle
insertion
site

FIGURE 13.1: Entry site at the proximal tibia. (From Hodge D III. Intraosseous infusion. In: Henretig FM, King C, eds. *Textbook of pediatric emergency medicine procedures*. Philadelphia: Williams & Wilkins; 1997:292, with permission.)

- Insert the IO needle either perpendicular (90 degree) to the tibial surface, or angled 60 to 75 degree caudad to avoid the growth plate. Using firm, constant pressure and a twisting motion, puncture the bone.
- The resistance suddenly decreases once the marrow cavity is entered. It is rarely more than 1 cm from the skin through the cortex. Excessive force may cause puncture through the posterior cortex.
- Remove the stylet.
- Use a 5- to 10-mL syringe to aspirate blood for confirmation of placement.
- If no aspirate is obtained, carefully infuse 3 mL of normal saline. Palpate the area for any signs of extravasation.
- Secure the needle and immobilize extremity.

Complications
- Undetected extravasation of fluid into the surrounding tissue leading to compartment syndrome

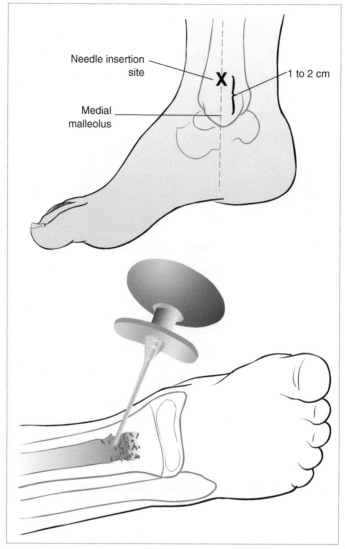

FIGURE 13.2: Entry site at the distal tibia. (From Hodge D III. Intraosseous infusion. In: Henretig FM, King C, eds. *Textbook of pediatric emergency medicine procedures*. Philadelphia: Williams & Wilkins; 1997:293, with permission.)

- Extravasation of medications into the surrounding skin leading to skin necrosis
- Localized bleeding
- Fat embolization (rare complication only reported in adults)
- Iatrogenic fractures
- Cellulitis and osteomyelitis
- Growth plate injuries possible (no report of permanent growth plate or bone damage reported)

Common Pitfalls
- Applying excessive force on the needle during insertion causing penetration through the posterior cortex

▪ Incomplete insertion of needle into the bone, thereby not penetrating the marrow space

Pearls

▪ Most medications can be given safely through the IO line, including crystalloid solutions, blood products, resuscitation medications, succinylcholine, antibiotics, and diazepam.

▪ Blood from the IO access site may be sent for type and screen and serum chemistries. Complete blood count of marrow aspirate is not a reliable representation of peripheral blood.

▪ If unsuccessful, move to opposite leg or alternative site because even if successful with second attempt, first puncture site will allow fluid to extravasate into surrounding tissue.

▪ Infusion rates are three to four times faster with pressure infusions when compared to gravity infusions. Therefore, use a 30- to 60-mL syringe to give fluid boluses or use pressure bags for rapid infusion of fluid or blood products.

▪ Blood clots may block the needle opening. Frequent flushing of the line with 3 to 5 mL of saline or use of pressure infusions will prevent this from occurring.

▪ Remove the IO line once other vascular access has been established to reduce the risk of infection, extravasation, or dislodgement of needle.

Suggested Readings

Hodge D III. Intraosseous infusion. In: Henretig F, King C, eds. *Textbook of pediatric emergency procedures*. Baltimore: Williams & Wilkins; 1997.

14

Peripheral Venous Cutdown—Saphenous Vein

Amir Darvish

Indications
- Emergent venous access for fluid resuscitation or drug infusion if alternative peripheral or central access is either unattainable or contraindicated

Contraindications
- **Absolute Contraindications**
  - Major blunt, long-bone fracture or penetrating trauma proximal to site of cutdown
- **Relative Contraindications**
  - Suspected proximal vascular injury (in the extremity or inferior vena cava)
  - Overlying infection, burn, or skin damage at the site of cutdown
  - Coagulopathy

Risks/Consent Issues
- Pain (local anesthesia can be given)
- Local bleeding and hematoma
- Infection (sterile technique will be utilized)

Landmarks
Greater saphenous vein is most easily accessible 1 to 2 cm anterior and 1 to 2 cm superior to the medial malleolus. The vein may be palpable in a nonhypotensive patient.

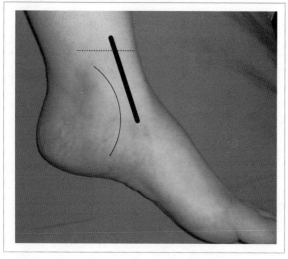

FIGURE 14.1: Saphenous vein runs vertically 2 cm anterior to the medial malleolus of the ankle. The ideal site of cutdown is 2 cm superior to the medial malleolus (*dotted lines*).

Technique
- **Patient Preparation**
  - Extend and externally rotate lower extremity.
  - Immobilize if needed, especially in children.
  - Sterilize entire ankle with povidone-iodine solution and drape.

  Note: Unless immediate emergent access is warranted the surgeons attempting procedure must wear cap, eye shields, and mask with sterile gown and gloves.
- **Procedure**
  - Analgesia: Use 25- or 27-gauge needle to anesthetize skin and subcutaneous tissue with 1% lidocaine.
  - Isolate the vein (see Fig. 14.2A–B)
    - Make skin incision *transversely* over saphenous vein landmark.
    - Apply traction to skin on either side of incision to expose subcutaneous tissue.
    - Dissect subcutaneous tissue using curved hemostat with tip facing downward, *parallel to the course of the vein.*
    - After exposing vein, pass hemostat under vein, turn tip upward, and spread to isolate vein above the hemostat.
  - Stabilizing the vein (Fig. 14.2C)
    - Pass 3-0 or 4-0 silk suture ties under the vein using curved hemostat.
    - Clamp each tie with hemostats, one proximally and the other distally.
    - Distal suture may be tied to ligate the vessel. This decreases bleeding, but also sacrifices the vessel.
    - Apply traction on each tie, thereby lifting the vessel and exposing the anterior surface of the vein.
  - Cannulating the vein (Fig. 14.2D–E)
    - With the tip of no.11 scalpel blade make a flap incision to the anterior surface of the vein, approximately one third the diameter of the vein.
    - A vein pick may be used to elevate the flap.
    - Carefully advance catheter through incision.
    - Flush catheter with saline solution and attach to intravenous line.
  - Secure catheter (Fig. 14.2F)
    - Tie the proximal suture around the vein and the IV catheter to secure in place.
    - Cut the ends of the proximal and distal ties.
    - Suture catheter to the skin and close the incision using 4-0 nylon sutures.
    - Cover skin insertion site with a sterile dressing.

Complications
- Injury to surrounding structures such as tibialis anterior tendon and saphenous nerve
- Vein transaction or laceration without ability to cannulate
- Hematoma formation
- Phlebitis
- Wound infection
- Wound dehiscence

Common Pitfalls
- Skin incision with scalpel should be superficial to only expose subcutaneous tissue. Deep incision may transect the vein.

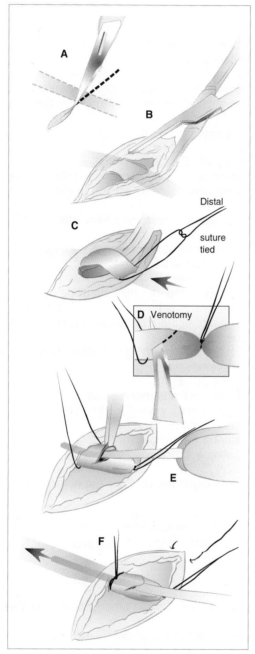

FIGURE 14.2: Procedures for venous cutdown catheterization. **A:** A transverse incision is made at the appropriate site. The incision should extend into the subcutaneous tissue but not deep enough to potentially lacerate the vein. **B:** The vein is isolated using blunt dissection. A suture is passed around the vein and cut to give two ligatures. **C:** The distal suture is tied and used to stabilize the vessel. **D:** Venotomy is performed to allow insertion of the catheter. Alternatively the surgeon may choose to insert the catheter over a needle without performing a venotomy, in a manner similar to percutaneous catheterization. **E:** The catheter is inserted into the vein. Placement within the vessel is confirmed by aspirating blood or infusing fluid. **F:** The proximal suture is tied and the wound is closed and dressed. (From Vinci RJ. Venous cutdown catheterization. In: Henretig FM, King C, eds. *Textbook of pediatric emergency procedures.* Philadelphia: Williams & Wilkins; 1997:284, with permission.)

▪ The incision on the anterior surface of the vein must be deep enough to fully enter the lumen of the vein. If too large (greater than 1/2 the diameter of the vein) the vessel may tear completely and cause significant bleeding.

▪ The catheter must be removed if it penetrates the posterior wall of the vessel.

Pearls

▪ The most difficult and time-consuming aspect is usually threading the catheter into the vein.

▪ The vein is very delicate. Do not force the catheter through the vein.

▪ Gently lifting up the proximal tie will help minimize back-flow bleeding.

▪ Do not tie the proximal suture too tight around the catheter for fear of occluding it.

▪ Early catheter removal will decrease incidence of phlebitis and infection.

Suggested Readings

Klofas E. A quicker saphenous vein cutdown and a better way to teach it. *J Trauma*. 1997;43(6):985–987.

Reichman EF, Simon RR, eds. *Emergency medicine procedures*. McGraw-Hill; 2004: 331–336.

Vinci R. Venous cutdown catheterization In: Henretig F, King C, eds. *Textbook of pediatric emergency procedures*, Baltimore: Williams & Wilkins; 1997.

15

Radial Arterial Cannulation

Ashley Shreves

Indications
- Direct arterial blood sampling
- Continuous arterial blood pressure monitoring

Contraindications
- Absolute: None
- **Relative Contraindications**
  - Coagulopathy or recent thrombolysis
  - Overlying infection, burn, or skin damage
  - Severe peripheral atherosclerosis

Risks/Consent Issues
- Thrombosis and occlusion of the vessel are common (30%–40%) but almost all resolve spontaneously without requiring intervention, and ischemic complications are rare/case-reportable.
- Risk of bleeding and infection are low.

Landmarks
- Radial artery cannulation site is just medial and proximal to the radial styloid on the volar surface of the wrist.

Technique
- Position the patient's supinated wrist in 60 degree of extension. Placement of a gauze or towel under the dorsal surface of the wrist and taping wrist in extension may facilitate positioning.
- Prepare and drape the area in a sterile manner.
- Anesthetize the skin over the radial artery with a small wheal of 1% lidocaine.
- Open the packaging and remove unit. Remove the protective shield. To ensure proper feeding, advance and retract the spring-wire guide through the needle via the lever. Then retract the wire proximally as far as possible before using.
- Palpate the course of the artery with the middle and index fingers of the nondominant hand. Hold the needle at a 45-degree angle to the skin, pointing cephalad and puncture the skin. Advance the needle until a flash of bright red blood is seen in the clear hub of the needle.
- Decrease the angle of the needle to 20 degrees and advance the guide-wire (via actuating lever) into the artery. **Do not force the wire if resistance is encountered**.
- Hold the clear transducer needle and advance the catheter forward into the vessel. A rotating motion can be applied to the catheter if resistance is encountered.

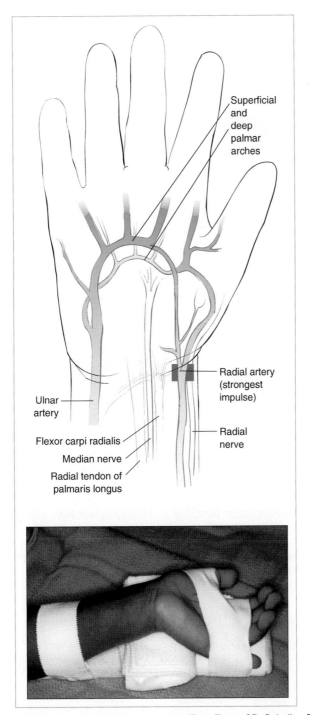

FIGURE 15.1: Radial artery anatomy. (From Torrey SB, Saladino R. Arterial puncture and catheterization. In: Henretig FM, King C, eds. *Textbook of pediatric emergency procedures*. Philadelphia: Williams & Wilkins; 1997:784, with permission.)

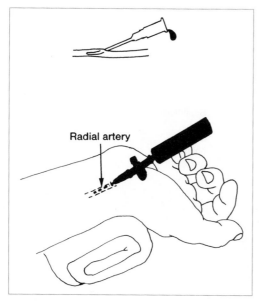

FIGURE 15.2: Radial artery cannulation. Secure the hand and wrist to the arm board, with the wrist placed in extension as shown. (From Simon RR, Brenner BE. *Emergency procedures and techniques.* Philadelphia: Lippincott Williams & Wilkins; 2002:505, with permission.)

- Holding the catheter in place, remove the introducer needle, guide-wire, and feed tube assembly. Pulsatile flow indicates successful cannulation.
- Attach a stopcock and injection tubing to the catheter hub. Suture into place. Apply dressing.

Complications
- Radial artery thrombosis and subsequent occlusion ranges from 4% to 40%, and resolution of thrombosis may take weeks. However, permanent ischemic damage is extremely rare. The Allen test is not a valid predictor of ischemic injury to the hand.
- Cerebral embolization is theoretically possible and could result from rapid, large-volume, arterial catheter irrigation.
- Ecchymoses and minor hematomas at the cannulation site are common (up to 80%) but almost always asymptomatic. If patient is anticoagulated, compression neuropathy can develop from larger hematomas.
- Infection (line sepsis and cellulitis) is very uncommon (0.6%).

Common Pitfalls
- Puncture of both walls of the vessel with cannulation deep to the artery
- Advancement of wire through resistance with subsequent damage to the vessel

Pearls
- Use of a 20-gauge Teflon catheter has been associated with the least complications. Larger catheters have greater risk for thrombosis.
- Make sure the target wrist is not rotated as this can shift the location of the vessel.

- Apply a three-way stopcock to the catheter hub to facilitate easy blood gas draws.
- Saline (versus heparin) is sufficient for flushing the catheter, especially during the patient's stay in the emergency department (ED).

Suggested Readings

Bedford RF, Wollman H. Complications of percutaneous radial-artery cannulation: An objective prospective study in man. *Anesthesiology*. 1973;38:228.

Davis FM, Stewart JM. Radial artery cannulation: A prospective study in patients undergoing cardiothoracic surgery. *Anesthesiology*. 1980;52:41.

Downs JB, Rackstein AD, Klein EF, et al. Hazards of radial-artery catheterization. *Anesthesiology*. 1973;38:283.

Roberts JR, Hedges JR. *Clinical procedures in emergency medicine*, 4th ed. Philadelphia: WB Saunders; 2004.

Wilkins RG. Radial artery cannulation and ischemic damage: A review. *Anesthesiology*. 1985;40:896.

Section Editor: Joshua Quaas

16

Paracentesis

Brian Kwong and Mark Clark

Indications
- Diagnostic: To analyze abnormal fluid collection in peritoneal space to determine etiology or pathologic conditions (e.g., infection)
- Therapeutic: To evacuate ascites for symptomatic relief, usually of shortness of breath

Contraindications
- **Absolute Contraindications**
  - Disseminated intravascular coagulopathy
- **Relative Contraindications**
  - Intra-abdominal adhesions
  - Abdominal wall cellulitis
  - In second or third trimester pregnancy, an open supraumbilical or ultrasound-assisted approach is preferred
  - Exercise caution in coagulopathic patients

Landmarks
- Preferred approach: 4 to 5 cm superior and medial to the anterior superior iliac spine
  - Stay lateral to the rectus sheath to avoid the inferior epigastric artery.
  - The abdominal wall is thinner in this location.
- Alternative approach: 2 cm below the umbilicus in the midline
  - Avoid if the patient has a midline surgical scar.

Technique
Commercial paracentesis kits containing rigid plastic sheath cannulas are available. However, standard steel needles can be left in the peritoneal cavity for intervals of over an hour without significant risk of injury.
- **Patient Preparation**
  - Direct patient to urinate or empty the bladder via urinary catheterization.
  - Sterilize the area where the needle will be inserted with copious povidone-iodine solution or similar surgical prep.
  - Drape the area with sterile towels or sterile fenestrated drape.

- **Patient Positioning**
  - If there is a large amount of ascites, the patient may be placed in a supine position with the head of the bed slightly elevated.
  - Patients with lesser amounts of ascites may be placed in a lateral decubitus position for optimal pooling of fluid.
- **Ultrasonography** (preferred but not essential)
  - Bedside ultrasonography is used to verify if the chosen site has a large fluid pocket with no bowel adhesions
- **Paracentesis**
  - Analgesia
    - Produce local anesthesia using up to 5 mg/kg of 1% lidocaine with epinephrine.
    - Raise a subcutaneous wheal with a small-bore (27-gauge) needle, then generously infiltrate the deeper tissues in the area of the paracentesis needle's eventual passage using a larger-bore needle.
    - Anesthetize to the depth of the peritoneum.
  - Needle insertion
    - Standard-sized (1.5 in.) metal needle will be sufficient in most cases. A longer (3.5 in.) spinal needle may be necessary in obese patients.
    - For diagnostic taps, a smaller gauge needle (22–20 gauge) should be utilized to decrease the chance of postprocedural fluid leak. For therapeutic taps, a larger (18 gauge) needle may be used to hasten fluid evacuation.
    - Attach needle to a 60-mL syringe.
    - Advance the needle in slow, controlled 5-mm increments with continuous gentle aspiration of the syringe.
    - A "Z-tract" method may be employed to decrease the risk of postprocedural fluid leak.
    - Overlying skin is pulled by an assistant or by the non–needle bearing hand 2 cm in the caudal direction.
    - After penetrating the peritoneum and obtaining fluid return, the skin is released.
    - Upon removal of the needle, skin will slide and return to original positioning, sealing the needle tract.
  - Fluid drainage
    - Metal needles should be stabilized to the patient's skin with a thick stack of commercial tube sponges, or with 4-in. gauze pads secured with tape.
    - If flow ceases, the needle should be gently rotated and/or advanced in 1-mm increments.
    - IV tubing and a three-way stopcock may be attached to facilitate drainage of larger quantities.
    - Vacuum bottles may be utilized to facilitate drainage; however, use caution because the continuous suction provided may attract bowel or omentum to the end of the paracentesis needle with resultant occlusion.
- **Ascitic Fluid Analysis**
  - Order the following standard tests (see "Pearls" section for additional tests)
    - Culture and sensitivity
    - Gram stain
    - Cell count
    - Albumin level

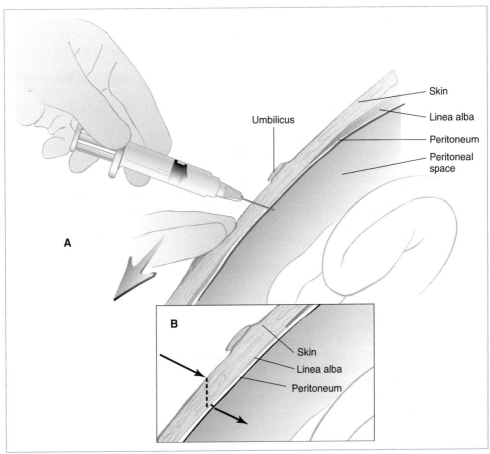

FIGURE 16.1: Z-track formation and controlled removal of ascetic fluid. **A:** Needle insertion with caudal traction on overlying skin. **B:** Z-track formation after release of skin and removal of needle. (From Lane NE, Paul RI. Paracentesis. In: Henretig FM, King C, eds. *Textbook of pediatric emergency procedures*. Philadelphia: Williams & Wilkins, 1997:924, with permission.)

Complications

- Persistent ascitic fluid leak at the puncture site (rectified with single suture)
- Trauma: Puncture of vasculature, organs, or hollow viscera
- Infection: Cellulitis, abdominal wall abscess, peritonitis
- Dilutional hyponatremia
- Hypotension with large volume paracentesis (>4 L). An uncommon, poorly documented complication. Colloid or albumin infusion to prevent this should be considered (mixed literature support).

Common Pitfalls

- Use of inadequate local anesthesia
- Failure to use ''Z-tract'' method to prevent persistent ascites leak
- Failure to correctly interpret fluid values (see ''Pearls'' section)

Pearls

- Bedside ultrasonography may be employed to confirm presence of ascites before needle placement and may help in identifying anatomic anomalies such as bowel adhesions.
- Consider the following additional ascites fluid tests (based on clinical suspicion):
  - Bilirubin (bowel or biliary perforation)
  - Protein and glucose (spontaneous bacterial peritonitis [SBP] or gut perforation)
  - Lactate dehydrogenase (LDH) (SBP or malignancy)
  - Amylase/triglyceride (chylous ascites)
  - Cytology (malignancy)
  - Tuberculosis smear/culture
- Ascites can be classified based on the **serum-ascites gradient (SAAG)**. The SAAG is the difference between the measured serum and ascitic albumin concentrations. A SAAG of 1.1 or greater correlates with conditions that increase portal pressure (transudates), while a SAAG of <1.1 correlates with conditions that produce exudates:
  - High gradient ($\geq$1.1 g/dL): Transudative
    - ▸ Cirrhosis
    - ▸ Heart failure
    - ▸ Budd-Chiari syndrome
    - ▸ Constrictive pericarditis
  - Low gradient (<1.1 g/dL): Exudative
    - ▸ Cancer (primary peritoneal carcinomatosis or metastases)
    - ▸ Tuberculosis peritonitis
    - ▸ Pancreatic ascites
    - ▸ Nephrotic syndrome
    - ▸ Serositis in connective tissue diseases
- Strongly suspect **SBP** if there are >250 neutrophils/μL or >500 white blood cells (WBCs)/μL.
  - Correct for a hemorrhagic tap by subtracting one WBC for every 250 red blood cell (RBC)/mm^3
  - Fluid should also be sent for total protein, LDH, and glucose to distinguish between SBP and secondary bacterial peritonitis

Suggested Readings

Marx JA. Peritoneal procedures. In: Roberts JR, Hedges J, eds. *Clinical procedures in emergency medicine*, 4th ed. Philadelphia: WB Saunders; 2004:851–856.

Runyon B. Ascites and spontaneous bacterial peritonitis. In: Feldman M, Friedman LS, Sleisenger MH, eds. *Sleisenger and Fordtran's gastrointestinal and liver disease*, 7th ed. Philadelphia: WB Saunders; 2002:1517–1542.

17 Gastroesophageal Balloon Tamponade (GEBT) or Sengstaken-Blakemore Tube

Mitchell Adelstein and Jennifer Kaufman

Indications
- Temporary control of variceal hemorrhage
- Massive upper gastrointestinal blood loss in the setting of known portal hypertension or prior variceal hemorrhage in the absence of endoscopy

Contraindications
- Availability of endoscopy
- Hemorrhage controlled with nonselective vasoconstrictors (octreotide or somatostatin)
- Spontaneous resolution of hemorrhage

Technique
- **Check Equipment**
  - Verify patency of both esophageal and gastric tamponade balloon tubes by progressive inflation of air in 100 mL increments.
  - Deflate fully, clamp, and coat all balloons with water-soluble gel.
  - Nasogastric tube (if a 3-lumen gastroesophageal balloon tamponade [GEBT] is used) attachment is optional (see Fig. 17.2).
    - Tie tube along the course of the GEBT with silk sutures.
    - Tube tip should sit 3 to 4 cm proximal to the esophageal balloon.
- **Patient Preparation**
  - Analgesia, sedation, and soft restraints should be used as needed because procedure is uncomfortable.
  - Consider endotracheal intubation in those unable to maintain airway protection.
  - With patient lying supine, elevate head of bed to approximately 45 degrees (left lateral decubitus is an acceptable alternative).
  - Apply topical anesthetic to the posterior pharynx.
  - Remove existing nasogastric tube if present (stomach should be evacuated before GEBT).
- **Tube Placement**
  - Pass fully deflated GEBT through the mouth (preferred over nasal passage) to the 50-cm mark.
  - Apply suction to the gastric and esophageal aspiration lumens.
  - Position must NOW be confirmed radiographically (inflation of the gastric balloon with 50 mL of air can assist in radiographic confirmation).
  - Inflate gastric balloon with increments of 100 mL air to volume of approximately 500 mL (or to your specific GEBT recommendation).
  - Clamp both the air inlet and pressure monitoring outlet of the gastric balloon.
- **Securing the Tube**
  - Proximal end of the tube must be secured through a traction device.

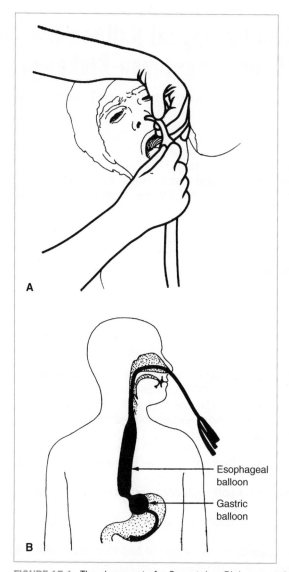

FIGURE 17.1: The placement of a Sengstaken-Blakemore tube. **A:** To pass the tube, fold the empty balloon around itself, and give the patient appropriate analgesia. **B:** The gastric and esophageal balloons are shown inflated in proper position. (From Simon RR, Brenner BE. *Emergency procedures & techniques*, 4th ed. Philadelphia: Lippincott Williams & Wilkins; 2002:11, with permission.)

> ▷ Sponge rubber cuff for nasal passage
> ▷ External traction pulley for oral passage

- Once GEBT is secured in place, the gastric aspiration port is connected to high intermittent suction (60–120 mm Hg).
- Consider reconfirming placement.

■ **Inflating the Esophageal Balloon**

- Inflate esophageal balloon to 30 to 45 mm Hg (no more than 45 mm Hg).
- Balloon pressure should be set at the lowest level required to stop bleeding from aspiration suction port.

- Once the desired pressure is reached, the esophageal balloon port is clamped.
- If bleeding is detected from the gastric aspiration port despite fully inflating both gastric and esophageal balloons, the source is usually a gastric rather than esophageal varix.
- Increase external traction either by pulling to a more taut position and re-fixing to the nasal cuff or by adding 0.45 to 0.91 kg (1–2 lb) of weight to the external traction pulley in incremental steps.
- The esophageal aspiration port (4-lumen tube) or the attached NG tube should be connected to continuous suction.
- **Tube Maintenance**
  - Once balloon tamponade has achieved hemostasis, the esophageal balloon pressure is decreased by 5 mm Hg every 3 hours until a balloon pressure of 25 mm Hg is reached.
  - Maintain adequate analgesia and sedation as the GEBT is very uncomfortable.

Complications
- Aspiration
- Asphyxia in unintubated patients
- Pressure necrosis of lips, nose, esophagus, gastric mucosa
- Esophageal rupture due to inflation of misplaced gastric balloon

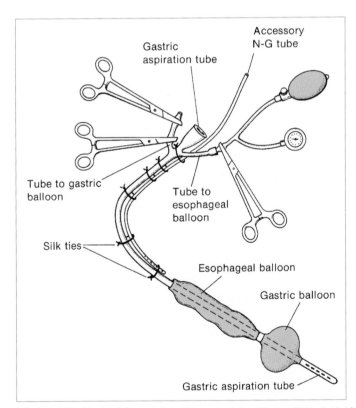

FIGURE 17.2: Modified Sengstaken-Blakemore tube. Also available is the Minnesota tube, which has a built-in esophageal port. (Reused with permission from Yamada T. *Textbook of gastroenterology*, 4th ed., Vol. 1. Philadelphia: Lippincott Williams & Wilkins; 2003:707.)

Common Pitfalls

- Use of inadequate local anesthesia and general sedation
- Failure to add standard nasogastric tube to 3-lumen GEBT for suction of oropharyngeal secretions
- Failure to verify placement of gastric balloon before inflation

Pearls

- Threshold for endotracheal intubation should be very low before placement of GEBT.
- Since the advent of endoscopic sclerotherapy, the GEBT is rarely used and it is not considered the standard of care that all emergency physicians have experience in placing the GEBT.
- The GEBT is meant solely for temporary control of bleeding.
- Consultation for more definitive endoscopic therapy should be obtained as soon as possible.

Suggested Readings

Yamada T. *Textbook of gastroenterology*, Vol. 1. Philadelphia: Lippincott Williams & Wilkins; 2003:707.

18

Hernia Reduction

Melissa Rockefeller and Eric Perez

Indications
- Incarcerated hernias of the groin and abdominal wall

Contraindications
- **Strangulated Hernia**
  - Signs and symptoms include extreme tenderness, blue discoloration, erythema, peritoneal signs, free air on x-ray, fever, elevated while blood cell (WBC) count, signs of bowel obstruction, and shock
  - Surgical emergency
- Presence of bowel obstruction in children younger than 2 years

Risks/Consent Issues
- Mild pain and discomfort are likely.
- Written consent is generally not needed.

Landmarks
- **Groin Hernias**
  - Both indirect and direct hernias occur superior to the inguinal ligament.
  - An indirect hernia passes through the internal inguinal ring and into the inguinal canal.
  - A direct hernia passes through the muscular and fascial wall of the abdomen and does not travel into the inguinal canal.
  - A pantaloon hernia is a combination of a direct and indirect hernia.
  - A femoral hernia occurs inferior to the inguinal ligament and travels into the potential space of the femoral canal medial to the femoral vein.
- **Pelvic Floor Hernias**
  - Occurs in the perirectal area.
- **Ventral Hernias**
  - Occurs due to weakening of the diastases of the anterior abdominal wall.
  - Ventral hernias include incisional, umbilical, epigastric, and Spigelian hernias.

Technique
- **Positioning**
  - Place the patient so that gravity assists the reduction.
  - Place the patient with an inguinal hernia in Trendelenburg position (20 degrees) and in unilateral frog-leg position.
  - Place the patient with an abdominal hernia in supine position.
  - Maintaining the position for 10 minutes will often allow for spontaneous reduction.

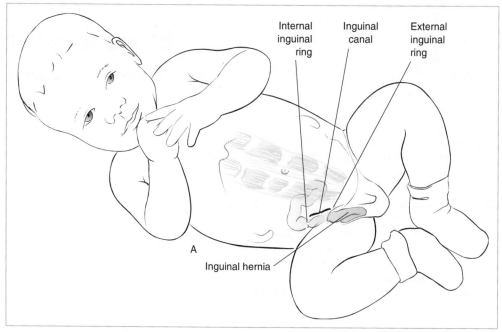

Internal
inguinal
ring

Inguinal
canal

External
inguinal
ring

A
Inguinal hernia

FIGURE 18.1: Anatomy of an inguinal hernia. (From Clark MC. Hernia reduction. In: Henretig FM, King C, eds. *Textbook of pediatric emergency procedures*. Philadelphia: Williams & Wilkins; 1997:931, with permission.)

- **Patient Preparation**
  - Provide appropriate analgesia and sedation.
  - Apply cool compresses to the hernia to reduce vasodilatation and intraluminal bowel gas.
- **Reduction**
  - Find the edge of the defect in the abdominal or groin wall and place your nondominant hand at this site to prevent ballooning of the hernia around the defect.
  - Gently guide the proximal portion of the hernia with slow, steady pressure through the defect and end with the contents most distal.
  - Repeated failed attempts or worsening pain should prompt surgical consultation.

Complications
- Injury to underlying bowel caused by excessive force
- Reduction of bowel into a preperitoneal location

Common Pitfalls
- Failure to find the defect through which to reduce the hernia
- Failure to appropriately position the patient
- Failure to appropriately administer analgesia/sedation
- Partial reduction of hernia left unrecognized due to patient's body habitus
- Failure to recognize ischemic/strangulated bowel

Pearls

- A gentle approach in a well-positioned, comfortable patient will yield the best results.
- Consult surgery if there are signs of strangulation.
- Ultrasonography may help identify ischemic bowel or determine alternate etiology of the mass.

Suggested Readings

Knoop K, Stack LB, Storrow AB. *Atlas of emergency medicine*, 2nd ed. New York: McGraw-Hill; 2002:207–208.

Manthey DE. Abdominal hernia reduction. In: Roberts, JR, Hedges J, eds. *Clinical procedures in emergency medicine*, 4th ed. Philadelphia: WB Saunders; 2004:860–867.

Tintanalli J, Kelen GD, Stapczynski JS. *Emergency medicine: A comprehensive study guide*, 6th ed. New York: McGraw-Hill; 2004:527–530.

19

Diagnostic Peritoneal Lavage

Laura Withers and Raymond Wedderburn

General

Diagnostic peritoneal lavage (DPL) is a sensitive (~95%) means to rapidly evaluate for intra-abdominal injury in the trauma patient.

Indications

- **In Blunt Trauma**
  - Unexplained hypotension
  - Patient with an equivocal examination, altered sensorium, or who is otherwise difficult to assess (especially if computed tomography [CT] is unavailable)
  - Patient taken emergently to the operating room (OR) for extra-abdominal procedure, who requires further abdominal assessment or who will not be a candidate for serial examinations because of anesthesia
- **In Penetrating Trauma**
  - A hemodynamically stable, asymptomatic patient with an anterior abdominal wall stab wound and evidence of fascial penetration but no obvious indication for laparotomy

Contraindications

- **Absolute Contraindications**
  - Meets indications for exploratory laparotomy
- **Relative Contraindications**
  - Prior abdominal surgery—consider open technique
  - Pregnancy—consider open technique with supraumbilical approach
  - Morbid obesity
  - Ascites or advanced cirrhosis
  - Coagulopathy

Risks/Consent Issues

- In patients who require DPL because of altered sensorium, consent is implied. Discussion with the patient and/or family should be held when possible.
- The incidence of complications may be lower for open diagnostic peritoneal lavage compared with the percutaneous technique; however, the percutaneous technique is somewhat faster.

Landmarks

The incision or puncture site is in the midline, one-third of the distance from the umbilicus to the symphysis pubis. In the pregnant patient or the patient with a pelvic fracture, the incision should be made just above the umbilicus.

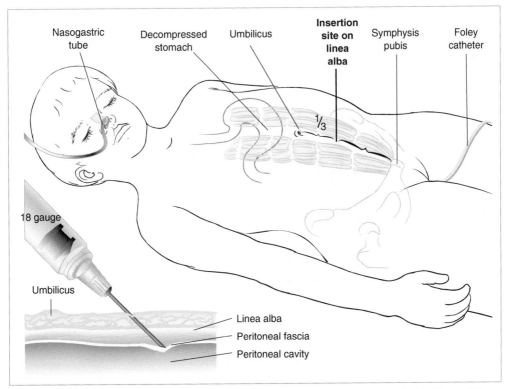

FIGURE 19.1: Anatomical landmarks for diagnostic peritoneal lavage. (From VanDevander PL, Wagner DK. Diagnostic peritoneal lavage. In: Henretig FM, King C, eds. *Textbook of pediatric emergency procedures.* Philadelphia: Williams & Wilkins; 1997:358, with permission.)

Technique
■ **Patient Preparation**
- Place a urinary catheter to empty the bladder (if not contraindicated).
- Place a nasogastric tube (if not contraindicated) and keep it connected to suction to decompress the stomach.
- Gather instruments, sterile supplies, and appropriate sterile gown.
- Prepare the abdomen from costal margin to pubis and from flank to flank with povidone/iodine solution (Betadine) or chlorhexidine and create a sterile field with towels or drapes.
- Inject local anesthesia (1% lidocaine with epinephrine is preferred) in the skin area where the incision will be made.

■ **Open Technique**
- Using a no. 10, 11, or 15 blade scalpel make a 2- to 4-cm incision in the vertical direction at a site one-third of the distance from the umbilicus to the pubis.
- Divide the subcutaneous tissue down to the level of the fascia.
- Grasp the fascia with clamps and elevate it. Incise it sharply.
- Grasp the peritoneum with two clamps, release one and re-grasp so that the bowel that may be caught can fall away. Repeat with the second clamp. Incise peritoneum sharply.
- Insert a peritoneal dialysis catheter into the abdomen directing it gently toward the pelvis.

- Follow directions under "Common Technique for Aspiration and Lavage" section.
- At the conclusion of the procedure (after the catheter is removed), the fascial incision should be closed with no. 0 or no. 1 PDS or nylon suture. Skin can be closed with staples.

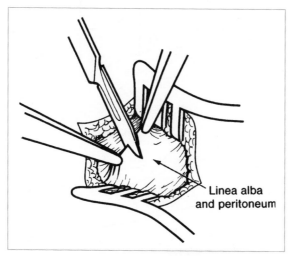

FIGURE 19.2: Make an incision between two hemostats that pick up the peritoneum and fascia as shown. (From Simon RR, Brenner BE. *Emergency procedures and techniques.* Philadelphia: Lippincott Williams & Wilkins; 2002:17, with permission.)

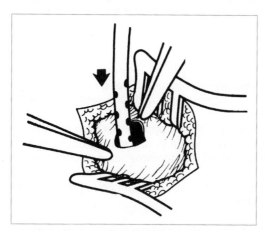

FIGURE 19.3: Pass a catheter through a 2-cm incision and direct it toward the pelvis. (From Simon RR, Brenner BE. *Emergency procedures and techniques.* Philadelphia: Lippincott Williams & Wilkins; 2002:17, with permission.)

Percutaneous Technique
- Elevate the skin on either side of the needle insertion site, between clamps.
- Insert an 18-gauge beveled needle in a syringe through the skin and soft tissue. The fascia will cause resistance, which will be felt to release when the needle enters the abdomen. Advance the needle 0.5 to 1 cm into the abdomen. Draw back on the needle. Easy aspiration confirms abdominal location.

- The J-shaped or flexible side of a guide-wire is threaded through the needle. STOP if resistance is met or when approximately 5 cm of wire remains outside the abdomen.
- Leaving the wire in place, remove the needle.
- Make a 0.5- to 1-cm incision at the insertion site.
- Insert a dialysis catheter over the wire into the abdomen in the direction of the pelvis (dilatation with a dilator may be required as a separate step before catheter insertion).
- Remove the wire.

Common Technique for Aspiration and Lavage
- Connect the dialysis catheter to a syringe and aspirate.
  - ▸ If 10 mL of gross blood is aspirated, the DPL is positive and the patient should undergo immediate laparotomy.
  - ▸ If bile, enteric contents, or food particles are aspirated, the DPL is positive and the patient should undergo immediate laparotomy.
- If aspiration yields less than 10 mL of blood, instill 10 mL/kg (up to 1 L) of warm normal saline into the abdomen. Shift the abdomen gently (i.e., place in Trendelenburg, then reverse Trendelenburg positions) and allow the fluid to remain for 5 to 10 minutes.
- Place the empty infusion bag or container on the floor below the patient to allow the fluid to drain. The container should be vented to promote drainage of the fluid. Drain at least half of the infused fluid.
- Send a sample of 20 mL to the laboratory for red blood cell (RBC) and white blood cell (WBC) counts.

Complications
- Local wound complications such as infection, dehiscence, and hematoma may be higher with open technique.
- Intraperitoneal injury to solid organs, bowel, bladder, and vasculature may be more common with the percutaneous technique.
- Procedure can cause pain.

Common Pitfalls
- False-positives may occur in the presence of pelvic fractures.
- If resistance is encountered when placing the catheter or infusing fluid, stop and check the catheter position. If the catheter is preperitoneal, DPL can be reattempted.
- If adequate fluid cannot be siphoned, the catheter may be obstructed and can be gently manipulated. Gently changing the patient's position or shifting the abdomen may release compartmentalized fluid.

Pearls
- DPL does not evaluate the retroperitoneum. It should be evaluated by CT scan in the stable patient.
- DPL may be falsely positive, particularly in the presence of pelvic fractures. A positive DPL does not mandate laparotomy. Stable patients with positive DPL may be candidates for nonoperative management.
- DPL, CT, and focused abdominal sonogram for trauma (FAST) can substitute or augment each other. The particular clinical situation, capacity of the particular institution, and skills of the providers are important considerations.
- Infusion of fluid can confound future CT and US findings.

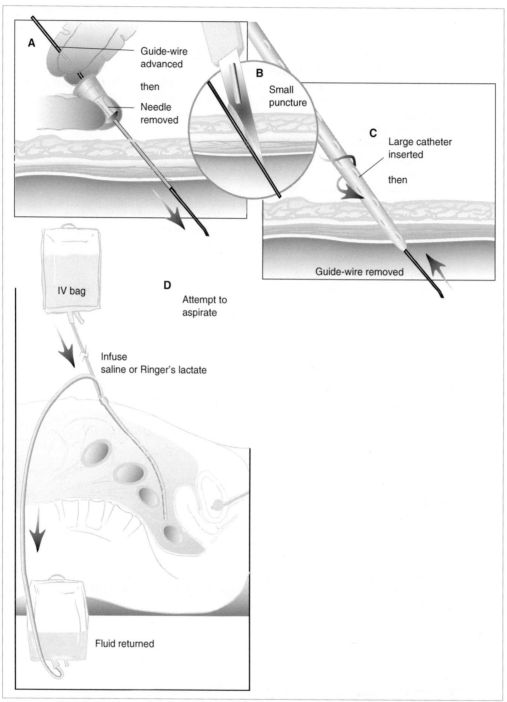

FIGURE 19.4: **A:** Guide-wire advanced through needle. **B:** Small puncture with scalpel. **C:** Lavage catheter advanced into the peritoneal cavity over the guide-wire. **D:** An initial attempt is made to aspirate blood from the peritoneal cavity; 10–15 mL/kg normal saline or Ringer's lactate is infused via the lavage catheter; the bag is dropped to a level below the abdomen and the fluid is recovered by gravity. (From VanDevander PL, Wagner DK. Diagnostic peritoneal lavage. In: Henretig FM, King C, eds. *Textbook of pediatric emergency procedures*. Philadelphia: Williams & Wilkins; 1997:362, with permission.)

TABLE 19.1: Interpretation and appropriate action based on lavage findings

Findings	Interpretation	Action
>100,000 RBC	Positive for **blunt** trauma	Laparotomy
20,000–100,000 RBC	Indeterminate for **blunt** trauma	Consider further imaging; correlate clinically
>10,000 RBC	Positive for **penetrating** trauma	Laparotomy
<10,000 RBC	<2% chance of missed injury	May still need to evaluate for diaphragmatic injury in penetrating trauma
>500 WBC	Positive	Laparotomy

RBC, red blood cell; WBC, white blood cell.

Suggested Readings

Marx JA. Peritoneal procedures. In: Roberts, JR, Hedges J, eds. *Clinical procedures in emergency medicine*, 4th ed. Philadelphia: WB Saunders; 2004:841–851.

20

Nasogastric Tube Placement

William Bagley and Jennifer Stratton

Indications

- Diagnosis and evaluation of upper gastrointestinal (GI) bleeding
  - Is melena or bright red blood per rectum (BRBPR) a result of gastric bleeding?
  - Is there persistent bleeding in patients presenting with coffee-ground emesis?
- Decompression of obstructed GI tract, such as, small bowel obstruction (SBO)
- Lavage or removal of toxins (e.g., overdose, poisonings)
- Prevention of aspiration and gastric dilatation (e.g., in intubated patients)

Common Reasons for NGT Placement

Melena

Bright red blood per rectum (BRBPR)

Coffee-ground emesis

Small bowel obstruction (SBO)

Intubated patient

Contraindications

- **Absolute Contraindications**
  - Facial trauma with possible cribriform-plate fracture
    - Concern for passage into intracranial space
- **Relative Contraindications**
  - Severe coagulopathy
    - If critical, consider orogastric tube placement
  - Alkali ingestions or esophageal strictures
    - Placement may cause esophageal rupture

Technique

- **Patient Preparation**
  - Elevate the head of the patient's bed to upright position (if possible).
  - Place emesis basin on the patient's lap.
  - Select the more patent nostril for tube placement.
    - Have the patient occlude one nostril at a time and sniff.
    - It may be necessary to switch to the opposite nostril if one side proves to be too difficult.
  - In awake patients, anesthetize both nares at least 5 minutes before attempting tube placement.
    - Inject lidocaine gel (5 mL of 2% viscous lidocaine) via 10 mL syringe.
    - Use benzocaine (Cetacaine) spray for oropharynx.
    - Consider nebulized lidocaine (2.5 mL of 4% lidocaine) via face mask as alternative to gels and sprays.

- Immediately after opening the nasogastric tube (NGT) package, place the small (easily misplaced) "connector" in your pocket or a safe place; it is frequently missing/lost when you want to connect the NGT to suction.
- Estimate tube insertion distance.
  - Measure the tube from the patient's xiphoid process to the earlobe through to the tip of the nose. Add 15 cm to this distance and mark on the NGT with a small amount of tape.
- Lubricate NGT.

Insertion
- Insert tube (usual adult size 16 Fr or 18 Fr) into selected nostril aiming along the floor of the nose, posteriorly and caudally.
- Once in nasopharynx, have the patient flex his head forward to aid tube placement into the esophagus.
- Pause as tube enters oropharynx and have the patient swallow water either via straw or syringe to aid in the passage of tube, and then rapidly advance the tube into the stomach to the predetermined depth.

Confirmation of Placement
- Patient is able to speak clearly.
  - If the patient is unable to speak, the tube is likely in the trachea and needs to be removed.
- Aspirate the gastric contents.
- Insufflation of air through a 50- or 60-mL syringe into the end of the NGT while auscultating over the stomach should reveal borborygmi (gurgling in stomach).
  - If the patient burps after insufflation, the tube is likely in the esophagus and needs to be advanced.
- Order chest x-ray.
  - It is not standard to routinely confirm NGT placement with chest x-ray.
  - If a chest x-ray is planned for endotracheal tube placement and so on, consider obtaining after NGT placement.
  - If the patient is unconscious, consider x-ray confirmation, especially if charcoal is to be administered through the NGT.

Secure the Tube
- Clean and dry the tube, if necessary.
- Tape NGT at nose entry site with emphasis of alleviating pressure of the tube on the nose.
- Secure the tube to the patient's gown for added stability.

Complications
- Epistaxis
- Tracheal intubation
- Esophageal/gastric perforation
- Aspiration
- Sinusitis or otitis media
- Ulceration of mucosa
- Esophageal stricture

Common Pitfalls
- Use of inadequate local anesthesia
- Pulmonary placement of the NGT
- Esophageal placement of NGT
- Curling of the NGT in the patient's mouth

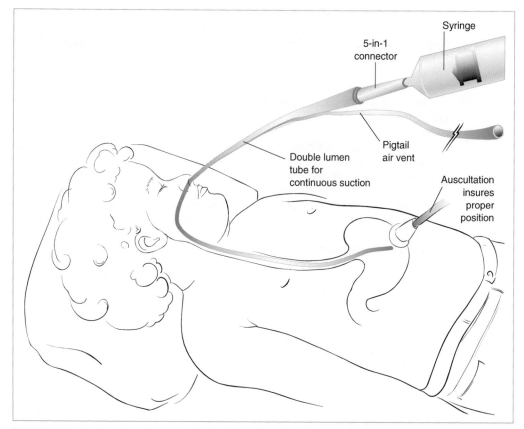

FIGURE 20.1: Confirmation of nasogastric tube placement. (From Simon HK, Lewander W. Gastric intubation. In: Henretig FM, King C, eds. *Textbook of pediatric emergency procedures*. Philadelphia: Williams & Wilkins; 1997:912, with permission.)

- Leaving the NGT on constant suction, leading to gastric mucosal damage
- NGT secured too tightly to medial or lateral aspect of nostril, leading to necrosis or bleeding

Pearls
- Most NGT complications occur with prolonged nasogastric intubation.
- NGT placement might require multiple attempts.
  - Larger-sized NGTs may be difficult to pass in narrow nasal passages.
  - Smaller-sized tubes may bend too easily and curl in the patient's mouth.
- In the intubated, nonagitated, and noncombative patient, gently lifting the jaw forward or pushing the trachea to the patient's left can ease passage of the NGT.
  - If there are any concerns that the patient may bite down DO NOT place your fingers in the mouth.
- In patients who are unconscious or have an altered mental status, consider airway protection via intubation before NGT insertion to prevent aspiration.
- If the NGT has been confirmed to be in the stomach and there is minimal return during lavage, the drainage holes may be clogged.

- Consider decreasing the vacuum pressure setting or you can attempt to push air into the venting lumen with a 50- or 60-mL syringe.
- In patients vomiting blood (bright red or coffee-ground), NGT lavage is not used for diagnostic purposes but rather to remove the blood irritating the stomach and to determine if bleeding persists (consult a gastroenterologist if lavage does not clear).

21 Anorectal Foreign Body Removal

Heather Huffman-Dracht and Wendy Coates

Indications
- Anorectal foreign body (FB) in a stable, cooperative patient, which is:
  - Palpable by rectal approach
  - Without sharp edge/broken glass

Contraindications
- Obtain surgical consult immediately in following instances:
  - Signs of perforation, obstruction, or severe abdominal pain
  - Nonpalpable FB
  - Broken glass in rectum
  - Uncooperative or intolerant patient
  - Lack of equipment necessary for retrieval

Key Elements of History
- Ingestion (e.g., bones, toothpicks) versus rectal insertion
- Size and composition of foreign body
- Time of ingestion/insertion
- Attempts made to remove FB
- Assess for red flags—fever, abdominal pain, hematochezia
- Assess for sexual/physical assault, sexually transmitted disease (STD) risk

Landmarks
- Determine the orientation, location, and composition of the anorectal FB and, thereby the appropriate approach to removal by the following:
  - Detailed history
  - Radiography
    - Kidney, ureter, and bladder (KUB) x-ray
    - Chest x-ray for free air detection (if concerned about perforation)
  - Physical examination, including digital rectal examination
- Visualization of the anorectum is enhanced with the patient in the lateral decubitus position, lithotomy position, or prone with knees tucked into chest.

Technique
- **Equipment**
  - Depends on the composition and locale of the FB but may include:
    - Anesthesia/analgesia
    - Light source

- Speculum—such as vaginal speculum, anoscope, Parks retractor—to improve visualization
- Ring and/or tenaculum forceps
- Foley catheter and/or endotracheal tube
- Vacuum extractor

Patient Preparation
- Get informed consent detailing risks, benefits, and alternatives.
- Order KUB x-ray to localize and define FB, and to assess for obstruction or perforation.
- Parenteral sedation and analgesia to enable relaxation and tolerance of the procedure. Avoid oversedation because the patient must be alert to assist in delivery of foreign body.
- Place patient in preferred position.
- A perianal block may facilitate further sphincter relaxation. This is achieved by superficial injection of local anesthetic ($\leq$1.5 mg/kg of 0.5% bupivacaine or $\leq$7 mg/kg of 1% lidocaine with 1:100,000 epinephrine) in a ring around the anus.

Examination
- External examination: Assess for signs of trauma
- Digital rectal examination (DRE)
  - Gauge location and orientation of FB
  - Assess for discharge or bleeding
  - Small, blunt foreign bodies may be removed during DRE
- Anoscopy
  - Assess for mucosal injury
  - Visualize FB

Removal of Foreign Body
- Attempt delivery of FB by applying suprapubic pressure in synchrony with the patient bearing down (i.e., Valsalva maneuver).
- If unsuccessful, digitally guide the presenting part of the FB anteriorly (away from the sacrum) and attempt delivery again.
- If still unsuccessful, directly visualize the anorectum via speculum or anoscopy. Use forceps to grasp the presenting portion and apply gentle traction in conjunction with the Valsalva maneuver. Goal is removal of speculum/anoscope, forceps, and foreign body as a single unit.
- Glass FBs may prove difficult to remove by traction alone due to the vacuum created by the glass in conjunction with the proximal bowel. The following two additional techniques may prove helpful in the removal of glass FBs:
  - Pass two Foley catheters or endotracheal tubes (ETT) just beyond the FB on opposite sides and inflate the balloons. Attempt removal of FB by gentle traction on the catheters/ETTs.
  - Utilize rigid sigmoidoscopy (or Foley catheter) to insufflate air in the rectum proximal to the FB, thereby releasing the vacuum and allowing removal by traction with plastic, rubber, or gauze-tipped forceps.

Follow-up
- Postprocedure sigmoidoscopy is mandated in following instances:
  - Rectal bleeding/mucosal damage
  - Worsening of rectal pain
- Surgical consult and admission warranted in following instances:
  - Failed retrieval/uncooperative patient
  - Postretrieval abdominal pain, fever, hematochezia
  - Shattering of glass FB

Complications
- Mucosal damage
- Bowel perforation
- Shattering of glass within the anorectum
- Infection

Common Pitfalls
- Inadequate local anesthesia and sedation
- Attempting removal of nonpalpable FB
- Failure to directly visualize (i.e., via anoscopy/speculum) FB while applying forceps
- Attempting removal of glass FB without ensuring forceps tips covered with protective gauze, plastic, or rubber
- Failure to screen for STDs

Pearls
- Take time to plan your approach based on the orientation and composition of the FB and prepare accordingly.
- Postprocedure concern for mucosal damage requires sigmoidoscopy before disposition.
- All discharged patients must understand the importance of immediate return if signs of infection, rectal bleeding, or perforation occur.

Suggested Readings

Coates WC. Anorectum. In: Marx JA, Hockberger RS, Walls RM, eds. *Rosen's emergency medicine*, 6th ed. St. Louis: Mosby; 2006:1521–1522.

Strear CM, Coates WC. Anorectal procedures. In: Roberts JR, Hedges JR, eds. *Clinical procedures in emergency medicine*, 4th ed. Philadelphia: WB Saunders; 2004:874–876.

22

Rectal Prolapse Reduction

Kari Scantlebury

Indications
- Prolapse of one or all layers of the rectal mucosa through the anal opening.
  - *Complete prolapse* occurs when all layers of the rectum protrude through the anal opening.
  - *Incomplete prolapse* refers to an internal prolapse that does not project through the anal opening and does not need an emergent reduction.
  - *Mucosal prolapse* is a protrusion of only the rectal mucosa.

Contraindications
- Any of the following conditions require an emergent surgical consultation:
  - Irreducible prolapse
  - Strangulation or gangrene of the rectal tissue
  - Perforation or rupture of the rectal tissue
  - Anal incontinence

Landmarks
- A thick muscle layer palpable between the thumb and forefinger suggests a complete prolapse.
- The mucosal folds originate from the central lumen of the protrusion and extend outward in a radial manner.
- Mucosal prolapses tend to extend not beyond 4 cm from the anus, whereas complete prolapses may extend up to 15 cm from the anal verge.

Technique
- **Patient Preparation**
  - Analgesia/sedation may be necessary for relief of anxiety and full relaxation of sphincter muscles.
  - Place patient in the prone or lateral decubitus position.
    - Children may be allowed to remain in parent's lap to aid in relaxation.
  - Tape buttocks apart or have an assistant hold, to facilitate reduction.
  - If significant edema is present, plain sugar or salt may be applied to the prolapsed tissue to reduce the swelling.
- **Reduction**
  - Place thumbs on either side of the lumen, and the fingers should grasp the exterior of the protrusion.
  - Gentle, constant circumferential pressure is applied from the thumbs at the portion closest to the lumen to guide the walls inward as the prolapse is rolled back through the anal opening.
- **Postreduction Care**
  - After complete reduction, perform a digital rectal examination to evaluate for a mass that may have been the lead point for the prolapse.

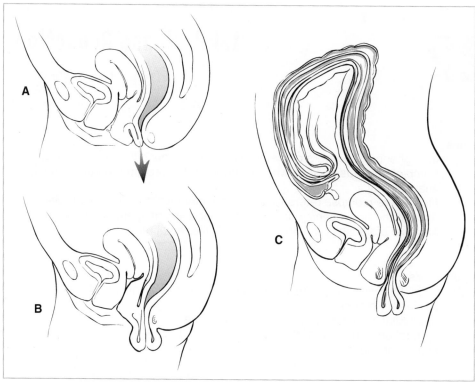

FIGURE 22.1: Anatomy of a rectal prolapse. **A:** Partial prolapse. **B:** Complete prolapse. **C:** Prolapsed intussusception. (From Schwartz G. Reducing a rectal prolapse. In: Henretig FM, King C, eds. *Textbook of pediatric emergency procedures*. Philadelphia: Williams & Wilkins; 1997:948, with permission.)

- Surgical follow-up should be arranged following a successful reduction.
- Patient education regarding dietary fiber, adequate fluid intake, and stool softeners should be provided to reduce likelihood of constipation and straining.

Complications
- Failure of reduction
- Mucosal ulceration
- Necrosis of the rectal wall
- Bleeding
- Incontinence

Common Pitfalls
- Inadequate analgesia resulting in failure of reduction
- Misdiagnosis of hemorrhoids, polyps, cystocele, or carcinoma as a rectal prolapse

Pearls
- Successful reduction is dependent upon analgesia/sedation and constant, slow, steady pressure.

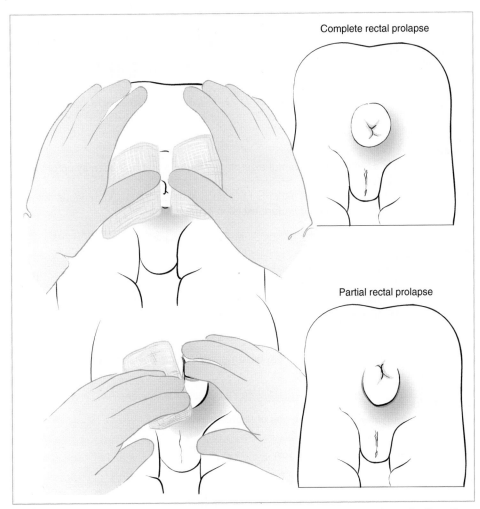

FIGURE 22.2: Rectal prolapse reduction. (From Schwartz G. Reducing a rectal prolapse. In: Henretig FM, King C, eds. *Textbook of pediatric emergency procedures*. Philadelphia: Williams & Wilkins; 1997:949, with permission.)

- Rectal prolapse in children is often associated with cystic fibrosis, parasitic infection, and malnutrition in addition to constipation.
- Loss of anal sphincter tone and incontinence are associated with delays in reduction.

Suggested Readings

Wolfson AB, Hendey GW, Hendry PL, et al. *Harwood-Nuss' clinical practice of emergency medicine*, 4th ed. Philadelphia: Lippincott Williams & Wilkins; 2005.

Stear CM, Coates WC. Anorectal procedures. In: Roberts JR, Hedges JR, eds. *Clinical procedures in emergency medicine*, 4th ed. Philadelphia: WB Saunders; 2004: 877–880.

23 Excision of Acutely Thrombosed External Hemorrhoids

Laura Withers and Mitchell Bernstein

Indications

- Used for a thrombosed, painful external hemorrhoid that has been symptomatic for less than 72 hours.
  - After 72 hours most patients have decreased pain and spontaneous resolution of their acute thrombosis, therefore excision is not indicated.

Contraindications

- **Relative Contraindications**
  - Crohn disease—referral to specialist as there is a high rate of fistula formation.
  - Pregnant women—most cases can be managed medically using Sitz baths, increased dietary fiber, and PO fluids.
    - Excision is necessary only for severe pain as most hemorrhoids resolve after delivery.
  - Uncooperative patients are best managed in the operating room.

Landmarks

- Hemorrhoids represent a mass of dilated venules.

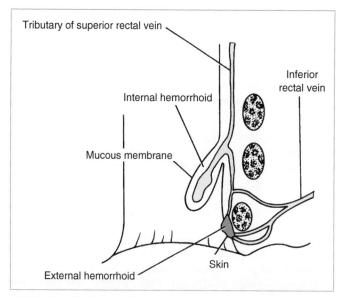

FIGURE 23.1: Varicosed tributary of the superior rectal vein forming the internal hemorrhoid. (From Snell RS. *Clinical anatomy*, 7th ed. Philadelphia: Lippincott Williams & Wilkins; 2004:427, with permission.)

- Internal hemorrhoids originate above the dentate line.

> They can prolapse and extend below the dentate line outside the rectum.
- External hemorrhoids originate below the dentate line.

Technique
Patient Preparation
- Place the patient in the prone or left lateral decubitus position.
  > Have an assistant spread the patient's buttocks, or gently spread the buttocks and maintain the positioning with tape.
- Consider anoscopy before the procedure to evaluate for other lesions.
- Prepare the area with povidone-iodine solution (Betadine) using sterile gloves and universal precautions attire.
- Inject 1% lidocaine with epinephrine or 0.5% bupivacaine into the base of the thrombosed hemorrhoid.
  > A topical lidocaine gel can be used in the anal canal to supplement local anesthesia.
  > Intravenous analgesia is also recommended before administration of local anesthetic.
  > Avoid multiple injection sites because this increases bleeding.
Incision
- Test the adequacy of the local anesthesia by grasping the hemorrhoid with forceps.
- Using a no. 11 scalpel blade, make an *elliptical incision* around the thrombosis with the long axis in the radial direction relative to the anus.
  > Never incise in a circumferential axis.
  > Control bleeding with direct pressure.
- Elevate skin edges with forceps and excise to expose the underlying thrombosis.
- Dissect the clot under direct visualization and completely remove it and any overlying skin using forceps or by applying pressure.
  > After initial clot is removed, have an assistant spread the incision to expose the base of the hemorrhoid and allow removal of further clots.
- Pack the wound loosely with standard cotton gauze to prevent skin edges from reapproximating prematurely.
- Tape buttocks together with gauze to create a pressure dressing.
Follow-up Care
- Counsel patient to apply direct pressure if bleeding or spotting occurs.
- Dressing may be removed after 12 hours. At this time, the patient should begin taking Sitz baths and applying soothing cream to the area (e.g., Preparation H, Anusol HC, or lidocaine ointment).
- Patient should be started on stool softeners and fiber supplements and told to drink additional fluid.
- Patient should be instructed to follow-up in 2 to 4 weeks.

Complications
- Pain
- Bleeding
- Infection
- Anal stenosis that is associated with circumferential excision around the entire anus
- Deep incision can damage the external anal sphincter

Pearls
- After resolution of an acute episode, a skin tag will often be left behind. Reassure patients that this is normal.

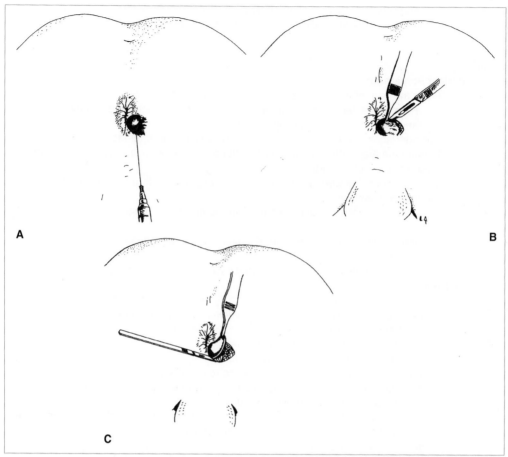

FIGURE 23.2: Anesthetize an external thrombosed hemorrhoid with 1% lidocaine with epinephrine **(A)** with a 15 or no. 11 blade, excise the hemorrhoid in an elliptical fashion at its base **(B)**. Be certain also to excise a wedge of skin and the subcutaneous tissue that contain additional clots, as shown above **(C)**. (From Simon RR, Brenner BE. *Emergency procedures & techniques*, 4th ed. Philadelphia: Lippincott Williams & Wilkins; 2002:28, with permission.)

- Refer lesions suspicious for carcinoma to a colorectal surgeon for treatment.
- Thrombosis of external hemorrhoids may recur or occur synchronously with prolapse and strangulation of internal hemorrhoids. Surgical intervention to excise the underlying vein or decrease blood flow to the hemorrhoidal tissue should be considered for these patients.

Section Editor: Ari M. Lipsky

24

Testicular Torsion

Julie Kasarjian and Clint J. Coil

Indications

Manual detorsion in the emergency department is a safe, noninvasive method for rapid derotation of the spermatic cord and salvage of the testis. It can serve as a temporizing measure to attempt to reperfuse the testis while the patient is awaiting definitive surgical management.

- Testicular torsion must be suspected in any patient presenting with acute scrotal pain/swelling or history of intermittent testicle pain.
- **Signs and Symptoms**
  - Testicular tenderness
  - High-riding testis with horizontal lie
  - Absent cremasteric reflex on the affected side
  - Negative Prehn sign (no relief of pain upon elevation of the testis)
- The most common misdiagnosis assigned to true testicular torsion is epididymitis. Epididymitis is more likely to be associated with epididymal tenderness, an intact cremasteric reflex on the affected side, a positive Prehn sign (relief of pain upon elevation of the testis), a positive urinalysis, and a history of sexually transmitted diseases (STDs).

An urologist or general surgeon should be consulted immediately when torsion is suspected to prepare for emergency surgery.

Contraindications

- Manual detorsion should not delay scrotal exploration and bilateral orchiopexy in the operating room (OR).
- Spermatic cord anesthesia should be used only after discussing with the consulting urologist because it may blunt the subjective endpoint of detorsion efforts (relief of pain).

Risks/Consent Issues

- Pain and discomfort (may be decreased by sedation and local anesthesia)
- Local bleeding and/or potential for infection secondary to spermatic cord anesthesia (sterile technique must be used)
- Manual detorsion does not replace the absolute need for surgical scrotal exploration/orchiopexy

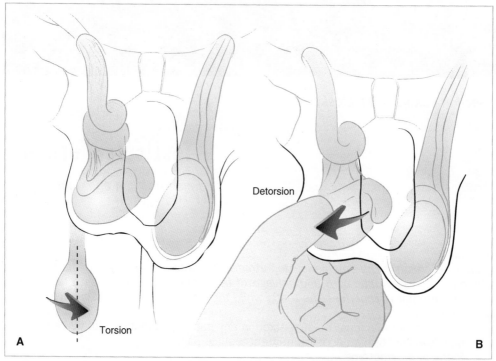

FIGURE 24.1: Manual detorsion. **A:** Torsion of the testis with two inward twists has resulted in a new high-lying position. **B:** The testis is grasped with the fingers and rotated outwardly with two full 360-degree twists. (From Cronan KM, Zderic SA. Manual detorsion of the testes. In: Henretig FM, King C, eds. *Textbook of pediatric emergency procedures.* Philadelphia: Williams & Wilkins; 1997:1005, with permission.)

Landmarks
- If considering spermatic cord anesthesia/block, identify the spermatic cord at the external inguinal ring. Alternatively, if severe edema is present, palpate cord at pubic tubercle over pubis.

Technique
- **Patient Preparation**
  - Place patient in reclining, supine, or lithotomy position.
  - Sterilize skin before administering local anesthesia.
- **Anesthesia/Analgesia**
  - Consider systemic analgesia and/or light sedation.
  - Consider spermatic cord block using 10 mL of 1% plain lidocaine (maximum 3 mg/kg), after discussing first with urologist or general surgeon.
    - ▶ Insert small (27-gauge) needle directly into spermatic cord.
    - ▶ Slowly inject the anesthetic after aspirating for blood first to assure the needle is not intravascular.
- **Detorsion**
  - The most common direction for torsion to occur is laterally to medially.
  - The initial attempt at detorsion should therefore be medial to lateral (Fig. 24.1). Imagine you are "opening a book."
  - Multiple rotations of the testicle may be necessary for complete detorsion.
  - A small percentage of cases are torsed in the opposite direction. If detorsion efforts appear ineffective/painful, attempt to detorse in the opposite direction.

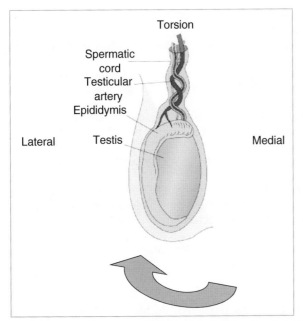

FIGURE 24.2: Right spermatic cord torsion. Manual detorsion using 180 degrees or more of medial to lateral ("opening a book") rotation, lifting slightly upward to release the cremasteric muscle (caudal to cranial). To detorse left testis, use similar, medial to lateral, rotation. (From Porth CM. Disorders of the male genitourinary system. In: *Pathophysiology. Concepts of altered health states*. Philadelphia: Lippincott Williams & Wilkins; 2004. Accessed August 18, 2006, at http://connection.lww.com/Products/porth7e/Imagebank.asp.)

■ **Confirmation**
  ○ Relief of pain
  ○ Restoration of anatomy (vertical lie of testicle)
  ○ Eventual return of cremasteric reflex
  ○ Color Doppler ultrasonogram shows return or improvement of flow
  ○ If the maneuver fails to relieve or worsens pain and/or appears to be shortening the cord, detorsion in the opposite direction should be attempted

Complications
  ■ Unsuccessful manual detorsion
  ■ Patient unable to tolerate procedure (consider procedural sedation)
  ■ Testicular loss due to prolonged ischemia

Common Pitfalls
  ■ Misdiagnosis/delay in manual detorsion
  ■ Failure to make arrangements for surgical consultation and intervention immediately
  ■ Rotation in wrong direction
  ■ Use of inadequate sedation and anesthesia

Pearls
  ■ Testicular torsion is considered a surgical emergency. A urologist or general surgeon should be consulted without delay for any suspected testicular torsion.

- Although torsion can occur at any age, the most common presentation is either during the first year of life or at puberty.
- Some patients with torsion will give a potentially misleading history of minor trauma.
- Ultrasonography may assist in the diagnosis, but results can be misleading, and should therefore not substitute for definitive diagnosis through operative exploration.
- Manual detorsion should not be attempted if it leads to a delay in operative management. Manual detorsion should not be considered an alternative to surgery.
- In the OR, usually both testicles are secured to the scrotal wall (orchiopexy) to prevent recurrence.
- Delays in presentation or diagnosis of >12 hours usually result in testicular loss. Operative exploration and detorsion within 6 hours of symptom onset is a frequently cited goal for management of suspected torsion and is usually associated with salvage of the testicle.
- Presence of a testicular tumor may predispose to torsion.

Suggested Readings

Kahler J, Harwood-Nuss AL. Selected urologic problems. In: Marx JA, Hockberger RS, Walls RM, eds. *Rosen's emergency medicine: Concepts and clinical practice*, 6th ed. Philadelphia: Elsevier Science; 2005.

Perron CE. Pain—scrotal. In: Fleisher GR, Ludwig S, Henretic FM, eds. *Textbook of pediatric emergency medicine*, 5th ed. Philadelphia: Lippincott Williams & Wilkins; 2006.

Schneider RE. Urologic procedures. In: Roberts JR, Hedges JK, eds. *Clinical procedures in emergency medicine*, 4th ed. Philadelphia: WB Saunders; 2004.

Schneider RE. Acute scrotal pain. In: Wolfson AB, ed. *Harwood-Nuss' clinical practice in emergency medicine*, 4th ed. Philadelphia: Lippincott Williams &Wilkins; 2005.

25

Phimosis Reduction

Richard G. Newell and Dan Chavira

Indications
▪ Phimosis requires emergent treatment when it results in urinary retention.

Contraindications
▪ None

Risks/Consent Issues
▪ Procedure can cause pain (local anesthesia will be given)
▪ Instruments may cause local bleeding
▪ There is potential for introducing infection, however sterile technique will be used
▪ Possibility of scar at site of incision/dilation (however definitive treatment will likely be circumcision, thereby removing the scarred tissue)
▪ Possibility of damage to glans penis and urethral meatus

Technique
▪ **Patient Preparation**
  ○ Inform patient/parent regarding plan of action.
  ○ Position: Supine with legs slightly abducted.
  ○ Clean penis and surrounding region with antiseptic solution.
  ○ Sterile drape revealing only the genital region.
  ○ It may be helpful to provide light sedation with an orally delivered benzodiazepine.
▪ **Local Anesthesia:** Use 1% or 2% lidocaine (without epinephrine)
  ○ Local: Beginning proximally at the coronal sulcus, infiltrate lidocaine into the medial aspect of the dorsum of the foreskin proceeding distally to the tip of the foreskin (see Fig. 25.1)
  ○ Dorsal nerve block: Provides anesthesia only to the dorsum of the penis (see Fig. 25.2)
    ▸ Using a 27-gauge needle, inject the lidocaine subcutaneously at the base of the dorsum of the penis just inferior to pubic symphysis.
    ▸ Begin on one side of the base of the penis and inject 3 to 5 mL and then withdraw the needle back to the surface of the skin (without coming out of the skin) and direct the needle to the opposite side and again inject 3 to 5 mL.
  ○ Penile ring block: Provides anesthesia to the entire distal penis (see Fig. 25.3)
    ▸ Perform the dorsal nerve block as above.
    ▸ Using the same technique as above, *ventrally* infiltrate lidocaine, thereby producing a ring of subcutaneous lidocaine at the base of the penis.
▪ **Dilation Only:** Oftentimes the scarred opening of the foreskin can be dilated, thereby allowing for immediate urination and prompt outpatient referral to urologist for definitive treatment.

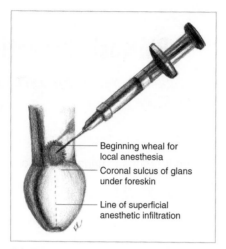

FIGURE 25.1: Local anesthesia. Courtesy of Kim Kiser.

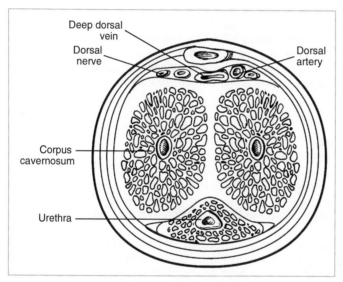

FIGURE 25.2: Dorsal nerve block. Courtesy of Kim Kiser.

- With a hemostat, test and ensure adequate anesthesia (likely a penile block will be the most effective type of anesthesia for this procedure).
- With the penis in the anatomical position, carefully pull the foreskin distally (away from the glans) to ensure that the glans and urethral meatus are not damaged.
- Slowly advance a hemostat or Iris scissors through the foreskin opening and gradually dilate by opening the instrument.
- Expect some bleeding and do not be afraid if you cut/tear the foreskin somewhat—the urologists are much more aggressive than you will ever be!
- Ensure that the patient can urinate easily.
- Consider placing a Foley catheter until a urologist can see the patient.

■ **Dorsal Slit**
- With a hemostat, test and ensure adequate anesthesia (whether a penile block or local anesthesia is used).

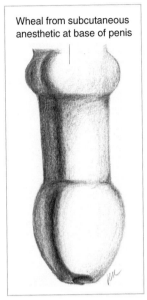

Wheal from subcutaneous anesthetic at base of penis

FIGURE 25.3: Penile ring block. Courtesy of Kim Kiser.

- Insert a closed straight hemostat dorsally between the glans penis and foreskin all the way to the coronal sulcus (take care not to injure the urethral meatus).
- Carefully separate any adhesions that may be present by opening the instrument.
- Insert *one* jaw of the open hemostat to the coronal sulcus, along the path taken previously (between the glans and overlying foreskin).
- Ensure that there is tenting of the foreskin caused by the inner jaw of the hemostat (ensures that inner jaw is not in urethral meatus).
- Close and latch the hemostat, effectively crushing the dorsal foreskin between the jaws (leave in place for ~5 minutes).
- Cut the crushed foreskin with straight scissors (expect some minor bleeding).
  - If the inner and outer foreskin layers separate and continue to bleed, absorbable sutures may be used to obtain hemostasis.
- Retract the foreskin and clean the glans penis and urethral meatus with antiseptic solution.
- Inspect the glans and urethral meatus for any injuries.
- Ensure that the patient can urinate easily.

Complications
- Urethral meatus or glans penis injury may occur if care is not taken to visualize (or at least anatomically locate) these two structures throughout the procedure
- Bleeding from cut/dilated tissue

Common Pitfalls
- Inadequate anesthesia (allow 10–15 minutes for lidocaine to work)
- Lidocaine containing epinephrine should never be used because of the potential for vasoconstriction and subsequent penile necrosis
- Physician anxiety about dilating/cutting the foreskin

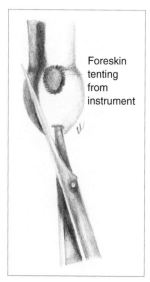

Foreskin tenting from instrument

FIGURE 25.4: Dorsal slit. Courtesy of Kim Kiser.

Pearls

- Adequate anesthesia/sedation is likely the most important component of this procedure.
- Do not be afraid to damage the foreskin because this will be removed with circumcision.

Suggested Readings

Cantu S. *Phimosis and paraphimosis*. Accessed April 11, 2006, at http://www .emedicine.com/emerg/topic423.htm. 2006.

McCollough M, Sharieff G. Renal and genitourinary tract disorders. In: Marx JA, Hockberger RS, Walls RM, eds. *Rosen's emergency medicine: Concepts and clinical practice*, 6th ed. Philadelphia: Elsevier Science; 2005.

Santucci RA. Phimosis, adult circumcision, and buried penis. (Accessed August 15, 2006, at http://www.emedicine.com/med/topic2873.htm.)

Schneider RE. Male genital problems. In: Tintinalli JE, Kelen GD, Stapczynski JS, eds. *Emergency medicine: A comprehensive study guide*, 6th ed. New York: McGraw-Hill; 2004.

Schneider RE. Urologic procedures. In: Roberts JR, Hedges JK, eds. *Clinical procedures in emergency medicine*, 4th ed. Philadelphia: WB Saunders; 2005.

26

Paraphimosis Reduction

Richard Newell and Dan Chavira

Indications
- Paraphimosis is a urologic emergency, and reduction is always indicated when the condition is present.

Contraindications
- None

Risks/Consent Issues
- Procedure may cause pain (local anesthesia will be given)
- Instruments may cause local bleeding
- There is potential for introducing infection (sterile technique will be used)
- Possibility of scar at site of incision/dilation (however, definitive treatment will likely be circumcision, thereby removing the scarred tissue)
- Possibility of damage to glans penis and urethral meatus

Technique
- **Patient Preparation**
  - Inform patient/parent regarding plan of action.
  - Position: Supine with legs slightly abducted.
- **Anesthesia**
  - A topical anesthetic may be all that is necessary.
    - Apply viscous lidocaine or eutectic mixture of local anesthetics (EMLA) to the inner layer of the foreskin.
    - This will also serve as a lubricant.
  - If further anesthesia is necessary, progress from local, to dorsal nerve block, and finally, to penile ring block.
    - See Chapter 25 for details and pictures of penile nerve blocks.
    - When providing local anesthesia with 1% or 2% lidocaine (without epinephrine), be sure to infiltrate into the constricting ring as well.
    - Consider light sedation with an oral benzodiazepine also.
- **Manual Reduction**
  - Using your hands or an elastic bandage, manually compress the glans and foreskin for 3 to 5 minutes to remove as much edema as possible.
  - Place both thumbs on the glans penis and apply slow, steady pressure while using your other fingers just proximal to the phimotic ring to pull the foreskin over the glans penis (see Fig. 26.2).
  - Successful reduction occurs when the phimotic foreskin is reduced back to normal position over the glans.
  - If unsuccessful, proceed to assisted manual reduction methods.
- **Assisted Manual Reduction**
  - Iced-glove method

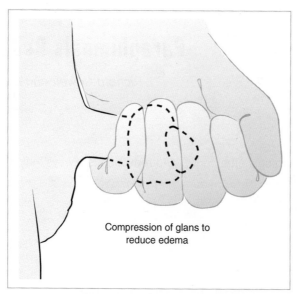

FIGURE 26.1: Technique for compression of glans to reduce edema and allow for manual reduction of paraphimosis.

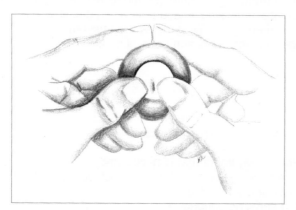

FIGURE 26.2: Manual reduction of paraphimosis. With the thumbs on the glans penis and the fingertips on the tight band of foreskin, the glans is pushed as the foreskin is pulled over the glans. Courtesy of Kim Kiser. (From Green M, Strange GR. Paraphimosis reduction. In: Henretig FM, King C, eds. *Textbook of pediatric emergency procedures*. Philadelphia: Williams & Wilkins; 1997:1008, with permission.)

- ▷ Place a mixture of crushed ice and cold water in a glove and tie closed the cuffed end.
- ▷ Invert the thumb of the glove by pushing it into the glove/ice water mixture, thereby producing a condomlike apparatus surrounded by ice water.
- ▷ Place as much of the penis as possible into the thumb of the glove which will provide compression and vasoconstriction (both decreasing edema).
- ▷ Allow to sit for 10 minutes.
- ▷ Attempt manual reduction as outlined earlier.
- ▷ If unsuccessful proceed to the Babcock clamp method.
- • Babcock clamp method (see Fig. 26.3)
  - ▷ Ensure adequate anesthesia (e.g., penile ring block as described in Chapter 25).

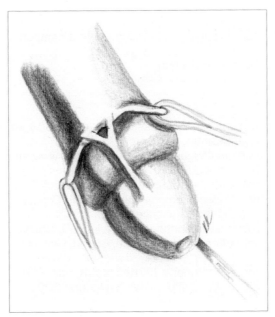

FIGURE 26.3: Babcock clamp method. Courtesy of Kim Kiser.

- ► Use six Babcock clamps (no serrated edges) to evenly and circumferentially grasp the phimotic ring.
- ► Apply slow, steady, distal traction on the Babcock clamps while using your thumbs to apply proximal pressure to the glans.
- ► If reduction is unsuccessful proceed to phimotic ring incision.
- ▪ **Phimotic Ring Incision**
  - ◦ Usually recommended to be performed by a urologist in the operating room, but may be performed by an emergency physician comfortable with this procedure, if instructed to do so by urology.
  - ◦ Ensure adequate anesthesia and sedation.
  - ◦ Place sterile drapes to reveal only the genital region.
  - ◦ Clean penis and surrounding region with antiseptic solution.
  - ◦ Using Iris scissors or a no. 15 blade incise the dorsal skin, subcutaneous tissue, and the constricting ring.
  - ◦ When the phimotic ring is incised, it will spring open revealing a diamond shaped defect.
  - ◦ Reduce the foreskin over the glans penis and complete the dorsal slit by extending the incision as needed (see Chapter 25 for dorsal slit technique).

Complications
- ▪ Laceration or tear to the skin of the penile shaft (suture if needed with 3–0 or 4–0 absorbable material)

Common Pitfalls
- ▪ Inadequate anesthesia (not allowing 10–15 minutes for lidocaine to work)
- ▪ Lidocaine containing epinephrine should not be used because of the potential for vasoconstriction and subsequent penile necrosis
- ▪ Physician anxiety about cutting the foreskin or accidentally cutting the penis

Pearls

- Adequate anesthesia/sedation is likely the most important component of this procedure.
- Slow, steady pressure is best for reduction.

Suggested Readings

Cantu S. *Phimosis and paraphimosis*. Accessed April 11, 2006 at http://www .emedicine.com/emerg/topic423.htm, 2006.

Donohoe JM. *Paraphimosis*. Accessed August 25, 2006 at http://www.emedicine.com/ med/topic2874.htm, 2006.

McCollough M, Sharieff G. Renal and genitourinary tract disorders. In: Marx JA, Hockberger RS, Walls RM, eds. *Rosen's emergency medicine:Concepts and clinical practice*, 6th ed. Philadelphia: Elsevier Science; 2005.

Schneider RE. Male genital problems. In: Tintinalli JE, Kelen GD, Stapczynski JS, eds. *Emergency medicine: A comprehensive study guide*, 6th ed. New York: McGraw-Hill; 2004.

Schneider RE. Urologic procedures. In: Roberts JR, Hedges JK, eds. *Clinical procedures in emergency medicine*, 4th ed. Philadelphia: WB Saunders; 2005.

27

Suprapubic Catheterization

Neil Patel and Amy H. Kaji

Indications
- Urethral trauma
- Urethral stricture
- Chronic urethral infection
- Urinary retention (e.g., prostate obstruction, gynecologic malignancy, spinal cord injury)
- Urinalysis or urine culture in children younger than 2 years
- Phimosis

Contraindications
- An empty or nonpalpable urinary bladder
- History of previous lower abdominal surgery
- Lower abdominal wound or cellulitis
- Previous pelvic radiation with resultant scarring
- Known bladder cancer

Landmarks
- In the adult, the urinary bladder is a pelvic organ located immediately posterior to and extending slightly above the symphysis pubis (see Fig. 27.1)
- In the child, the urinary bladder is still an abdominal organ, located in the midline, slightly superior to the symphysis pubis

Technique
- **Gather Equipment**
  - Povidone-iodine antiseptic solution
  - Sterile gloves and drapes
  - Suprapubic catheterization kit (e.g., Cook cystostomy kit) which typically includes:
    - Local anesthetic (1% lidocaine), 10-mL syringe, 25-gauge needle
    - 22-gauge, 1.5-in. (for children) or 3-in. (for adults) spinal needle
    - 4 × 4-cm gauze pads
    - J-tip guide-wire
    - Scalpel (no. 11 blade)
    - Dilator
    - Introducer sheath
  - Foley catheter (size should be 1F smaller than the diameter of the introducer sheath)
  - Sterile, closed system urinary drainage bag
  - Sterile dressing
- **Patient Preparation**
  - Place the patient in the supine position with the abdomen and pubic region exposed.

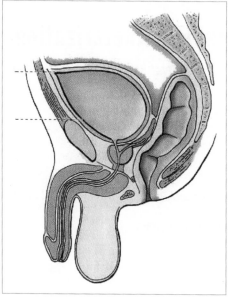

FIGURE 27.1: Relationship of bladder to symphysis pubis. (From Moore KL, Dalley AF. *Clinically oriented anatomy*, 5th ed. Maryland: Lippincott Williams & Wilkins; 2006:406, with permission.)

- Place small children in the frog-legged supine position; a parent or guardian may hold and help calm the child in his or her lap.
- Sterilize, prepare, and drape the lower abdomen and pubic region with povidone-iodine solution.
- Shave the hair in the suprapubic region beforehand, if necessary.
- Observe sterile technique throughout the remainder of the procedure.

- **Localization of the Urinary Bladder**
  - Palpate the bladder 1 to 2 cm above the symphysis pubis in the midline.
  - To facilitate bladder localization, ensure that the patient is well hydrated and has not recently voided.
  - If available, use bedside ultrasonography to identify the bladder, which appears as an anechoic mass in the lower abdomen when full (see Fig. 27.2)

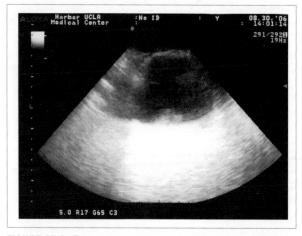

FIGURE 27.2: Transverse sonogram of urinary bladder. (Courtesy of Dr. Patel and Dr. Kaji.)

- If the bladder cannot be located or appears to be empty, delay the procedure until the bladder is distended.

Insertion of Needle

- Identify the needle insertion point at the midline by measuring 1 to 2 cm cephalad to the superior aspect of the symphysis pubis.
- Using a 25-gauge needle and 1% lidocaine, raise a small wheal at the needle insertion site.
- Attach a 22-gauge spinal needle of appropriate length (1.5 in. for children and 3 in. for adults) to a 10- or 20-mL syringe containing 1% lidocaine.
- Enter the insertion point at a 20- to 30-degree angle *caudad* from the perpendicular in adults, and 20 to 30 degrees *cephalad* from the perpendicular in small children.
- Inject 5 mL of 1% lidocaine while advancing the needle toward the bladder, intermittently pausing to aspirate for urine.
- Once urine is aspirated, the needle should be advanced no further.
- If no urine is aspirated, withdraw the needle to just below the skin and redirect either 10 degrees cephalad or caudad.
- A maximum of three attempts should be made before the procedure is terminated.

Seldinger Technique for Foley Insertion (see Fig. 27.3)

- Keeping the spinal needle in place, unscrew the syringe and advance a J-tipped guide-wire through the needle into the bladder.

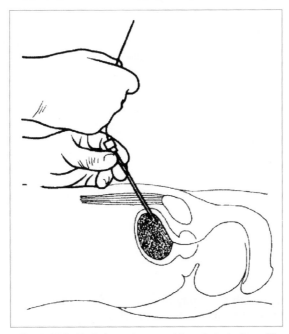

FIGURE 27.3: Technique of suprapubic catheterization with a small-gauge intracath. (From Simon RR, Brenner BF. *Emergency procedures and techniques*, 4th ed. Philadelphia: Lippincott Williams & Wilkins; 2002:434, with permission.)

- Remove the needle over the guide-wire, leaving the guide-wire in place.
- Use a no. 11 blade to make a stab incision adjacent to the guide-wire.
- Advance a dilator and introducer sheath into the bladder over the guide-wire.
- Remove the dilator and guide-wire, leaving only the sheath in place.
- Advance a Foley catheter through the introducer sheath.

> The size of the Foley catheter should be 1F smaller than the diameter of the introducer.

- Inflate the Foley balloon with 10 mL of normal saline (NS) or sterile water and attach the catheter to a reservoir bag.
- Remove the peel-away introducer sheath. Pull back on the Foley catheter until resistance is met, which indicates that the balloon is against the inner wall of the bladder.

- **Secure the Tube** (see Fig. 27.4)
  - Place sterile dressing around the catheter insertion site and affix the tube to the lateral aspect of the patient's abdomen or thigh with cloth tape to prevent kinking of the tube.

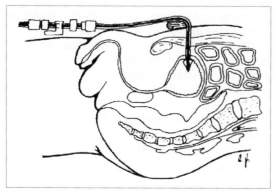

FIGURE 27.4: Trocar taped over 4 × 4-cm gauze pads after insertion. (From Simon RR, Brenner BF. *Emergency procedures and techniques.* 4th ed. Philadelphia: Lippincott Williams & Wilkins; 2002:434, with permission.)

Complications

- Hematuria (usually transient)
- Hematoma
- Infection (intra-abdominal, bladder, or skin)
- Abscess formation
- Peritoneal perforation
- Bowel perforation
- Leakage around the catheter site
- Bladder stones

Common Pitfalls

- Attempting the procedure with an empty or near-empty bladder
- Failure to note the presence of abdominal wounds or infection
- Inadequate anesthesia
- Failure to observe sterile technique

Pearls

- Whenever possible, use ultrasonography to guide aspiration or catheter placement.
- In nonemergent situations, wait until the bladder is full before attempting catheterization.

▪ If a formal suprapubic catheterization kit (Cook cystostomy kit) is not available, a single-lumen central venous catheter kit may be substituted as a temporizing measure.

Suggested Readings

Gochman RF, Karasic RB, Heller MB. Use of portable ultrasound to assist urine collection by suprapubic aspiration. *Ann Emerg Med*. 1991;20:631–635.

Moore KL, Dalley AF. *Clinically oriented anatomy*, 5th ed. Maryland: LWW, Inc.; 2006: 406.

Nomura S, Ishido T, Teranshi J, et al. Long term analysis of suprapubic cystostomy drainage in patients with neurogenic bladder. *Urol Int*. 2000;65:185–189.

O'Brien WM. Percutaneous placement of a suprapubic tube with peel-away sheath introducer. *J Urol*. 1991;145:1015–1016.

Roth DR, Choi HK. Suprapubic catheterization and aspiration. Accessed August 28 at http://www.emedicine.com/proc/fulltopic/topic82964.htm. 2006.

Simon RR, Brenner BF. *Emergency procedures and techniques*, 4th ed. Baltimore: Lippincott Williams & Wilkins; 2002:432–434.

Vilke GM. Bladder aspiration. In: Rosen P, ed. *Atlas of emergency procedures*. St. Louis: Mosby; 2001:130–131.

28 Priapism: Intracavernous Aspiration

Timothy Horeczko and Ari M. Lipsky

Indications

- To alleviate compartment syndrome in ischemic low-flow (veno-occlusive) priapism
- May be caused by:
  - Trauma (genital, pelvic, perineal)
  - Thromboembolism (sickle cell disease, leukemia)
  - Medications (cyclic guanosine monophosphate [cGMP] inhibitors, neuroleptics, erectile-dysfunction injectables, cocaine/marijuana/ecstasy, and others)
  - Neoplasm (primary or metastatic)
  - Neurologic disorders (spinal cord injury, spinal stenosis)
  - Infection (recent infection with *Mycoplasma pneumoniae*, malaria)

Contraindications

- **Absolute Contraindications**
  - Nonischemic high-flow (arterial) priapism
    - See "Technique" section for differentiation
  - Priapism relief with medical management
    - Treatment of underlying etiology
    - Ice packs to the groin
    - "Steal phenomenon" by having patient run or climb stairs
    - Oral medications recommended by some experts but the literature does not clearly support its efficacy
      - Terbutaline 5 mg PO followed by second dose 5 mg PO 15 minutes later, if necessary
      - Pseudoephedrine 60 to 120 mg PO
- **Relative Contraindications**
  - Coagulopathy
  - Thrombocytopenia

Risks/Consent Issues

- Major risk of priapism with or without treatment is long-term impotence. This should be explained clearly to the patient and documented.
- Procedure may cause pain (local anesthesia will be given).
- Needle puncture may cause local bleeding and scarring.
- Whenever the skin is punctured, there is potential for infection (sterile technique will be used).

Landmarks

- Needle aspiration/irrigation of the cavernosa is performed laterally and dorsally on the shaft of the penis, that is, at 2 or 10 o'clock position. This technique avoids the corpus spongiosum and urethra ventrally and the neurovascular bundle and penile vein dorsally.

Technique

- **Distinguish Ischemic Low-Flow (Veno-Occlusive) Priapism from Nonischemic High-Flow (Arterial) Priapism**
  - Detailed history and physical examination
    - High-flow priapism is often not painful
  - **Penile blood gas**
    - Clean with povidone-iodine solution. Infiltrate 1 mL of 1% lidocaine with a tuberculin syringe for local anesthesia. Use a 19- or 21-gauge scalp vein ("butterfly") needle attached to syringe to puncture perpendicularly at 2 or 10 o'clock position on penile shaft to draw blood gas (see Fig. 28.1).

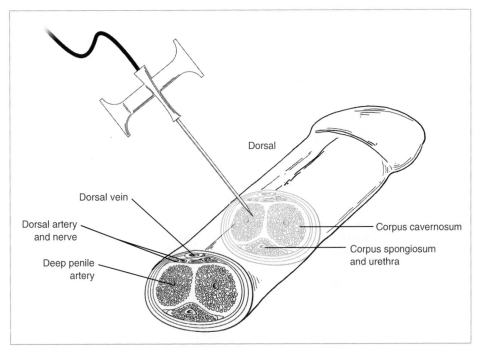

Dorsal

Dorsal vein

Dorsal artery and nerve

Deep penile artery

Corpus cavernosum

Corpus spongiosum and urethra

FIGURE 28.1: Cross-section of penis and placement of needle. Courtesy of Tim Horeczko.

- Note color of aspirated blood. As a guideline, low-flow priapism is more consistent with pH <7.0 to 7.25, Po_2 <30 mm Hg, and Pco_2 >60 mm Hg. A high-flow lesion will more closely reflect normal arterial values.
  - Penile Doppler ultrasonography may be considered, if available, to aid in distinguishing high- from low-flow priapism.
  - Consider complete blood cell (CBC) count (leukemia, platelets), reticulocyte count (sickle cell), urinalysis/Gram stain (infection), and coagulation panel.
    - Treat the underlying disorder (e.g., hydration, pain control, and possible transfusion for sickle cell disease).
  - Penile aspiration is indicated only for low-flow priapism (see Fig. 28.2).
- **Patient Preparation for Aspiration**
  - Establish IV access and place patient on oxygen and monitor.
  - Consider procedural sedation for patients unable to tolerate procedure.

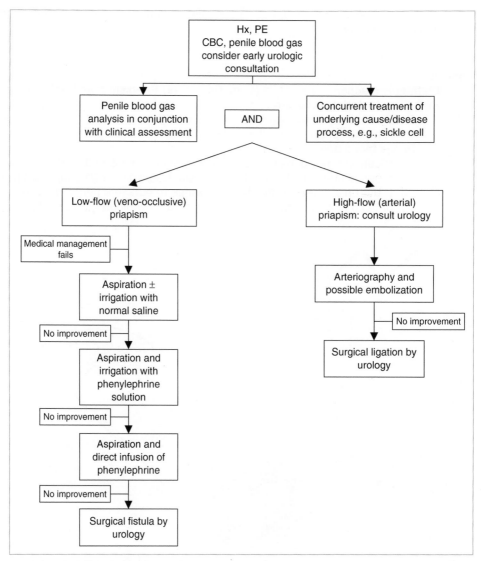

FIGURE 28.2: Priapism algorithm. Hx, history; PE, physical examination; CBC, complete blood count.

- Assemble the following supplies: Povidone-iodine or chlorhexidine, 1% lidocaine, 27-gauge needle (for penile block), sterile field supplies, sterile gloves, 19- or 21-gauge scalp vein ("butterfly") needle, three-way stopcock, 10 mL empty syringe, 10 mL syringe with normal saline (NS), 10 mL syringe with phenylephrine solution (see subsequent text), 4 × 4-cm gauze, and Kerlix gauze.
- Prepare sterile field; swab copiously with antiseptic solution from glans to base of penis.
- Perform penile nerve block: Use 1% lidocaine and 27-gauge needle to form ring block around entire base of penile shaft (see Chapter 25 for details).
- **Penile Aspiration** (for low-flow priapism *only;* see algorithm in Fig. 28.2)
  - Palpate either of the paired, engorged corpora cavernosa at 2 or 10 o'clock position (avoiding the dorsal penile vein at 12 o'clock position).

- Attach 19- or 21-gauge scalp (''butterfly'') needle and 10 mL empty syringe to three-way stopcock.
- Place needle into one corpus cavernosum perpendicularly at 2 or 10 o'clock position midshaft, aspirating on insertion (Fig. 28.1). Advance needle only enough to ensure blood return.
  - ▸ If there is inadequate return of blood or lack of initial detumescence, irrigate with a small amount (1 mL) of NS to flush the clot and to allow for further aspiration.
  - ▸ Aspirate blood while milking shaft until penis detumesces, taking care not to dislodge needle or cause laceration.
  - ▸ It is necessary to aspirate only from one corpus cavernosum as there is communication between the two corpora.
- If there is minimal response to direct aspiration, begin irrigation with dilute phenylephrine solution—mix 1 mg phenylephrine in 100 mL of NS ($10\mu g$/mL); irrigate the cavernosum with 10 mL ($100\mu g$) at a time, every 3 to 5 minutes. Aspirate the solution back after each infusion. It is helpful to attach both the syringe for aspiration and the NS syringe to the stopcock to facilitate aspiration and irrigation.
- If unable to irrigate or if there is no result with dilute phenylephrine solution, use nondiluted phenylephrine to inject directly in 200- to 500-μg aliquots every 3 to 5 minutes. Do not exceed a total maximum dose of 1,500μg.
- After the procedure, remove needle, hold pressure for 5 minutes, and wrap with compression dressing to avoid hematoma formation.
- Consider placing rubber band at base of penis as a temporizing measure to avoid retumescence after procedure.

Complications
- Erectile dysfunction or impotence
  - Both of these may also result if the procedure is *not* performed
- Infection
- Systemic reaction to sympathomimetic injection, including dysrhythmia

Common Pitfalls
- Delay in differentiation between low- and high-flow priapism and not recognizing that they have different treatments
- Inadequate anesthesia and analgesia
- Failure to hold pressure after cavernosal puncture in order to avoid hematoma formation
- Failure to determine cause of priapism and treat underlying condition simultaneously

Pearls
- Advise the patient that impotence is a frequent complication of priapism with or without treatment, regardless of the length of symptoms or success of intervention.
- Low-flow priapism is more common, characterized by prolonged and painful erection. Sickle cell disease is the most common cause of priapism in children. Prompt aspiration of the corpora is essential to minimize ischemia.
- The risk of priapism with the use of sildenafil (Viagra) is very low.

- High-flow priapism is rare, and is usually due to penile, perineal, or pelvic trauma. Less common causes are malignancy (primary and metastatic), Fabry disease, and Peyronie disease. Aspiration is not recommended in arterial priapism because it is not effective and may be harmful.
- Patients should be monitored during and following intracavernous injection of sympathomimetic drugs for acute hypertension, reflex bradycardia, tachycardia, palpitations, and cardiac dysrhythmia.
- Surgical shunts for the treatment of low-flow priapism should be considered only after trial of intracavernous injection of sympathomimetics has failed.
- Piesis sign: In young children, perineal compression with the thumb causes prompt detumescence in high-flow priapism.

Suggested Readings

Cherian J, Rao AR, Thwaini A, et al. Medical and surgical management of priapism. *Postgrad Med J.* 2006;82:89–94.

Ciampalini S, Savoca G, Buttazzi L, et al. High-flow priapism: Treatment and long-term follow-up. *Urology.* 2002;59:110–113.

Dougherty CM, Richard AJ, Carey MJ. *Priapism.* Accessed September 26, at http://www .emedicine.com/emerg/topic486.htm, 2006.

Mantadakis E. Outpatient penile aspiration and epinephrine irrigation for young patients with sickle cell anemia and prolonged priapism. *Blood.* 2000;95:78–82.

McCollough M, Sharieff G. Renal and genitourinary tract disorders. In: Marx JA, Hockberger RS, Walls RM, eds. *Rosen's emergency medicine: Concepts and clinical practice*, 6th ed. St Louis: Mosby; 2006.

National Guideline Clearinghouse (NGC). *Guideline summary: The management of priapism (2003).* Rockville: National Guideline Clearinghouse (NGC). Accessed September 26, at http://www.guideline.gov; 2006.

Section Editor: Jerrica L. Chen

29 Perimortem Cesarean Section

Armin Perham Poordabbagh and Penelope Chun

Indications
- Gravid patient with a potentially viable fetus of ≥24 weeks gestational age and imminent maternal death or unresponsive to cardiopulmonary resuscitation (CPR) for 5 minutes.

Survival of mother and infant is greatest when procedure is performed within 5 minutes of maternal arrest.

Contraindications
- Patient with fetus <24 weeks gestational age.
- Lower limit of fetal viability varies depending on institution and available resources.

Risk/Consent Issues
- Verbal consent from family when possible.

Technique
- **Patient Preparation**
  - Procedure should be performed by the most experienced person available.
  - Contact all essential personnel (i.e., neonatology/pediatrics, obstetrics).
  - Continue CPR on maternal patient throughout entire procedure.
- Estimate fetal age/maturity (if unknown from history):
  - Height of uterine fundus reaches the umbilicus at 20 weeks gestational age and increases approximately 1 cm for each additional week.
  - Four finger breadths above the umbilicus is approximately 24 weeks gestational age.
- **Incision**
  - Use a scalpel with a no. 10 blade.
  - Make a midline vertical incision on the abdomen from just above the symphysis pubis extending to the umbilicus along the linea nigra/linea alba.
  - Incise through all layers of the abdominal wall to the peritoneal cavity.
  - Use retractors (if available) to retract abdominal wall and expose the uterus.
- **Reflect Bladder Inferiorly**
  - If a full bladder obstructs view of the uterus, decompress bladder with a puncture incision and deflate with either pressure or suction.

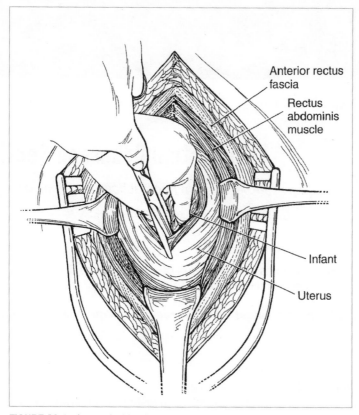

Anterior rectus
fascia

Rectus
abdominis
muscle

Infant

Uterus

FIGURE 29.1: Anatomical landmarks.

- Bladder repair may be done later (if mother survives).
- Make a small vertical incision (2 to 5 cm) along the lower uterine segment until amniotic fluid is encountered.
  - Be careful not to cause inadvertent injury to the underlying fetus.
- Insert index finger into incision and lift the uterus away from the fetus.
- Use bandage (blunt-ended) scissors to extend the incision either transversely or vertically.
  - Avoid tearing the uterine vessels located along the lateral margins of the uterus when making a transverse incision.
  - Incision should be large enough for delivery of the fetal head and body.
- **Deliver Baby**
  - Place hand into the uterus and gently deliver the infant's head. Check for nuchal cord.
  - If the infant's feet are first encountered, continue as a breech delivery.
- Suction the mouth and nares with bulb suction.
- Complete delivery of the infant's shoulders and thorax.
- Clamp and cut the umbilical cord.
- Continue neonatal resuscitation as necessary.
- Check maternal pulses and continue CPR.
  - Relief of aortocaval compression by the uterus improves maternal hemodynamics.
  - Cases of maternal survival have been reported.

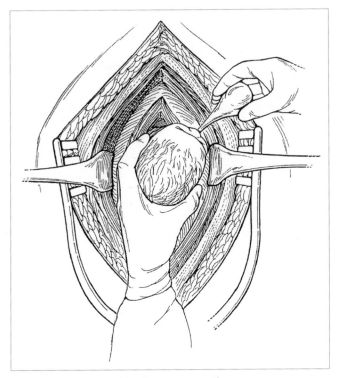

FIGURE 29.2: Delivery through cesarean section.

Complications
- Bladder injury
- Bowel injury
- Fetal lacerations and injury
- Neonate with neurologic deficits and/or demise
- Maternal bleeding and infection
- Maternal morbidity

Common Pitfalls
- Use of fetal Doppler or ultrasonography—not practical before procedure and creates unnecessary time delay!

Pearls
- Fetal survival is dependant on time from maternal cardiac arrest to fetal delivery.
- Begin cesarean delivery within 4 minutes of cardiopulmonary arrest and complete delivery of infant within 5 minutes of arrest.
- Prognosis of fetal survival is greater with the sudden death of a previously healthy mother or in those fetuses with later gestational age.
- Continue CPR throughout procedure and reassess maternal vital signs after delivery. Maternal survival after relief of aortocaval compression has been reported.
- Neonatologist/pediatrician and obstetrician should be present when possible.

Suggested Readings

Benrubi GI. *Handbook of obstetric and gynecologic emergencies*, 3rd ed. Philadelphia: Lippincott Williams & Wilkins; 2005.

Roberts JR, Hedges JR. *Clinical procedures in emergency medicine*, 4th ed. Philadelphia: WB Saunders; 2004:1137–1139.

Wolfson AB, Hendey GW, Hendry PL, et al. *Harwood-Nuss' clinical practice of emergency medicine*, 4th ed. Philadelphia: Lippincott Williams & Wilkins; 2005:521.

30

Shoulder Dystocia

Shadi Kiriaki and Ted Korszun

Definition
- Impaction of the fetal shoulders in the pelvic outlet occurring after delivery of the head in the vertex presentation.
  - Prohibits adequate fetal respiration.
  - Compromises fetal circulation.
- These maneuvers in general are intended to disimpact the shoulders by adducting the shoulders with direct pressure or rotating the trunk.

Contraindications
- Immediate availability of obstetric services for cesarean section.

Risks/Consent Issues
- Brachial plexus injury
- Humeral/clavicular fractures
- Hypoxic brain injury
- Fetal demise
- Maternal hemorrhage

Techniques:
More than one maneuver may be required.
- **Patient Preparation**
  - IV, oxygen, and maternal and fetal monitor must be available.
  - Call for assistance and obstetric, anesthesia, and pediatric backup.
  - Drain bladder if distended.
  - Avoid maternal pushing while attempts are made to reposition fetus.
  - Avoid excessive head and neck traction or uterine fundal pressure.
- **Manzanti Maneuver**
  - Adduct shoulders by applying downward or oblique suprapubic pressure to dislodge anterior shoulder from pubic symphysis.
- **McRoberts Maneuver**
  - Hyperflex maternal hips to a knee to chest position.
  - This flattens the lumbar spine and rotates the pelvis toward the head, which frees the impacted anterior shoulder.
- **Woods Screw Maneuver**
  - Rotate the fetus 180 degrees by applying pressure to the clavicular surface of the posterior shoulder in an attempt to dislodge anterior shoulder.
  - Do not twist the head and neck.
- **Rubin Maneuver**
  - Place one hand behind the posterior shoulder and adduct shoulder while rotating it anteriorly.

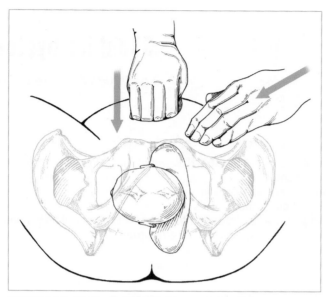

FIGURE 30.1: Manzanti maneuver.

- **Gaskin Maneuver**
  - Mother is repositioned on her hands and knees (on "all fours") and gentle downward traction is applied to posterior shoulder or upward traction applied to the anterior shoulder.
- **Delivery of the Posterior Arm**
  - Locate the posterior arm in the vagina.
  - Apply pressure to the antecubital fossa to flex the elbow and bring the forearm across chest.
  - Locate the forearm and hand and pull through the vagina to deliver the posterior shoulder.
- **Clavicular Fracture**
  - Fracture the clavicle intentionally to decrease bisacromial diameter by pulling anterior clavicle outward away from the lung to avoid causing a pneumothorax.
- **Zavanelli Maneuver** (cephalic replacement)—in preparation for cesarean section
  - Relax the uterus with terbutaline (0.25 mg SC) or nitroglycerin (50 to 200 μg/minute IV).
  - Reverse the cardinal movements of labor.
  - Rotate fetal head to occiput anterior position.
  - Flex fetal neck and apply gentle cephalad pressure to fetal head to replace the fetus back into the pelvis.
  - Prepare for cesarean section.
- **Symphysiotomy**—use as last resort, if all other techniques fail and cesarean delivery is unavailable.
  - Sterilize the skin over the pubic symphysis area with povidone-iodine solution.
  - Infiltrate skin and fibrocartilaginous area with local anesthetic.
  - Displace urethra laterally.
  - Incise skin and fibrocartilage of pubic symphysis.

Complications
- **Fetal**
  - Brachial plexus injury due to excessive head and neck traction

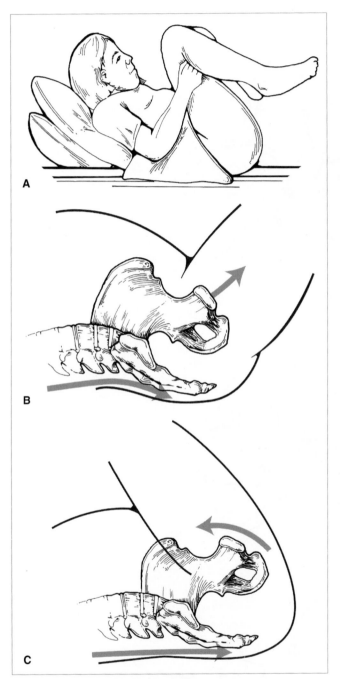

FIGURE 30.2: McRoberts maneuver.

- Fractures of humerus and clavicle
- Pneumothorax
- Hypoxic brain injury
- Fetal death
- **Maternal**
  - Hemorrhage

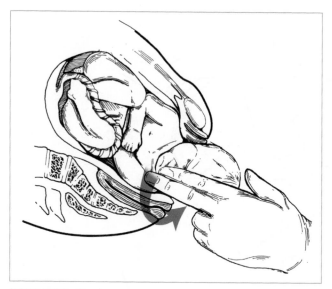

FIGURE 30.3: Woods screw maneuver.

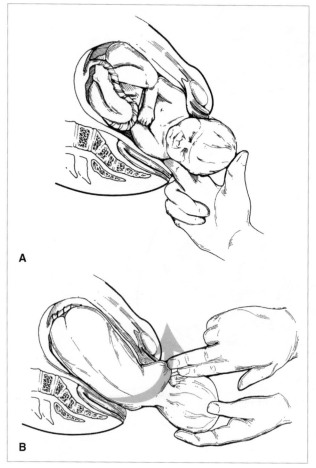

FIGURE 30.4: Rubin maneuver.

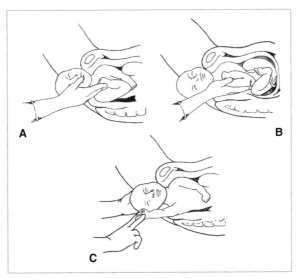

FIGURE 30.5: Delivery of posterior arm. (From Simon RR, Brenner BE. *Emergency procedures and techniques,* 4th edition. Philadelphia: Lippincott Williams & Wilkins; 2002:214, with permission.)

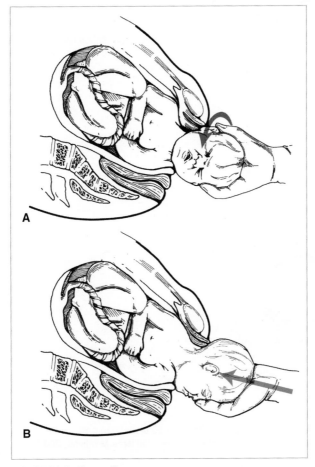

FIGURE 30.6: Zavanelli maneuver.

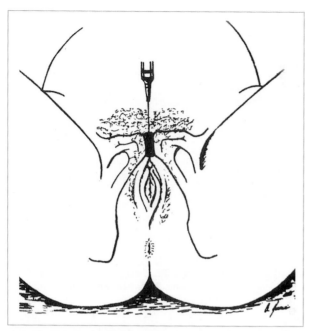

FIGURE 30.7: Infiltration of anesthetic solution over the symphysis pubis. (From Simon RR, Brenner BE. *Emergency procedures and techniques,* 4th ed. Philadelphia: Lippincott Williams & Wilkins; 2002:220, with permission.)

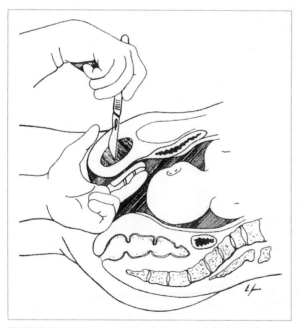

FIGURE 30.8: Make an incision into the symphysis pubis with a no. 10 blade. (From Simon RR, Brenner BE. *Emergency procedures and techniques,* 4th ed. Philadelphia: Lippincott Williams & Wilkins; 2002:221, with permission.)

- Severe perineal lacerations
- Uterine atony

Common Pitfalls
- Failure to approach shoulder dystocia methodically
- Excessive traction on the fetal head and neck
- Prolong dystocia

Pearls
- Consult obstetrics EMERGENTLY to assist with delivery and prepare for possible cesarean section.
- A combination of McRoberts and Manzanti maneuvers is most often used and effective; however, more than one maneuver may be required depending on the severity of the dystocia.
- Never rotate the head and neck or use excessive traction.
- Approach dystocia methodically.
- Be aware of how much time has lapsed since delivery of head; fetal morbidity and mortality is significantly increased with dystocia >7 minutes.
- Document, document, document.
  - Maneuvers used during delivery
  - Time of delivery of head, shoulder, and infant
  - All associated injuries
- Send umbilical blood for pH analysis.

Suggested Readings
Benrubi GI. *Handbook of obstetric and gynecologic emergencies*, 3rd ed. Philadelphia: Lippincott Williams & Wilkens; 2005.

Roberts JR, Hedges JR. *Clinical procedures in emergency medicine*, 4th ed. Philadelphia: WB Saunders; 2004:1128.

Simon RR, Brenner BE. *Emergency procedures and techniques*, 4th ed. Philadelphia: Lippincott Williams & Wilkins; 2002:213.

31

Vaginal Breech Delivery

Lekha Ajit Shah and Resa Lewiss

Indications

- Imminent vaginal delivery without obstetrical backup
  - Buttocks or feet of the fetus appear at the vulva
  - Development of fetal distress

Contraindications

- Placenta previa
- Immediate availability of obstetric services

Risk/Consent Issues

- Peripartum fetal and maternal morbidity or mortality
- Maternal bleeding and pain
- Breech position may result from underlying fetal or uterine abnormalities

Presentation Types

- Frank breech—fetus with bilateral hip flexion and knees extended with lower extremities opposite the head.
- Footling (incomplete) breech—one or both hips or knees extended and presenting before buttocks.
- Complete breech—bilateral hip and knee flexion with feet opposite the trunk.

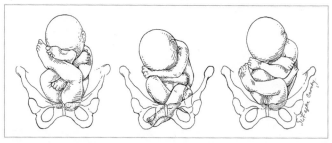

FIGURE 31.1: Fetal attitude in frank, incomplete, and complete breech presentations. (From Cruikshank DP. Breech, other malpresentations, and umbilical cord complications. In: Scott JR, Gibbs RS, Karlan BY, et al. *Danforth's obstetrics and gynecology*, 9th ed. Philadelphia: Lippincott Williams & Wilkins; 2003:382, with permission.)

Techniques

- Examine the vagina to determine the presenting part.
- Use ultrasonography or Leopold maneuver to determine fetal lie.

- Consult obstetrics EMERGENTLY to assist with delivery and prepare for possible cesarean section.
- Place the mother in the lithotomy position with a wedge under her buttocks.
- Consider episiotomy with local perineal anesthesia once the fetal anus has appeared at the vulva (see Chapter 32).
- Allow maternal effort to spontaneously deliver the fetal buttocks, flexed knees, and lower limbs.
- Avoid excessive premature traction of the fetus, which can cause undesirable positioning of the head resulting in head and nuchal arm entrapment.
- If knees are extended, the physician may flex each knee (Pinard maneuver—see Fig. 31.2) to facilitate delivery.

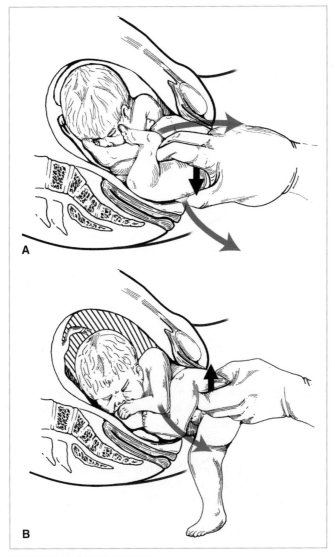

FIGURE 31.2: Pinard maneuver.

- Grasp the infant's bony pelvis during vaginal delivery.
- Rotate the fetus in the anteroposterior plane to deliver each shoulder.

- Shoulder delivery may be expedited by flexing the fetal elbow or adducting the extended elbow by placing a finger in the antecubital fossa.
- When delivering the head, attempt to flex the neck by holding the chin and applying suprapubic pressure (see Fig. 31.3) or use the Mauriceau maneuver.
  - The middle finger of one hand is placed in the mouth, and the second and fourth fingers on the malar eminences to promote flexion and descent while counterpressure is applied to the occiput with the middle finger of the other hand.
- Use forceps if needed.
- Consider symphysiotomy as a last resort (see Chapter 30 for description).

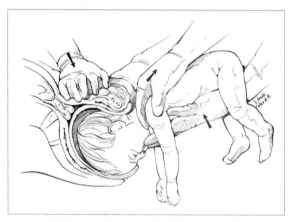

FIGURE 31.3: Breech delivery of fetal head performed by flexing the head while applying suprapubic pressure. (From Benrubi GI. *Handbook of obstetric and gynecologic emergencies,* 3rd ed. Philadelphia: Lippincott Williams & Wilkins; 2005:187.)

Complications
- Prolapsed cord
- Shoulder dystocia
- Head entrapment
- Fetal ischemia due to excessive traction on the cord
  - This may be prevented by checking cord pulsations and forming a small loop of cord.
- Neurologic injuries due to excessive traction or neck hyperextension during delivery
- Visceral injuries due to excessive pressure on the abdomen during delivery

Common Pitfalls
- Confusion of malar/face presentation with breech presentation
- Grasping the fetal abdomen instead of the bony pelvis
- Hyperextension of the neck when delivering the head
- Excessive traction on the presenting part
- Rupturing of membranes prematurely

Pearls
- Breech presentation occurs in 4% of term pregnancies.
- Spontaneous version may occur at any point during delivery.

■ For head entrapment, attempt to facilitate delivery by administering terbutaline (0.25 SC) or nitroglycerin (50 to 200 μg/minute IV) to achieve uterine relaxation.

■ Leave membranes intact when possible to prevent cord prolapse, head entrapment, and fetal injury.

Suggested Readings

Benrubi GI. *Handbook of obstetric and gynecologic emergencies*, 3rd ed. Philadelphia: Lippincott Williams & Wilkins; 2005.

Roberts JR, Hedges JR. *Clinical procedures in emergency medicine*, 4th ed. Philadelphia: WB Saunders; 2004:1128–1132.

Scott JR, Gibbs RS, Karlan BY, et al. *Danforth's obstetrics and gynecology*, 9th ed. Philadelphia: Lippincott Williams & Wilkins; 2003.

Simon RR, Brenner BE. *Emergency procedures and techniques*, 4th ed. Philadelphia: Lippincott Williams & Wilkins; 2002:215–221.

32

Episiotomy

Annie Akkara and Jennifer Stratton

Indications
- To increase the diameter of the soft tissue outlet to relieve shoulder dystocia
- To facilitate delivery of fetus having nonreassuring fetal heart-rate tracings
- To facilitate delivery in malpresentations including breech and occiput posterior presentations
- To prevent severe spontaneous perineal lacerations

Contraindications
- Not recommended for routine delivery, especially in the primiparous patient

Landmarks

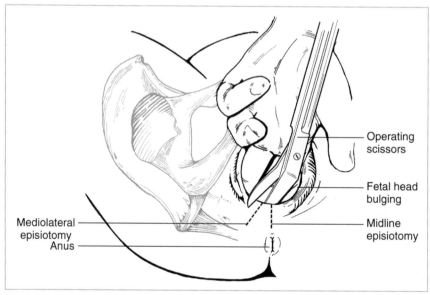

Operating scissors

Fetal head bulging

Mediolateral episiotomy

Midline episiotomy

Anus

FIGURE 32.1: Episiotomy landmarks.

Technique
- **Supplies**
  - A 3-0 or 2-0 absorbable suture (polygalactin preferred or chromic catgut) on atraumatic needle
  - Needle holder
  - Tissue scissors or scalpel
  - Suture scissors

- Gauze
- Local anesthesia and injection materials

Initiation of Procedure
- For vertex presentations, episiotomy is started when the fetal head begins to stretch out of the perineum and when 3 to 4 cm diameter of the caput is visible during a contraction.
- For breech presentations, episiotomy is started just before extraction of the fetus.
- Inject 1% or 2% lidocaine locally in the perineum where episiotomy is planned.

Median or Midline Technique
- Most commonly performed
- As the head crowns, two fingers are placed inside the vaginal introitus to expose the mucosa, posterior fourchette, and the perineal body.
- Tissue scissors are used to make a vertical incision beginning at the fourchette and extending caudally in the midline. The goal is to release the constriction caused by the perineal body.
- Incision should be directed internally to minimize the amount of perineal skin incised.
- Incision includes the vaginal mucosa, perineal body, and the junction of the perineal body with the bulbocavernosus muscle in the perineum.

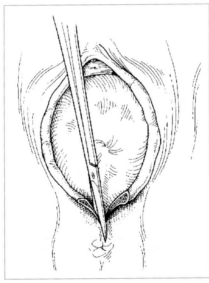

FIGURE 32.2: Midline episiotomy. As the fetal head distends, with the perineum under adequate anesthesia, the episiotomy is cut through the perineal body and the tissues of the vagina and the rectovaginal septum. (From Rouse DJ, St. John E. Normal labor, delivery, newborn care, and puerperium. In: Scott JR, Gibbs RS, Karlan BY, et al. eds. *Danforth's obstetrics and gynecology*, 9th ed. Philadelphia: Lippincott Williams & Wilkins; 2003:44, with permission.)

Mediolateral Technique
- As the head crowns, two fingers are placed inside the vaginal introitus to expose the mucosa, posterior fourchette, and the perineal body.
- Tissue scissors are used to make a 4- to 5-cm incision directed downward and outward toward the lateral margin of the anal sphincter in a 45-degree angle. This incision may be either to the left or the right.
- Incision includes the vaginal mucosa, transverse perineal and bulbocavernosus muscles, and the perineal skin.

Repair: Layer Closure

- A 2-0 or 3-0 absorbable suture is used.
- Initial step is to close the vaginal mucosa using a continuous suture from just above the apex of the incision to the mucocutaneous junction.
- Burying the closing knot minimizes the amount of scar tissue and prevents pain and dyspareunia.
- Large actively bleeding vessels may require ligation with separate absorbable sutures.
- The perineal musculature is reapproximated using three to four interrupted sutures.
- Closure of the superficial layers is done with several interrupted sutures through the skin and subcutaneous fascia that are loosely tied. The skin can also be closed using a running subcuticular suture.

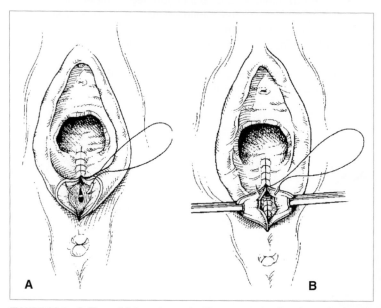

FIGURE 32.3: A: The episiotomy is repaired by reapproximating the vaginal mucosa in a running manner with a delayed absorbable suture. **B:** The submucosal tissue of the vagina and the subcutaneous tissue, and the fascia of the perineal body are then closed. (From Rouse DJ, St. John E. Normal labor, delivery, newborn care, and puerperium. In: Scott JR, Gibbs RS, Karlan BY, et al. eds. *Danforth's obstetrics and gynecology,* 9th ed. Philadelphia: Lippincott Williams & Wilkins; 2003:44, with permission.)

Complications

- Hemorrhage (more common with mediolateral technique)
- Hematoma formation
- Postpartum episiotomy pain
- Infection
- Third- and fourth-degree lacerations causing damage to the anal sphincter and rectum, respectively
- Rectovaginal fistula formation
- Incontinence
- Dyspareunia
- Sexual dysfunction

Common Pitfalls

  ▪ Performing episiotomy too early causes excessive blood loss.
  ▪ Performing episiotomy too late compromises protection of the maternal perineum because the fetal head may have already torn the perineal muscle and fascia.

Pearls

  ▪ Episiotomy should not be routinely performed.
  ▪ Begin performing episiotomy after the head has thinned out the perineum and the fetus is expected within the next three to four contractions.
  ▪ If a scalpel is used, place a tongue blade between the infant's head and the maternal perineum before making incision to avoid trauma to the infant.
  ▪ Perform thorough examination of the wound to evaluate for injuries to the anal sphincters and rectum.
  ▪ Third- and fourth-degree lacerations involving the anal sphincters and rectal mucosa respectively should be repaired in the operating room.
  ▪ Begin repair after the placenta is delivered and after full inspection and repair of the cervix and upper vaginal canal.
  ▪ Median episiotomy is more commonly associated with third- and fourth-degree lacerations; however, it is the easiest type to perform, results in less blood loss, and heals rapidly with minimal discomfort.
  ▪ Mediolateral episiotomy is associated with a lower risk of third- and fourth-degree lacerations; however, there is greater blood loss, repair is more difficult, and painful healing is more likely to result.

Suggested Readings

Roberts JR, Hedges JR. *Clinical procedures in emergency medicine*, 4th ed. Philadelphia: WB Saunders; 2004:1132–1135.

Scott JR, Gibbs RS, Karlan BY, et al. *Danforth's obstetrics and gynecology*, 9th ed. Philadelphia: Lippincott Williams & Wilkins; 2003.

Simon RR, Brenner BE. *Emergency procedures and techniques*, 4th ed. Philadelphia: Lippincott Williams & Wilkins; 2002:215.

Section Editor: Jonathan A. Edlow

33 Emergency Bedside Craniotomy (Burr Holes)

Michael Woodruff

Indications

- Suspected or confirmed epidural hematoma with evidence of **impending herniation or rapid neurologic deterioration**
  - Temporal bone fracture
  - Ipsilateral dilated pupil
  - Computed tomography confirmation recommended
  - Unresponsive to mannitol

Signs of Herniation

- ▷ Cushing response: Hypertension and bradycardia
- ▷ Ipsilateral pupillary dilatation (''blown'' pupil)
- ▷ Contralateral pupillary dilatation (Kernohan notch phenomenon)
  - ◈ The rare exception to the rule
- ▷ Rapid neurologic deterioration (extensor posturing)

Contraindications

- Availability of a neurosurgeon

Risks/Consent Issues

- Hemorrhage with uncontrollable meningeal bleeding
- Cerebral contusion/laceration
- Infection
- This is a last-resort procedure with serious, life-threatening complications.
  - Should be performed only in dire situations where direct neurosurgical intervention is not available.
  - Should be performed only in consultation with a neurosurgeon.
  - This is a rare procedure that is usually performed in rural/remote regions where long transport times to tertiary centers will condemn the patient to brain death if no intervention is made.

Landmarks

- Burr the hole in the temporal region on the same side as the "blown pupil."
    - Two finger breadths anterior to tragus
    - Two to three finger breadths superior to auricle

Technique

- Rapidly assemble the needed equipment.
    - Local anesthetic with epinephrine
    - Rake-type or self-retaining retractors
    - Scalpel
    - Cautery device
    - Fine suction instrument
    - Gelfoam or other hemostatic agent
    - Cranial drill (usually a hand brace) and bits
- Prepare the temporal region with Betadine or other prep solution.
- Make a 3- to 4-cm incision two finger breadths anterior to tragus (see Fig. 33.1).

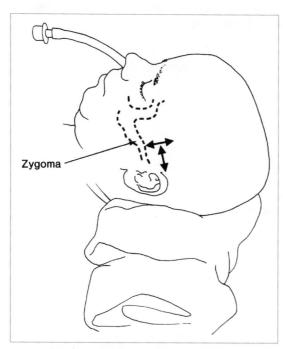

FIGURE 33.1: Burr hole is placed 2 finger breadths anterior to the tragus and 2–3 finger breadths superior to the zygoma or ear. (From Simon RR, Brenner BE. *Emergency procedures and techniques,* 4th ed. Philadelphia: Lippincott Williams & Wilkins; 2002:190, with permission.)

- Incise the temporalis muscle to the bone.
- Control muscle bleeding with cautery or retractors.
- Retract the skin to expose the skull (see Fig. 32.2).
- Use the drill to penetrate the outer table of the skull.
    - A pointed or "cutting" bit can be used for this step.
- Once the inner table of the skull is reached, switch to a conical "burr" to enlarge the opening and finish the burr hole.
    - Control bone bleeding with bone wax, if available.

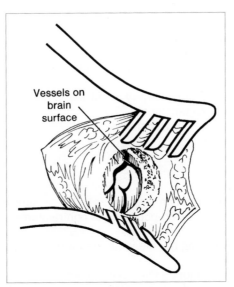

FIGURE 33.2: Retract temporalis muscle and then burr hole with drill to expose the bleeding blood vessels. (From Simon RR, Brenner BE. *Emergency procedures and techniques,* 4th ed. Philadelphia: Lippincott Williams & Wilkins; 2002:192, with permission.)

- Remove any extradural hematoma with careful suction.
  - Visualize the middle meningeal artery, and identify and cauterize or ligate briskly bleeding areas.
  - The burr hole may be enlarged with a rongeur if needed (see Fig. 33.3).

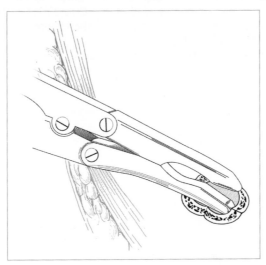

FIGURE 33.3: Enlarge burr hole with rongeur, if necessary.

- If subdural hematoma is noted and no epidural hematoma is present, the dura may be opened carefully and the clot evacuated with suction.
- If no hematoma is encountered, consider performing a burr hole on the contralateral side.
- Place Gelfoam or other hemostatic agent in the burr hole and close scalp in two layers.
- Transfer the patient for definitive care.

Precautions

- Care must be taken not to plunge the drill bit into the brain when penetrating the inner table of the skull.
- Bone and scalp bleeding can be brisk; the emergency physician must be prepared with some form(s) of hemostatic agent.
- If the bleeding branch of the middle meningeal artery is not found and cauterized/controlled, the patient may exsanguinate.
- This is not a definitive procedure; immediate transfer to a facility with neurosurgical capabilities is mandatory.

Pearls

- Kernohan notch phenomenon: When herniation causes pressure on Kernohan notch, the patient presents with a fixed dilated pupil on the contralateral side to the epidural hematoma.
- Bone bleeding can be controlled by rubbing the bleeding area with bone wax (available in most operating rooms).
- Carefully document the dire nature of patient's clinical condition, barriers to obtaining definitive neurosurgical care, and conversations with the consulting neurosurgeon.
- Physicians have been making burr holes with relatively unsophisticated tools for thousands of years, so take a deep breath and relax.

Suggested Readings

Donovan DJ, Moquin RR, Ecklund JM, et al. Cranial burr holes and emergency craniotomy: review of indications and technique. *Mil Med*. 2006;171(1):12–19.

Springer MF, Baker FJ. Cranial burr hole decompression in the emergency department. *Am J Emerg Med*. 1988;6(6):640–646.

World Health Organization. *Essential surgical care manual*. Chp 17.6. Access on July 16, 2007. http://www.who.int/surgery/publications/scdh_manual/en/print.html.

34

Epley Maneuver

Andrew Chang

Indications

- Used to treat posterior canal benign positional vertigo (BPV) that has been confirmed through a positive Hallpike test (upbeat, ipsilateral, and torsional nystagmus in the head-hanging position).
- This is also known as the *canalith repositioning maneuver* and the "modified" Epley maneuver (the originally described maneuver used premedication and had fewer steps).

Contraindications

- Unstable heart disease
- Ongoing stroke or transient ischemic attack (TIA)
- Severe neck disease
- High-grade carotid stenosis

Risks/Consent Issues

- There have been no reported serious adverse events, such as neck fracture or carotid artery dissection.
- Warn the patient that he will likely become symptomatic during the various head maneuvers, but that this will be transient.
- Rarely the patient may vomit. In general, premedication is not needed.

Landmarks

The Epley maneuver is a four- to five-step maneuver that moves the otoliths in the plane of the posterior semicircular canal back into the utricle where they belong (see Fig. 34.1).

Technique

- Patient is sitting upright in the gurney and positioned far enough back such that when he lies down, his head will overhang the edge of the gurney.
- Turn the patient's head 45 degrees to the side that was positive during the Hallpike test, which was performed to confirm the diagnosis of posterior canal BPV.
- Lower the guardrail of the gurney on the opposite side to which you have turned the patient's head. Warn the patient that you are going to lower him and that he may become symptomatic.
- Place the patient in the head-hanging position, supporting the patient's head with your hands. This does not need to be done rapidly. This step is identical to performing the Hallpike test.
- Keep the patient in the head-hanging position until his nystagmus and symptoms resolve, or at least for 30 seconds.

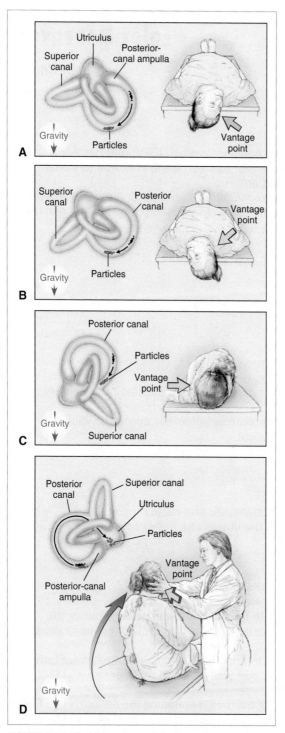

FIGURE 34.1: Bedside maneuver for the treatment of a patient with benign paroxysmal positional vertigo affecting the right ear. (Permission obtained from Furman JM, Cass SP. Benign paroxysmal positional vertigo. *N Engl J Med.* 1999;341:1590–1596.)

- Turn the patient's head 90 degrees to the other side. Again, hold this position for 30 seconds or until the nystagmus and vertigo resolve.
- Tell the patient to roll onto his side and turn his head so that he is looking at the floor. Try to keep the head in the dependent position throughout. Hold this position for at least 30 seconds or until his vertigo resolves.
- Sit the patient up with his legs extended over the side of the gurney (you previously lowered the guard rails on this side to allow for this) and tilt his head forward slightly.
    - You can tell the patient to put his hands on your shoulder in order to assist you in lifting him up to the sitting position.

Complications

- Rarely the patient may vomit.

Common Pitfalls

- Not sitting the patient far enough back in the gurney so that the head is overhanging the edge of the gurney
- Not warning the patient that he will become symptomatic and to keep his eyes open
- Performing the maneuver in a patient with vestibular neuritis or labyrinthitis

Pearls

- The amount of time recommended to keep the patient in the upright position after performing the Epley maneuver has changed drastically over the years. Currently, it is felt that 20 minutes is enough time for the otoliths to reattach themselves to a membrane within the utricle. Therefore, approximately 20 to 30 minutes after performing the Epley maneuver, the Hallpike test can be repeated in the patient. If it is still positive, the Epley maneuver can be repeated.

Suggested Readings

Chang AK, Schoeman G, Hill MA. A randomized clinical trial to assess the efficacy of the Epley maneuver in the treatment of acute benign positional vertigo. *Acad Emerg Med*. 2004;11:918–924.

Epley JM. The canalith repositioning procedure: For treatment of benign paroxysmal positional vertigo. *Otolaryngol Head Neck Sur*. 1992;107:399–404.

Furman JM, Cass SP. Benign paroxysmal positional vertigo. *N Engl J Med*. 1999;341: 1590–1596.

35 Hallpike Test (Dix-Hallpike, Nylan-Barany)

Andrew Chang

Indications

- Used to confirm the diagnosis of benign paroxysmal positional vertigo (BPPV, also known as BPV) of the posterior semicircular canal

Contraindications

- Unstable heart disease
- Ongoing stroke or transient ischemic attack (TIA)
- Severe neck disease
- High-grade carotid stenosis

Risks/Consent Issues

- There have been no reported serious adverse events, such as neck fracture or carotid artery dissection.
- Warn the patient that he will become symptomatic during the procedure, but that this will be transient. Inform the patient that this response is actually very useful.
- Rarely the patient may vomit. In general, premedication is not needed.

Landmarks

The Hallpike test diagnoses the inappropriate presence of otoliths in the posterior semicircular canal. This canal is oriented 45 degrees from the vertical (see Fig. 35.1).

Technique

- Patient is sitting upright in the gurney and positioned far enough back such that when he lies down, his head will overhang the edge of the gurney.
- Warn the patient that you are going to lower him and that he may become symptomatic. Instruct the patient to keep his eyes open as it is extremely important for you to document both the presence and direction of nystagmus.
- Turn the patient's head 45 degrees to one side. This is important to do from the start because it orients the posterior canal into the same plane as the upcoming movement into the head-hanging position. This is the most provocative way to make the otoliths move if they are truly present in the posterior semicircular canal.
- Have the patient lie in the head-hanging position, supporting the patient's head with your hands. This does not need to be done rapidly.
- If otoliths are present, there is usually a few seconds delay (but not longer than approximately 15 seconds).
- The patient will develop reproduction of his symptoms and usually, nystagmus.
- It is important to observe the direction of the nystagmus.
  - Nystagmus is defined as the direction of the fast phase.

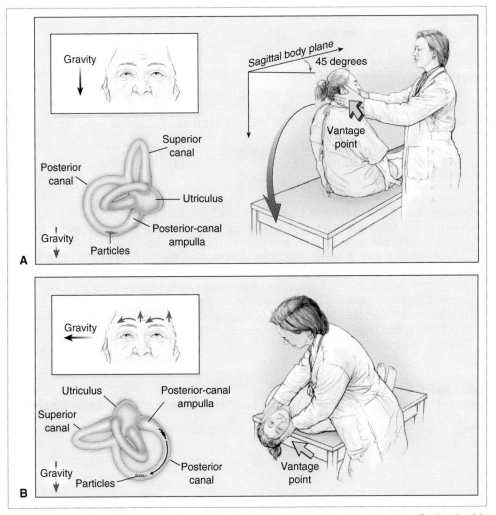

Gravity

Sagittal body plane
45 degrees

Superior canal

Posterior canal

Utriculus

Posterior-canal ampulla

Gravity

Particles

Vantage point

A

Gravity

Utriculus

Superior canal

Posterior-canal ampulla

Gravity

Particles

Posterior canal

Vantage point

B

FIGURE 35.1: The Dix-Hallpike test of a patient with benign paroxysmal positional vertigo affecting the right ear. (Permission obtained from Furman JM, Cass SP. Benign paroxysmal positional vertigo. *N Engl J Med.* 1999;341:1590–1596.)

- Classic nystagmus is upbeat (toward the forehead) and ipsilateral (toward the involved side), as well as torsional/rotatory.
- Downbeat or vertical nystagmus can indicate a central cause of vertigo and requires further evaluation.
  ▪ Sit the patient back up.
    - Most patients will become dizzy from orthostasis, and it is important to distinguish this from positional vertigo.
    - If a patient had a positive result on Hallpike test, the eyes usually reverse direction when the patient sits up.
  ▪ If the side you just tested is positive, then you can treat the patient with the Epley maneuver.
  ▪ If the side you just tested is negative, then test the other side in the same manner.

Complications
- Rarely the patient may vomit.

Common Pitfalls
- Not sitting the patient far enough back in the gurney so that the head is overhanging the edge of the gurney.
- Not warning the patient that he will become symptomatic and to keep his eyes open.
- Not observing the direction of the nystagmus.

Pearls
- Always start with the patient's head turned 45 degrees to one side and then lay him into the head-hanging position. Although it is possible to get a positive test result by lying the patient down and then turning his head 45 degrees to one side, this alternative way is not as provocative in moving the otoliths and is more likely to result in a false-negative test result.
- Although it is possible to have bilateral posterior semicircular canal BPV, in general only one side should test positive during the Hallpike test.
- It is important to note which side is positive during the Hallpike test as this will be the starting position for the Epley maneuver, which is used to treat BPV of the posterior semicircular canal.

Suggested Readings
Furman JM, Cass SP. Benign paroxysmal positional vertigo. *N Engl J Med*. 1999;341: 1590–1596.

36

Lumbar Puncture

Amy S. Hurwitz and Jonathan A. Edlow

Indications
- Used to obtain cerebrospinal fluid (CSF) and to measure the opening pressure of the subarachnoid space to aid in the evaluation and management of patients with acute headache or other symptoms of the following conditions:
  - Meningitis
  - Subarachnoid hemorrhage (SAH)
  - Carcinomatous meningitis
  - Pseudotumor cerebri
  - Occasionally for Guillain-Barré syndrome
  - Occasionally in cases of encephalitis

Contraindications
- Patients who need a lumbar puncture (LP) and have any of the following should first have a brain imaging study, indicating that it is safe to perform an LP:
  - Altered mental status
  - Papilledema
  - New focal neurologic examination abnormalities
  - Elevated intracranial pressure (ICP)
    - Exception, pseudotumor cerebri
- Suspicion of spinal cord mass, or epidural hematoma/abscess
- Skin or soft tissue infection overlying lumbar spine
- Anatomic abnormalities: for example, patients with lumbar hardware from prior spinal surgery
- Coagulopathic patients

Risks/Consent Issues
- Post-LP headache occurs in approximately 15% to 20% of patients. Multiple therapies exist to treat this specific type of headache.
- Procedure can cause local pain. Local anesthesia will be given.
- Needle puncture can cause local bleeding, which is usually minimal.
- Potential for introducing infection exists; however, this is extremely rare. Sterile technique will be utilized.
- Theoretical risk of damage to neural tissue exists. Such occurrences are also very rare, most often temporary, and affect spinal nerve roots, not the cord itself.

Landmarks
The transverse axis connecting iliac crests passes through L4 vertebral body, allowing for identification of the L4/5 and L3/4 interspaces (see Fig. 36.1).

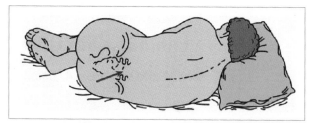

FIGURE 36.1: Anatomical landmarks. (From Fischbach FT. *A manual of laboratory and diagnostic tests,* 7th ed. Philadelphia: Lippincott Williams & Wilkins; 2003:295, with permission.)

Technique
- ### Patient Preparation
  - Explain procedure to patient and obtain patient consent.
  - Position patient in either lateral decubitus or sitting position.

  Lateral decubitus position
  - ▶ Have patient lie on one side, with knees to chest and head/shoulders curled toward knees as much as possible. Placing a pillow under the head helps reduce twisting of the shoulders.
  - ▶ Ensure that the lumbar spine lies parallel to the edge of the bed. (In an infant/child, or a poorly cooperative adult, it will be necessary to have an assistant hold the patient securely in the optimal position.) The top shoulder and hip should be directly above their bottom counterparts.
  - ▶ A cooperative patient can be asked to curve his/her lower back, out like an "angry cat" to optimally open the spinous processes.

  Sitting position
  - ▶ Have patient sit on side of the bed with the bed positioned below patient's midthigh and with feet of patient touching floor, if possible.
  - ▶ Ask patient to curve torso forward over a bedside table positioned in front of him/her; table height should be level with patient's upper abdomen. A pillow may be placed on the table for patient's comfort.
  - ▶ After positioning, but before prepping, mark the target for needle insertion with firm pressure from the Luer-lock (hub) end of a needle sheath against the skin (which will leave a mark for several minutes and provides a visual target).
  - ▶ Prepare a wide area with povidone-iodine or chlorhexidine gluconate solution.
    - ◆ Ensure the sterile field includes L4/5 and L3/4 interspaces. (Should first attempt at L4/5 be unsuccessful, the L3/4 interspace will be readily accessible.)
    - ◆ Use sterile drapes to frame workspace.
  - ▶ Reassess landmarks. It is crucial that the midline be defined.
    - ◆ Sometimes, in overweight patients, feeling the spinous processes in the thoracic spine (where they are easier to palpate) and marching down will help the surgeon ensure that they are in the midline.
    - ◆ Others have tried ultrasonography for this purpose but no convincing evidence exists yet.
- ### Insertion
  - Analgesia: Produce local anesthesia using 1% lidocaine.
    - ▶ Inject the subcutaneous area with a small-bore (27-gauge) needle, and then, using a larger-bore needle (22-gauge) infiltrate the prespinous soft tissues down to the supraspinous ligament. Massaging the area

afterward with your thumb will distribute the wheal and allow for reassessment of bony landmarks.

- Accessing subarachnoid space:
  - ▶ Place nondominant thumb on L4 spinous process.
  - ▶ Using dominant hand, insert 20- or 22-gauge spinal needle through the skin just caudal to your thumb. Take care to orient the bevel parallel to the long axis of the spinal column, as this will minimize trauma to the longitudinally arranged dural fibers.

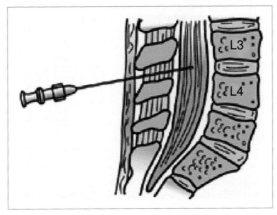

FIGURE 36.2: Needle insertion point. (From Fischbach FT. *A manual of laboratory and diagnostic tests,* 7th ed. Philadelphia: Lippincott Williams & Wilkins; 2003:295, with permission.)

  - ▶ Continue advancing needle with stylet in place until you meet resistance from the supraspinous ligament. Advance through the ligament and you will often feel a reduction in resistance (sometimes described as a slight ''pop'').
  - ▶ Remove the stylet. Watch the barrel of needle to look out for return of CSF as you advance very slowly.
- Measuring opening pressure:
  - ▶ Upon visualizing return of CSF, affix three-way stopcock to the needle hub, with chamber open to the vertically-oriented manometer.
  - ▶ With patient in lateral decubitus position, traditional doctrine mandates that you should have him/her slowly straighten legs and neck at this time.
  - ▶ Opening pressure is determined when CSF column ceases to climb, which usually takes approximately 1 to 2 minutes. Normal opening pressure is 6 to 20 cm H_2O in the lateral decubitus position.
  - ▶ Only recently has opening pressure been evaluated in the sitting position, with one study finding a 13-cm H_2O increase with patient sitting upright.
- Collecting CSF: You may either remove manometer or turn stopcock to allow for CSF to bypass manometer (see Fig. 36.3).
  - ▶ Collect 1 to 2 mL of CSF in each of four numbered tubes.
  - ▶ If the opening pressure was elevated, it is best to measure a closing pressure; this is particularly important in cases of likely pseudotumor cerebri.
- Removing needle: Replace stylet completely into needle hub. Inform patient the needle is being removed. Remove needle and place gauze over LP site for few seconds; then place a plastic adhesive dressing (e.g., Band-Aid).

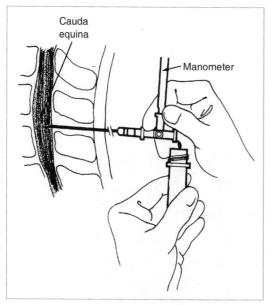

Cauda equina

Manometer

FIGURE 36.3: Turn stopcock to allow cerebrospinal fluid (CSF) to drain into collecting tubes. (From Simon RR, Brenner BE. *Emergency procedures and techniques,* 4th ed. Philadelphia: Lippincott Williams & Wilkins; 2002:199, with permission.)

- **Analyzing CSF**: Tightly screw the caps on the tubes of CSF to prevent loss *en route* to the laboratory. Most often, the following analyses are performed:
  - Tube no. 1: Cell count and differential
  - Tube no. 2: Gram stain and culture
  - Tube no. 3: Protein and glucose
  - Tube no. 4: Repeat cell count and differential

  Additional analysis may be performed on tube no. 4 if appropriate volume of CSF is included. Specific requests should be made, such as Lyme serology, HSV PCR (herpes simplex virus polymerase chain reaction), India ink preparation for Cryptococcus, cytologic evaluation for malignancy, or others, as indicated by your differential diagnosis.

Complications
- **Post-LP Headache**
  - Occurs in 15% to 20% of patients.
  - Therapies include hydration, caffeine, analgesics, and blood patch. Factors that correlate with increased incidence of post-LP headache include insertion of the needle perpendicular to the long axis of the cord, and use of a larger gauge needle. Young thin female patients also have a higher risk of post-LP headache.
- **Traumatic Tap**
  - Usually (but not always) caused by passing needle further than necessary, thereby disrupting the venous plexus at anterior aspect of canal.
- **Cerebral Herniation**
  - Occurs in the setting of elevated ICP before tap.
  - History, funduscopic examination, and/or computed tomography may be used to assess ICP before LP (see "Contraindications" section). Despite the severity of this complication, it is extremely rare.

- **Spinal Root Herniation**
    - Extremely rare; risk is minimized by replacing stylet before withdrawal of needle.
- Low back pain, seen in approximately 15% of patients, treated with analgesics.
- Serious bleeding is very rare.
- Infection, of any involved tissues is theoretically possible, but risk is minimized by sterile technique.

Common Pitfalls
- Inadequate use of local anesthesia
- Failure to place patient in fully tucked position (which maximizes interspace opening) or failure to have the upper shoulder and hip directly above their lower counterparts
- Failure to identify the midline
- Attempting to insert needle in L5/S1 interspace because of excessive concern for "going too high"
- Failing to obtain opening pressure
- Forgetting to replace stylet before removal of needle

Pearls
- Interpreting CSF data:
    - White blood cell (WBC) count
        - Zero to 5 WBCs is normal; higher values suggest an infectious process.
    - Red blood cell (RBC) count
        - Zero to 5 RBCs is normal in an atraumatic tap.
        - If traumatic, expect a marked diminution of RBCs from tube no. 1 to tube no. 4. If there is no clearing on successive tubes, RBCs are highly suggestive of SAH. There is no specific RBC threshold below which SAH can be completely excluded.
    - Xanthochromia
        - Pink or yellow tinge is present in the supernatant of "older" lysed RBCs, suggestive of SAH.
    - Glucose
        - Normal CSF glucose is two third of the serum glucose, and is usually 50 to 80 mg/dL.
        - Low CSF glucose is often seen in bacterial meningitis.
    - Protein
        - Normal CSF protein is 15 to 45 mg/dL.
        - Elevated protein level is nonspecific, but is seen in bacterial and aseptic meningitis, tuberculosis (TB) meningitis, Guillain-Barré syndrome, neoplastic disease, and multiple myeloma, among other pathologic processes.
- Remember to factor in timing from onset of symptoms to the LP being done. For example, xanthochromia may be absent in a SAH 4 hours old, or the number of cells in bacterial meningitis could be low in the first hours.
- Patient positioning is crucial for successful LP.
- The interspace and dural sac are wider at L3/4 than at L4/5. If LP fails at L4/5, you may be more successful at L3/4 interspace.
- In infants, the anatomical distances are remarkably smaller and the sensation of traversing different tissue densities is more subtle. Some practitioners will remove the stylet immediately after penetrating the skin and advance slowly, watching for CSF.

Suggested Readings

Abbrescia KL, Brabson TA, Dalsey WC, et al. The effect of lower-extremity position on cerebrospinal fluid pressures. *Acad Emerg Med*. 2001;8:8–12.

Edlow JA, Caplan LR. Avoiding pitfalls in the diagnosis of subarachnoid hemorrhage. *N Eng J Med*. 2000;342:29.

Evans RW. Complications of lumbar puncture. *Neurol Clin*. 1998;16:83–105.

Flaatten H, Thorsen T, Askeland B, et al. Puncture technique and postural puncture headache. A randomized, double-blind study comparing transverse and parallel puncture. *Acta Anaesthesiol Scand*. 1998;42(10):1209–1214.

Hasbun R, Abrahams J, Jekel J, et al. Computed tomography of the head before lumbar puncture in adults with suspected meningitis. *N Engl J Med*. 2001;345: 1727–1733.

O'Malley GF, Byers S, Dominici P. Cerebrospinal fluid opening pressure is constant and reproducible between the sitting and recumbent positions. *Acad Emerg Med*. 2006;13:S136.

Shah KH, Edlow JA. Distinguishing traumatic lumbar puncture from true subarachnoid hemorrhage. *J Emerg Med*. 2002;23:67–74.

Straus SE, Thorpe KE, Holroyd-Leduc J. How do I perform a lumbar puncture and analyze the results to diagnose bacterial meningitis? *JAMA*. 2006;296:2012–2022.

37

Occipital Nerve Block

Jay Smith and Jonathan A. Edlow

Indications

- Treatment of headache pain associated with occipital neuralgia.
    - Classically described as a persistent dull pain at the base of the skull with occasional, sudden shocklike pain or paresthesias radiating from the back of the head over the scalp to behind the eyes (follows distribution of the greater and lesser occipital nerves).
    - Thought to be caused by repetitive microtrauma to greater and lesser occipital nerves from hyperextension of the neck (i.e., computer monitors with focal point too high or activities like painting ceilings).
    - Usually unilateral, but rarely, bilateral.
    - This assumes that a complete history and physical examination do not suggest potential intracranial processes.

Contraindications

- Allergy to analgesic compounds or steroids
- Lack of a clear-cut diagnosis
    - Any suspected intracranial process or focal neurologic deficits

Risks/Consent Issues

- Risk of inadvertent injection of local anesthetic into occipital artery or one of its branches with secondary arrhythmias. Given the small dose of local anesthetic recommended, this is mostly a theoretical risk.
- Postblock ecchymosis or hematoma formation. This can be minimized by applying manual pressure or cold packs for 20 minutes over the injection site after the block is administered.
- Risk of inadvertent needle placement into the foramen magnum with subsequent total spine anesthesia.

Landmarks

- The greater occipital nerve is located medially to the palpated occipital artery at the level of the superior nuchal line which runs between the mastoid process and external occipital protuberance.

Technique

- In a 12-mL sterile syringe, draw up a total of 8 mL of local anesthetic (usually a long-acting agent such as bupivacaine) and 80 mg of methylprednisolone for a first time block or 40 mg of methylprednisolone for a repeat block.
    - Some authors endorse a mixture of 4 mL of a quick-acting local anesthetic, such as 1% lidocaine, with 4 mL of a longer-acting local anesthetic for more immediate observable results.

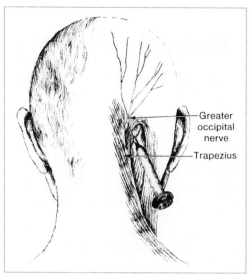

Greater
occipital
nerve

Trapezius

FIGURE 37.1: Block of the greater occipital nerve. (From Simon RR, Brenner BE. *Emergency procedures and techniques*, 4th ed. Philadelphia: Lippincott Williams & Wilkins; 2002:123, with permission.)

- Other injectable steroids, such as triamcinolone or betamethasone may be used.
- Place the patient in a sitting position, leaning over, with the forehead resting on a padded bedside table with the neck in a flexed position.
- Prepare the skin/hair with an antiseptic solution.
- Using a 25- or 27-gauge 1.5-in. needle, aim just medial to the occipital artery at the level of the superior nuchal line and advanced perpendicularly until the needle touches the skull or until a paresthesia is elicited (patient should be warned of this before starting). It should then be withdrawn approximately 2 to 4 mm and redirected superiorly.
- After gentle aspiration to confirm that the needle is not in a vessel, 5 mL of the previously prepared solution should be injected in a fanlike distribution. (Note: The solution should inject easily, resistance to injection is a sign of inappropriate needle positioning.)
- Further block of the lesser occipital nerve and several superficial branches of the greater occipital nerve can be achieved by directing the needle laterally and slightly inferiorly with injection of an additional 3 to 4 mL of solution, again, after gentle aspiration.

Common Pitfalls
- As noted in the preceding text, great care must be taken to use the appropriate landmarks and technique to avoid inadvertent needle placement in the foramen magnum.
- Although anticoagulation is not an absolute contraindication, the smallest needle possible should be used and postinjection manual compression and/or ice packs can help minimize hematoma formation.

Pearls
- Failure of an occipital nerve block to relieve headache is most commonly because the headache syndrome being treated is not occipital neuralgia.

- Stated another way, if the patient does not respond completely (or near completely) to an occipital nerve block, broaden your differential diagnosis.
- Patients who fail to respond to treatment should be followed up by a neurologist, and further imaging (computed tomography [CT] or magnetic resonance imaging [MRI]) of the head and neck should be considered for potential intracranial or vascular pathology.

Suggested Readings

Ashkenazi A, Levin M. Three common neuralgias: How to manage trigeminal, occipital, and postherpetic pain. *Postgrad Med*. 2004;116(3), http://www.postgradmed .com/issues/2004/09_04/ashkenazi.htm.

Ward JB. Greater occipital nerve block. *Semin Neurol*. 2003;23(1):59–62.

Section Editor: Ami Kirit Dave

38 Methylene Blue Injection/Open Joint Evaluation

Jennifer Teng and Kaushal Shah

Indications
- Clinical suspicion of open joint injury, for example, any situation where a wound is in close proximity to a joint, leading to suspicion that the joint could be exposed and contaminated
- Findings of intra-articular air or foreign body on biplanar radiographs

Contraindications
- Allergy to methylene blue
- Glucose-6-phosphate dehydrogenase (G6PD) deficiency secondary to anemia or methemoglobinemia
- Cellulitis overlying joint

Risks/Consent Issues
- Procedure can cause pain (local anesthesia will be used)
- Risk of introducing infection (sterile technique will be used)
- Risk of local bleeding

Landmarks
- Depending on joint, it is crucial to be familiar with joint anatomy and bony landmarks. Tendons, major vessels, and nerves should be avoided.
- For specific landmarks, see corresponding Arthrocentesis chapter.

Technique
- Prepare the methylene blue injection.
  - Methylene blue usually comes in 1-mL ampules. There are no exact dilutional guidelines; we recommend diluting 1 mL of methylene blue with 29 mL normal saline in a 30-mL syringe.
  - Attach an 18- or 20-gauge needle to the syringe.
- Prepare the joint before injection.
  - Prepare the skin using either a povidone-iodine solution or a chlorhexidine solution and a large sterile drape.
  - Using a small-gauge needle, deposit a small wheal of either 1% or 2% lidocaine (Xylocaine) for local anesthesia.

▪ Inject the joint.
  ° Enter the joint space using standard arthrocentesis technique.
  ° Inject the methylene blue solution into the affected joint space until the joint is fully distended or methylene blue exudes from the wound.
▪ The amount of solution necessary to fully distend the joint is mostly dependent on the joint in question.
  ° Knee joint—holds a maximum of approximately 60 mL.
  ° Shoulder joint—holds a maximum of approximately 30 mL.
▪ *If any extravasation of methylene blue solution is seen, this is a positive result and indicates probable open joint injury.*

Complications
▪ Septic joint can develop if sterile technique is not utilized
▪ Thrombophlebitis (resulting from injection of high doses of methylene blue; avoidable if adequately diluted)
▪ Necrosis (if extravasation occurs)
▪ Allergic reaction
▪ Contact of bone by the needle causes pain and can damage the articular surface, so avoidance of bony surfaces is imperative.

Common Pitfalls
▪ Failure to recognize that abrasions or lacerations in close proximity of a wound may indicate the presence of an open joint injury.
▪ Neurovascular structures are in close proximity to the major joints and may require vascular management and repair.

Pearls
▪ Always maintain a high clinical suspicion for possible open joint injuries—open fractures are orthopedic emergencies! Ideally, open joint injuries should be explored and treated within 6 hours to prevent infection and joint destruction.
▪ As with all orthopedic injuries, it is imperative to document a comprehensive neurovascular examination.
▪ Tetanus vaccination status should be obtained and provided if not up-to-date. Consider administration of tetanus immunoglobulin for large crush wounds.
▪ Wide-spectrum systemic antibiotics should be given promptly if open joint injury is confirmed. Classification of open fractures determines antibiotic coverage:
  ° **Grade I** (open fractures with a skin wound <1 cm)
    ▸ Cefazolin (1 g IV) is adequate for coverage. Clindamycin (900 mg IV) can be used for patients with allergies to penicillin or cephalosporins.
  ° **Grade II** (open fractures with a skin wound >1 cm)
    ▸ An aminoglycoside (i.e., Gentamycin 600 mg) should be added to the grade I regimen.
  ° **Grade III** (open fractures with extensive soft tissue damage/loss, segmental fractures, amputation)
    ▸ An aminoglycoside (i.e., Gentamycin 600 mg) should be added to the grade I regimen.
  ° If vascular injury or anaerobic contamination of joint is suspected (i.e., farm injury), penicillin (20 million units IV) should be added.
▪ Definitive treatment includes *immediate* surgical debridement, and irrigation of the joint and soft tissues to prevent infection and joint destruction.
▪ If in doubt, treat as an open joint injury.

Suggested Readings

Roberts JR, Hedges JR. *Clinical procedures in emergency medicine*, 4th ed. WB Saunders; (2004).

Hart RG, Rittenberry TJ, Uehara DT. *Handbook of orthopaedic emergencies*, 1st ed. Lippincott Williams & Wilkins; 1999.

Okike K, Bhattacharyya T. Trends in the management of open fractures. A critical analysis. *J Bone Joint Surg Am.* 2006;88(12):2739–2748.

Marx JA. *Rosen's emergency medicine: concepts and clinical practice*, 5th ed. CV Mosby; 2002.

39 Colles' Fracture Reduction with Hematoma Block

Turandot Saul and Ami Kirit Dave

Indications

- The Colles fracture is a transverse fracture through the distal 2 to 3 cm of the radial metaphysis
  - The most common mechanism is a fall on an outstretched hand.
  - The distal fragment is dorsally displaced and angulated.
  - The general plan of management and basic principles are:
    - Reduction of displaced fragments
    - Maintenance of reduction during healing
    - Functional rehabilitation of the limb
  - Displaced fractures of the distal radius are considered unstable when alignment cannot be maintained after closed reduction (this definition applies retrospectively).

Contraindications

- Do not perform hematoma block in following instances:
  - History of allergy to local anesthetics
  - Overlying infected or dirty skin
- Do not perform reduction if open fracture exists.
  - Cover with a sterile dressing.
  - Administer IV antibiotics and tetanus prophylaxis if necessary.
  - Consult orthopedic surgeon immediately.

Risks/Consent Issues

- Procedure can cause pain (local anesthesia will be given).
- Needle puncture can cause a small amount of bleeding.
- Sterile technique will be used but there is always risk of infection when skin is punctured.

Landmarks: Radiographic

- Standard radiographs should include a posteroanterior (PA) and a lateral projection.
- Fractures should be defined as: children or adult, extra-articular or intra-articular, comminuted or noncomminuted, angulated or not angulated.
- In adults, several measurements are used to determine the extent of deformity.
  - Radial height (PA view): Two parallel lines are drawn perpendicular to the long axis of the radius, one through the tip of the radial styloid and the other at the articular surface of the radius.
    - **Normal radial height is 9.9 to 17.3 mm.**

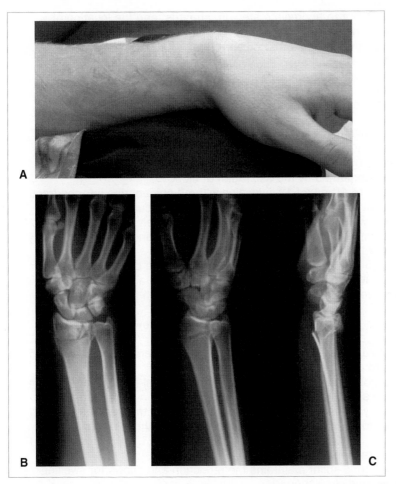

FIGURE 39.1: **A:** "Dinner-fork" deformity of Colles fracture. **B, C:** Colles fracture. (From Silverberg M. Colles' and Smith's fractures. In: Greenberg MI, ed. *Greenberg's text-atlas of emergency medicine*. Philadelphia: Lippincott Williams & Wilkins; 2005:483, with permission.)

- Radial inclination (PA view): A line is drawn through the articular surface of the radius, perpendicular to its long axis. A line is then drawn tangent from the tip of the radial styloid.
  ▸ **Normal radial inclination is 15 to 25 degrees.**
- Volar tilt (lateral view): A line is drawn perpendicular to the long axis of the radius. A line is then drawn tangent to it along the articular surface from the dorsal to palmar surface of the radius.
  ▸ **Normal volar tilt is 10 to 25 degrees.**

Technique
Clinical Assessment
- Inspection: Look for a break in the skin and skeletal deformity. The classic finding is the so-called "dinner-fork" deformity which is produced by dorsal displacement of the distal fracture fragments.

- Palpation: Attempt to appreciate step-off, crepitus, and the location of maximal tenderness.
- Testing of neurovascular status: Close attention must be given to finger sensation because acute median nerve compression is common in these injuries, especially in severely displaced, high-energy fractures.

■ **Hematoma Block**
- Prepare skin over the fracture site with povidone-iodine or chlorhexidine solution.
- Insert a 25-gauge needle dorsally into the hematoma at the fracture site approximately 30 degrees to the skin. Try to get the needle tip into the fracture space by touching the fractured surface of the distal fragment. Placement is confirmed by the aspiration of blood.
- Slowly inject 5 to 10 mL of 1% lidocaine without epinephrine into the fracture cavity and another 5 mL into the surrounding periosteum.
  ▷ Lidocaine will provide anesthesia for approximately 1 to 2 hours.
  ▷ Bupivacaine 0.5% may also be used if available and has a significantly longer duration of action (4 to 6 hours).
- Allow 10 to 15 minutes for the anesthesia to become effective.

■ **Reduction (Jones Method):** Goal is to restore the normal anatomy (restoring the radial height, volar tilt, and intra-articular step) through traction and manipulation.
- Place patient's fingers in a finger trap device with elbow in 90 degrees of flexion.
- Suspend 8 to 10 lb of weight from elbow (distal humerus specifically) for 5 to 10 minutes to disimpact fracture fragments.
- While in traction, apply dorsal pressure over the distal fragment with your thumbs while simultaneously applying volar pressure over the proximal segment with your fingers in an attempt to disimpact the fragments.
- Apply a volar force to the distal fragments to realign them into anatomic position.
- Remove the traction weight.

■ **Splinting:** A sugar-tong splint maintains the reduction and allows for swelling without compromising circulation.
- Extends from the dorsal metacarpal–phalangeal joints around the elbow to the midpalmar crease.
- The splint should be premeasured and created with six to eight layers of thickness.
- The elbow in placed in 90 degrees of flexion, the arm in pronation, and the wrist in slight flexion and slight ulnar deviation.
  ▷ Extensive flexion, >20 degrees, can cause median nerve compression.
  ▷ Some orthopedists prefer the forearm in neutral or in slight supination and some prefer a neutral wrist. The position of the forearm is controversial and the decision may be left to the orthopedic surgeon who will be following up the patient.
  ▷ The metacarpal–phalangeal joints should not be immobilized to reduce stiffness.
- Obtain postreduction x-rays to evaluate reduction.
  ▷ The volar tilt of the radius should be restored to anatomic position but neutral position or zero degrees are considered acceptable. The radial height should be within 2 mm of the ulna.
- Document neurovascular status after the procedure.

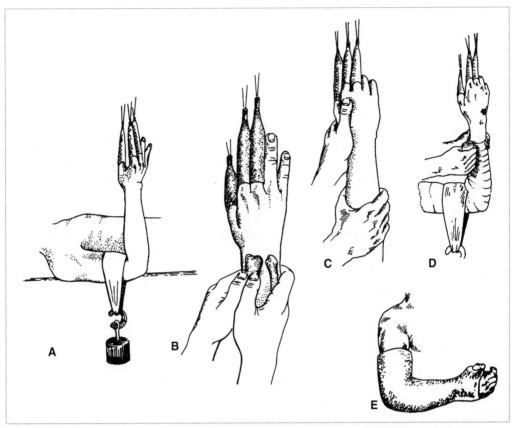

FIGURE 39.2: Colles fracture reduction. **A:** Fingers are placed in finger trap. **B:** After disimpaction of fragments with dorsal pressure, the fracture is reduced by applying a volar force to the distal segments. **C:** Adjust wrist into proper position for immobilization. **D:** Initial portion of splint is applied. **E:** Finished splint. (From Simon RR, Brenner BE. *Emergency procedures and techniques*, 4th ed. Philadelphia: Lippincott Williams & Wilkins; 2002:273, with permission.)

- Arrange follow-up:
  - Orthopedic follow-up within 3 days to assess reduction, need for surgical intervention, and eventual conversion to a short arm cast.
  - Repeat radiographs are recommended weekly for 2 to 3 weeks to ensure that there is maintenance of the reduction.

Complications
- Median/ulnar nerve injury or compression
  - May result from the original injury or after closed reduction from traction placed on the nerve, direct pressure from a splint or secondary to swelling
  - Carpal tunnel syndrome: Pain and paresthesias in median nerve distribution
- Compartment syndrome
- Loss of fracture reduction (more common with comminuted or severely displaced fractures)
  - Attempt restoration of volar tilt, radial inclination, and radial length
- Nonunion or malunion—angled, shortening

- Post-traumatic arthritis
- Tendon rupture (extensor pollicus longus)
- Reflex sympathetic dystrophy, a syndrome of paresthesias, pain, stiffness, and changes in skin temperature and color, complicates 3% of distal radius fractures

Common Pitfalls
- Use of inadequate local anesthesia
- Missing a distal radioulnar joint (DRUJ) dislocation
    - Injury disrupts the triangular fibrocartilage complex, which stabilizes the joint.
    - X-rays may be reported as normal; therefore physical examination is the key to diagnosis.
        - The wrist has limited range of motion, and crepitus on supination and pronation
        - There is loss of the ulnar styloid contour with volar ulna dislocation and prominence of the ulnar styloid with dorsal dislocation
        - More frequent if there is an associated ulnar styloid fracture
    - Orthopedic consultation is necessary for this injury.
- Missing a Salter-Harris type I fracture in pediatric patients
    - Tenderness over the distal radial physis
    - Only radiologic finding may be displacement or absence of the pronator quadratus fat pad sign
    - Splint, and arrange orthopedic follow-up
    - Rarely results in a growth disturbance
    - Consider child abuse in patients <1 year of age with this injury

Pearls
- Loss of reduction can occur in more unstable fractures. Risk factors for fracture instability include the following:
    - The pattern of the fracture (dorsal comminution beyond the midaxial plane of the radius, intra-articular fracture, associated ulnar fracture)
    - The severity of the primary displacement (dorsal angulation >20 degrees, radial shortening >5 mm)
    - Patient factors (age >60 years, quality of bone)
- Inadequate reduction can lead to radial shortening, limited range of motion, and chronic pain.
- Open fracture, inadequate reduction, or any neurovascular deficit requires immediate orthopedic consultation.
- Satisfaction with closed reduction outcomes and nonoperative management varies based on patient age, hand dominance, and functional demands and should be taken into consideration.
- Document neurovascular function both before and after the reduction, including symptoms of carpal tunnel syndrome.
- Motor function may be assessed by finger extension (radial nerve), thumb opposition (median nerve), and finger abduction (ulnar nerve).
- Instruct patient on range-of-motion exercises of fingers and shoulder to reduce stiffness.
- An aggressive course of management aiming for anatomic reduction and stable internal fixation may be indicated for the young patient, who is active and has an unstable, displaced, intra-articular fracture.

Suggested Readings

Berquist TH. *Imaging of orthopedic trauma*. New York: Raven Press; 1992.

Keats TE, Sistrom C. *Atlas of radiologic measurement*. St. Louis: Mosby; 2001.

Leventhal JM. The field of child maltreatment enters its fifth decade. *Child Abuse and Neglect*. 2003;27(1):1–4.

40 Extensor Tendon Repair

Faye Maryann Lee and Gregory S. Johnston

Indications
- For repair of partial or complete tendon injury
- Partial laceration of the extensor tendons proximal to the metacarpophalangeal (MCP) joint may or may not require repair; those at or distal to the MCP joint level must be repaired.

Contraindications
Delayed closure and or referral to a hand specialist or orthopedic surgeon may be more appropriate in these circumstances:
- Severe contamination or acute infection
  - In injuries due to human teeth (clenched fist injury or "fight bite")
- Delayed presentation of injury
- Extensive injury requiring prolonged use of tourniquet (longer than 20 to 30 minutes)
- Penetration of laceration into a joint capsule
  - These cases may be taken to the operating room for surgical exploration, irrigation, and IV antibiotics.

Risks/Consent Issues
- Pain (local anesthesia will be given)
- Bleeding
- Infection (thorough irrigation will be performed)
- Risk of injuring other structures—tendons, vessels, nerves
- Scar formation
- Laceration may need to be extended to allow adequate exploration or access to the surgical field

Landmarks
Treatment for open extensor tendon injuries and determination of emergency department (ED) management depends upon its anatomic location. The Verdan classification system divides the hand and wrist into eight zones (see Table 40.1 and Fig. 40.1).

Technique
- **Preparation**
  - Remove all rings immediately!
  - Radiographs, as indicated, should be employed to rule out associated fracture, foreign body, or joint space disruption.
  - Place the patient in a comfortable position, preferably supine, with the injury site easily accessible.

TABLE 40.1: The Verdan classification system

Zone	Finger	Thumb (T)
I	DIP joint	IP joint
II	Middle phalanx	Proximal phalanx
III	PIP joint	MCP joint
IV	Proximal phalanx	Metacarpal
V	MCP joint	CMC joint
VI	Metacarpals	
VII	Carpals	
VIII	Proximal wrist and distal forearm	

DIP, distal interphalangeal; IP, interphalangeal; PIP, proximal interphalangeal; MCP, metacarpophalangeal; CMC, carpometacarpal.

- Obtain proper lighting to optimize wound exploration, which should include thorough assessment for tendon injury and foreign bodies.
- Sterile conditions and technique should be employed.
- Adequate anesthesia should be administered once the initial neurovascular examination is complete. Lidocaine with epinephrine can be used in the hand except in areas supplied by end arteries. Local infiltration or the appropriate nerve block can be used.
- The wound should be thoroughly irrigated and free of contamination. Debridement of grossly contaminated tissue may be necessary.
- Good hemostasis is critical to wound exploration and tendon repair.
  - Elevate the arm for 1 minute to facilitate drainage of blood before applying a tourniquet.
  - Inflate a blood pressure cuff to 260 to 280 mm Hg and clamp the cuff tubes to avoid air leak. Apply the tourniquet for no longer than 20 minutes.
- **Materials:** Choice of suture material depends on the location of the tendon injury.
  - For repair of complete laceration injuries on the dorsum of the hand, nonabsorbable, synthetic (polyester) sutures are preferred (Ethilon).
    - Nylon sutures are acceptable, although colored nylon may be visible beneath the skin.
    - Chromic and plain gut should not be used in complete tendon laceration, as they will dissolve before adequate tendon healing has occurred.
    - Partial tendon injuries can be repaired with fine synthetic, absorbable sutures such as polyglactin (Vicryl).
    - Avoid silk sutures.
  - Size 4–0 sutures are appropriate for most extensor tendons; 5-0 sutures may be needed for smaller tendons. Smaller, tapered needles should be used to avoid tearing the tendon.
  - Instruments: Needle holder, two skin hooks and retractors, sharp and blunt-nosed scissors, hemostats, single-toothed forceps.
- **Procedure:** For open tendon injuries that will be repaired by a hand surgeon, primary skin closure and immobilization, unless otherwise noted, can be done outside of the operating room.
  - Zones VII (wrist) and VIII (distal forearm)

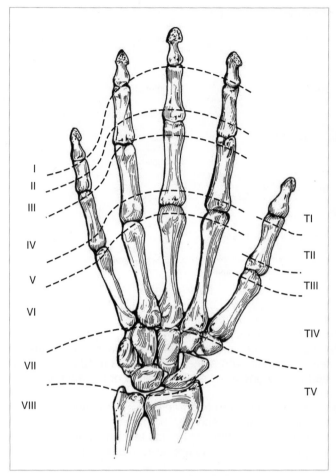

FIGURE 40.1: Extensor tendon repair landmarks.

▸ Extensor tendon lacerations in these areas are complex and should generally be repaired by an orthopedic/hand surgeon.
▸ Management includes irrigation, local wound care with primary repair of the skin, and the application of a volar splint with the wrist at 35 to 45 degrees of extension and the MCPs at 10 to 15 degrees of flexion.
▸ Outpatient follow-up with a hand surgeon should be arranged within 1 to 5 days.
  • Zone VI (metacarpal/dorsal hand)
▸ Most extensor tendon injuries in zone VI can be repaired outside of the operating room.
▸ The distal end of a severed tendon is usually found by passively extending the affected digit to bring the end into view.
▸ The proximal portion of a severed tendon may need to be retrieved; it may be necessary to extend the wound proximally with a scalpel (parallel to the course of the tendon) to obtain adequate exposure.
▸ Repair technique is based on size and shape of the tendon.
  ♦ Smaller tendons may be repaired using a figure of 8 or horizontal mattress suture.
  ♦ The modified Kessler or modified Bunnell techniques

◇ Using a small, tapered needle, insert the first suture into the exposed, cut end of the tendon
◇ Next weave the suture out, then back in through the lateral tendon margins, and then back out again through the exposed end.
◇ The same suture is then placed similarly through the end of the opposite half of the cut tendon.
◇ The suture ends are tied in a square knot between the cut ends, bringing the two halves together.

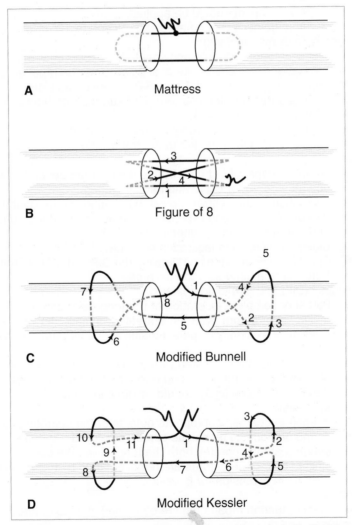

FIGURE 40.2: A: Horizontal mattress. **B:** Figure of 8 stitch. **C:** Modified Bunnell. **D:** Modified Kessler suture technique.

▷ All extensor tendon lacerations, repaired or unrepaired, should be immobilized and referred to a hand surgeon. Place a volar splint with the wrist in 45 degrees of extension, the affected MCP joint in neutral, and the unaffected MCP joints in 15 degrees of flexion. Allow the proximal interphalangeal (PIP) and distal interphalangeal (DIP) joints full range of motion.

- Zone V (MCP joint)
  - ▷ Owing to the complexities of a tendon injury in this region, repair should be done by an orthopedic/hand surgeon.
  - ▷ Open injuries should be considered secondary to a human tooth bite until proven otherwise.
    - ◆ Obtain radiographs.
    - ◆ Copiously irrigate the wound.
    - ◆ Leave the wound open unless completely certain that it did not enter a mouth.
    - ◆ A volar splint should be applied.
    - ◆ IV antibiotics with delayed closure in 5 to 10 days
- Zone IV (proximal phalanx)
  - ▷ Management is variable and should be discussed with a hand surgeon.
  - ▷ Lacerations of a single lateral slip can either be repaired or left unrepaired and splinted. Using 5-0 nonabsorbable suture material, a running suture or simple interrupted sutures with buried knots are appropriate for this area.
  - ▷ Apply splint from the forearm to the digit, leaving the DIP with full mobility. The PIP joint should be left in neutral position.
- Zone III (PIP)
  - ▷ Wounds suspected of penetrating the joint are generally taken to the operating room for exploration and irrigation.
  - ▷ Laceration of the central slip can result in long-term Boutonniere deformity (flexion of the PIP and hyperextension at the DIP due to unopposed flexion of the flexor digitorum superficialis [FDS]).
  - ▷ Close the open skin laceration primarily.
  - ▷ Splint the PIP in extension (leaving the DIP and MCP with full mobility).
  - ▷ Referred to a hand surgeon for repair.
- Zones I (DIP) and II (middle phalanx)
  - ▷ Partial or complete laceration of the tendons in zones I or II can result in mallet finger deformity. If left untreated, a mallet finger may develop a swan-neck deformity (hyperextension at the PIP and hyperflexion at the DIP).
  - ▷ Closed injuries are splinted with the DIP joint in extension and free range of motion of the PIP joint, and referred to a hand surgeon.
  - ▷ Repair of an open injury should be done in consultation with a hand specialist.
  - ▷ If repair is deemed appropriate outside of the operating room, the dermatotenodesis technique can be employed—the placement of a suture that incorporates both the tendon and the overlying skin into a single suture. The sutures are removed after 10 to 12 days and the finger splinted in extension for 6 weeks.
- **After-Care**
  - All extensor tendon repairs require some period of complete immobilization with splinting during tendon healing.
  - Patients should be advised to seek medical care for signs and symptoms of wound infection.
  - Timely follow-up with a hand specialist or orthopedic surgeon should be provided within 1 to 5 days.
  - Many clinicians and orthopedic surgeons will prescribe prophylactic antibiotics (with gram-positive coverage) if a tendon has been lacerated or sutured; however, prophylactic antibiotics have not been proven to reduce infection rates. No universally accepted standard of care exists.

Complications
- Wound infection
- Skin breakdown secondary to prolonged splinting
- Tendon rupture
- Tendon subluxation
- Loss of flexion may occur due to extensor tendon shortening
- Loss of flexion and extension can result from adhesions—this may be manifested by a weakened grip
- Deformity or dysfunction

Common Pitfalls
- Failure to recognize tendon injury because of incomplete assessment (can lead to deformity and/or loss of function)
- Neglecting to extend a laceration and attempting to examine, cleanse, or repair through a small laceration
- Neglecting to achieve adequate hemostasis with a tourniquet, resulting in failure to recognize an injured tendon
- Failure to adequately immobilize with a splint

Pearls
- Adequate anesthesia is critical for thorough assessment of injury, particularly strength of extension against resistance, which may be severely limited by pain.
- Adequate hemostasis is essential to complete tendon examination. A blood pressure cuff or other tourniquet should be employed.
- Wounds should be examined through a full range of motion and in the position of injury, because the site of tendon injury frequently does not lie directly beneath the site of the skin wound.
- Assess strength of active extension against resistance (and not just the presence of extension). Comparison with the uninjured hand can facilitate assessment.
- In combined (flexor and extensor) repairs, flexor tendon rehabilitation must take priority. Splinting extensor tendons even longer than the flexors is important to prevent damage to the repair by the more powerful flexor tendons.
- Little data exists on the optimal management of partial extensor tendon lacerations. It is considered optional to repair a laceration if less than 50% of the cross-sectional area is involved. Irrigation, skin closure, splinting, and timely follow-up with a hand surgeon are considered standard for unsutured partial tendon lacerations.

41

Digital Nerve Block

Tina Wu and Elizabeth M. Borock

Indications
- Used to provide local anesthesia to the digits for repair, reduction, or drainage
  - Lacerations
  - Nail bed injuries
  - Infections (i.e., felons, paronychias)
  - Amputations
  - Fractures or dislocations

Contraindications
- **Absolute Contraindications**
  - Transthecal technique contraindicated in cases of infection, including felon, tenosynovitis, and overlying cellulitis.
  - Allergy to lidocaine, bupivacaine or other selected anesthetic
- **Relative Contraindications**
  - Complex laceration or other injury involving multiple digits that can be more easily and adequately anesthetized with a nerve block at the wrist.

Risks/Consent Issues
- Needle puncture can cause pain and local bleeding
- Potential for introducing infection (sterile technique will be utilized)
- Potential for damage to neurovascular bundle
- Paresthesias
- Possible need for additional anesthetic or alternate procedures if the initial nerve block fails

Landmarks
- The common digital nerves divide into two pairs of nerves corresponding to the dorsal and palmar sides of the digits.
- **Palmar Nerve**
  - Located at the 4 and 8 o'clock positions when looking at a cross-section of the digit
  - Supplies the volar surface of the digit and the dorsal surface distal to the DIP joint for the middle three fingers
  - Blocking only the palmar nerves will provide adequate anesthesia on fingertip injuries distal to the DIP for the three middle fingers
- **Digital Nerve**
  - Located at the 2 and 10 o'clock positions when looking at a cross-section of the digit
  - Supplies the nail beds of the thumb, fifth digit and dorsal aspects of all three middle fingers up to the DIP
- For the thumb and fifth digit, all four nerves must be blocked for fingertip and nail bed anesthesia

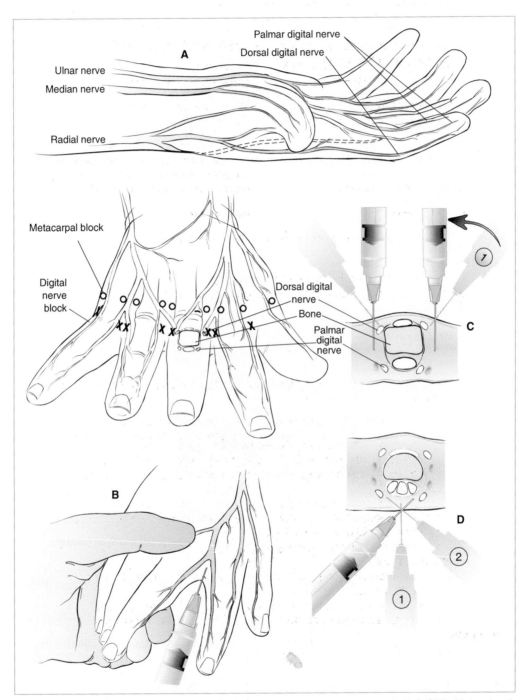

FIGURE 41.1: Dorsal technique for palmar and dorsal digital nerve block. (From Lewis L, Stephan M. Local and regional anesthesia. In: Henretig FM, King C, eds. *Textbook of pediatric emergency procedures*. Philadelphia: Williams & Wilkins; 1997:481, with permission.)

Technique: Three Approaches

- **Patient Preparation**
  - Document neurovascular examination before anesthesia.
  - Place patient's affected hand comfortably on bedside procedure table with palmar surface down (for traditional ring block and metacarpal nerve block) or palmar surface up (for transthecal approach).
  - Prepare the proximal finger and web space by using standard aseptic technique.
- **Equipment**
  - 1% Lidocaine (or 0.25% bupivacaine for longer, complicated procedures)
  - An 18-gauge needle for drawing up the anesthetic
  - A 25- or 27-gauge needle for the nerve block
  - A 5-mL syringe
  - Alcohol or povidone-iodine solution
  - Sterile gauze
  - Gloves
- **Traditional Ring Block**

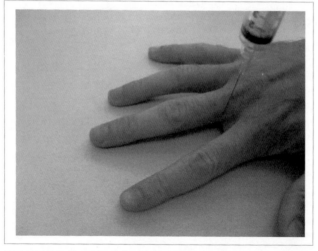

FIGURE 41.2: Traditional ring block. (Photo courtesy of Jayson Pereira, MD and Ryan Freidberg, MD.)

  - Give two injections of lidocaine, one on each side of the digit.
  - Locate dorsal-lateral aspect of proximal phalanx at the web space, just distal to MCP joint.
  - Advance needle until bone is struck, and aspirate and inject 0.5 mL of lidocaine to anesthetize the dorsal nerve.
  - Withdraw needle slightly and advance toward volar surface and inject 1 mL of lidocaine.
  - Repeat procedure on opposite side of finger.
  - Massage area of infiltrated skin for 15 seconds to ensure diffusion of the anesthetic.
  - Wait for 4 to 5 minutes to test for efficacy.
- **Transthecal Approach**
  - Advantages: Single injection and low risk of neurovascular bundle injury
  - Disadvantage: More painful to inject through volar surface
  - Anesthetic is infused directly into the flexor tendon sheath at the proximal digital crease on volar surface.

- Fill 5-mL syringe with lidocaine.
- Insert 25-gauge needle at a 90-degree angle at the midpoint of the proximal digital crease and advance until bone is struck.
- Withdraw needle approximately 2 to 3 mm (should be in flexor tendon sheath) and redirect at a 45-degree angle to the long axis of the digit.
- Aspirate and inject 1.5 to 3 mL lidocaine while palpating tendon sheath with other hand; continue until resistance is felt.
- After removing the needle, apply pressure over the tendon proximally to facilitate distal spread.
- Wait for 2 to 3 minutes to test for efficacy of anesthesia.
- Most effective for middle three fingers.

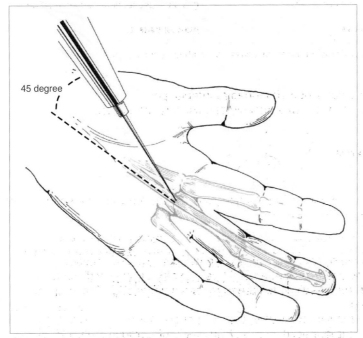

45 degree

FIGURE 41.3: Digital nerve block: Transthecal approach. The needle is directed into the proximal digital crease at a 45-degree angle to the long axis of the digit into the flexor tendon sheath where the lidocaine is deposited slowly.

- **Metacarpal Nerve Block (or common digital nerve block)**
  - Prepare skin over dorsal surface of web space between metacarpal heads.
  - Aspirate and inject subcutaneous wheal between metacarpal bones on dorsum of hand 1 to 2 cm proximal to web space.
  - Slowly advance needle through the wheal toward lateral volar surface of metacarpal head until slight tenting of the palmar surface is appreciated.
  - Aspirate and then inject 2 mL of anesthetic.
  - Repeat the process on the opposite side of the finger.
- **Thumb Block**
  - All four digital nerves must be blocked for complete anesthesia of the thumb.
  - Locate the flexor pollicis longus on the volar aspect of the thumb at the level of the proximal thumb flexor crease.
  - The nerves lie immediately adjacent to this tendon.
  - Aspirate and inject 1 to 2 mL of lidocaine along both sides of the tendon.

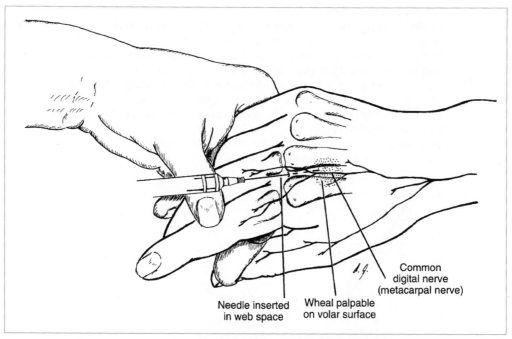

FIGURE 41.4: Block of common digital nerve. (From Simon RR, Brenner BE. *Emergency procedures and techniques,* 4th ed. Philadelphia: Lippincott Williams & Wilkins; 2002:135, with permission.)

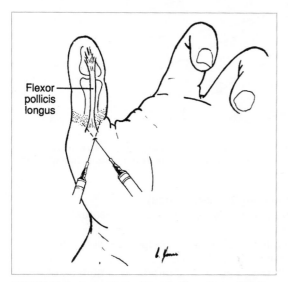

FIGURE 41.5: Nerve block of thumb. (From Simon RR, Brenner BE. *Emergency procedures and techniques,* 4th ed. Philadelphia: Lippincott Williams & Wilkins; 2002:136, with permission.)

Complications

- Laceration of digital nerve
- Intravascular injection may cause vasospasm and ischemia, suggested by blanching of digit
- Risk of flexor tendon injury with transthecal block
- Compartment syndrome

Common Pitfalls

- Use of inadequate local anesthesia
- Use of local anesthetic with epinephrine causing distal ischemia
- Relying on transthecal approach to achieve adequate anesthesia of the thumb and fifth finger for which additional blocking of the dorsal branches is required
- Injecting too lateral and missing the palmar sensory branches

Pearls

- Several studies have shown that the traditional ring block is better tolerated because of the thinner skin on the dorsal surface. However, single-injection techniques like the transthecal block are equally effective.
- The preferred site and technique should be tailored to the clinical situation.
- Only the palmar sensory branches need to be blocked to obtain full anesthesia of the middle three digits.
- When blocking the thumb, extend infiltration down to the edges of the flexor pollicis longus tendon to ensure anesthesia of palmar sensory branches.
- Massage the injected area for 30 seconds to improve diffusion process.

Suggested Readings

Chiu DTW. Transthecal digital block: Flexor tendon sheath used for anesthetic infusion. *J Hand Surg*. 1990;15A:471–473.

Dean E, Orlinsky M. Nerve blocks of the thorax and extremities. In: Roberts JR, Hedges JR, eds. *Clinical procedures in emergency medicine*, 3rd ed. Philadelphia: WB Saunders; 1998:484–490.

Hart RG, Fernandas FAS, Kutz JE. Transthecal digital block: An underutilized technique in the ED. *Am J Emerg Med*. 2005;23:340–342.

Hill RG Jr, Patterson JW, Parker JC, et al. Comparison of transthecal digital block and traditional digital block for anesthesia of the finger. *Ann Emerg Med*. 1995;25:604–607.

Sarhadi NS, Shaw-Dunn J. Transthecal digital nerve block, an anatomical appraisal. *J Hand Surg*. 1998;23:490–493.

Simon R, Brenner BE. *Emergency procedures and techniques*, 4th ed. Philadelphia: Lippincott Williams & Wilkins; 133–136.

Whetzel TP, Mabourakh S, Barkhordar R. Modified transthecal digital block. *J Hand Surg*. 1997;22A:361–363.

42 Fasciotomy

Gregory J. Lopez and Maurizio A. Miglietta

Indications
- For definitive treatment of compartment syndrome (see Table 42.1)
  - Common locations for compartment syndrome include the calf, anterior thigh and the forearm.
- Fasciotomy should be performed as soon as possible after compartment syndrome is diagnosed
  - Muscle death begins within 4 to 6 hours of vascular compromise; irreversible damage is achieved by 12 hours.
  - Some authors advocate early and even prophylactic fasciotomy, citing the risks of limb loss or dysfunction, rhabdomyolysis, lactic acidosis, and infection.
  - If available, early consultation is recommended with general surgery, orthopedics, vascular surgery, nephrology, or toxicology as relevant.

  For diagnosis of compartment syndrome, see "Pearls" section.

Contraindications
- There are no absolute contraindications to fasciotomy in the acute setting

Risks/Consent Issues
- Bleeding
- Infection
- Iatrogenic injury to nerve, muscle and vascular structures
- Continued muscle damage, despite intervention

TABLE 42.1: External and internal causes of compartment syndrome

External causes	Internal causes
Constrictive cast or dressing	Edema, inflammation, or hemorrhage within a fascial compartment following trauma, *closed or open* fractures, burns, frostbite, electrocution, rhabdomyolysis, infection, or envenomation
Tight fascial closure	Venous obstruction or ligation
Prolonged limb compression during unconsciousness, paralysis or surgery	Edema following revascularization or reperfusion
	Iatrogenic extravasation of fluids from IV catheter or arterial line

Adapted from Moore EE. *Trauma*, 5th ed. New York: McGraw Hill; 2005:903; table 41-1.

Landmarks

- The forearm—there are two compartments
  - The volar compartment of the arm is accessed through a volar-ulnar incision beginning 3 cm below the medial epicondyle and running down the volar-ulnar aspect of the arm, ending 5 cm proximal to the ulnar styloid. This incision allows for soft tissue coverage of the flexor tendons and ulnar and median nerves.
  - The dorsal compartment of the arm is accessed through a dorsal incision from 2 cm below the lateral epicondyle, cutting longitudinally to the midline of the dorsum of the wrist.

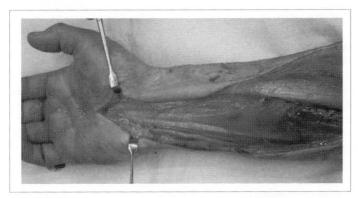

FIGURE 42.1: Fasciotomy of the forearm. (Reused with permission from Court-Brown C. *Trauma.* Philadelphia: Lippincott Williams & Wilkins; 2005:501.)

- The leg—there are four compartments accessible by two approaches
  - Double-incision fasciotomy; two approximately 8-cm incisions are made
    - Lateral incision 1 cm anterior to the fibula
      - Begin 2 cm below the fibular head and continue two-thirds of the length of the leg—this avoids peroneal nerve where it exits the fascia
      - Make two corresponding fascial incisions; one into the anterior compartment and one into the lateral compartment

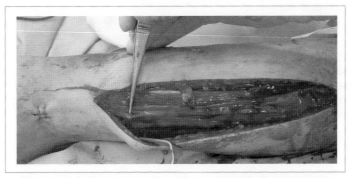

FIGURE 42.2: Anterior and lateral fasciotomy showing the superficial peroneal nerve. (Reused with permission from Court-Brown C. *Trauma.* Philadelphia: Lippincott Williams & Wilkins; 2005:500.)

    - Medial incision 2 cm posterior to the tibia; stay posterior incising over the gastrocnemius
      - Begin 2 cm below the tibial tuberosity continue two-thirds the length of the leg—this course avoids the saphenous vein and nerve

◆   Make two corresponding fascial incisions; one into the superficial posterior compartment and one into the deep posterior compartment

○ The perifibular approach has been shown to be less efficacious, requires more exposure, may require fibulectomy, and has generally fallen out of favor.

Technique

▪ Assemble your materials: Basic surgical tray, or minimally the following:
   ○ No. 10 blade scalpel
   ○ Blunt scissors
   ○ Two small tissue retractors or self-retaining retractors
   ○ Ten to 12 surgical sponges
   ○ Sponge forceps
   ○ Three to four hemostats
   ○ Needle driver and ligature
▪ Conscious sedation will be required for this procedure.
▪ The skin to be incised is prepped and draped in a sterile manner using 10% iodine solution or 2% chlorhexidine/70% ethyl alcohol (ChloraPrep). Allow to dry.
▪ Make your primary incision as above, initially incising the skin.
▪ Expose the outer investing layer of fascia.
▪ Make corresponding incisions through the fascia as described above using scissors.
▪ Control bleeding as necessary.
   ○ Direct pressure on the vessel should be the first means of hemostasis.
   ○ Ligature or clamping of the artery should be reserved for uncontrolled bleeding.
▪ Measure the compartment pressures to ensure that the fasciotomy has been therapeutic and extend fascial incision as needed until compartment pressures normalize.

Complications

▪ Hemorrhage
▪ Infection and sepsis
▪ Iatrogenic injury to superficial nerves or vascular structures

Common Pitfalls

▪ Failure to recognize the need for fasciotomy
▪ Failure to act promptly once the compartment syndrome is recognized
▪ Failure to check and recheck compartment pressures after fasciotomy

Pearls

▪ Routine antibiotic prophylaxis is not recommended, but may be given for other indications such as open fractures.
▪ Clinicians must maintain a low threshold for moving to measurement of compartment pressures and subsequent fasciotomy.
▪ If you suspect compartment syndrome, your first action should be to release any extrinsic compression of the limb—bivalve casts, remove restrictive or circumferential dressings and place leg at heart level.

■ Remember that compartment syndrome is a life- and limb-threatening condition; fasciotomy is generally well tolerated, and concerns regarding scar and damage to superficial nerves and vasculature should be of minimal concern.

Diagnosis of Compartment Syndrome

■ No single finding on clinical examination is diagnostic of compartment syndrome (see Tables 42.2 to 42.4).

■ The 5 P's—*pain, pallor, pulselessness, paralysis,* and *poikilothermia* are all late clinical findings and if all are present are clinically ominous, usually indicating severe damage to the limb.

■ Presence of pulses by palpation or Doppler ultrasonogram does not rule out compartment syndrome. Starling's law of the capillary predicts that nourishment of the tissues will cease long before pulses are impeded.

■ The clinical examination is more useful to rule out the diagnosis by the absence of signs; if there is reasonable suspicion, compartment pressures should be measured (see Chapter 43).

■ There is no agreed upon compartment pressure for which fasciotomy must be performed.

○ Normal tissue pressures are approximately 5 mm Hg.

○ Studies have utilized tissue pressures between 20 and 45 mm Hg as indication for fasciotomy.

TABLE 42.2: Performance characteristics of individual clinical examination findings for the diagnosis of compartment syndrome

	SN	SP	PPV	NPV
Pain	0.19	0.97	0.14	~1
Paresthesia	0.13	0.98	0.15	0.98
Pain on passive stretch	0.19	0.97	0.14	0.98
Paresis	0.13	0.97	0.11	0.98

SN, sensitivity; SP, specificity; PPV, positive predictive value; NPV, negative predictive value.
Adapted from Ulmer T. The clinical diagnosis of compartment syndrome of the lower leg: Are clinical findings predictive of the disorder? *J Orthop Trauma.* 2002;16:572.

TABLE 42.3: Performance characteristics of multiple clinical examination findings for the diagnosis of compartment syndrome

Number of clinical findings	Likelihood of compartment syndrome
Any one finding	~25%
Any two findings	68%
Any three findings	93%
All four findings	98%

Adapted from Ulmer T. The clinical diagnosis of compartment syndrome of the lower leg: Are clinical findings predictive of the disorder? *J Orthop Trauma.* 2002;16:572.

TABLE 42.4: Performance characteristics of the clinical examination for the diagnosis of compartment syndrome

	SN	SP	PPV	NPV
Clinical examination	0.20	0.97	0.15	0.98

Adapted from Velhamos GC, Toutouzas KG. Vascular trauma and compartment syndromes. *Surg Clin North Am.* 2002;82:1.

- Orthopedic literature cites compartment pressures of 20 or 30 mm Hg below diastolic pressure, or within 40 mm Hg of mean arterial pressure (MAP) as indication for fasciotomy.

Suggested Readings

Heppenstall RB. An update in compartment syndrome investigation and treatment. *Univ Penn Orthop J.* 1997;10:49–57.

McQueen MM, Court-Brown CM. Compartment monitoring in tibial fractures—the pressure threshold for decompression. *J Bone Joint Surg Am.* 1983;78–B:99–104.

Ulmer T. The clinical diagnosis of compartment syndrome of the lower leg: Are clinical findings predictive of the disorder? *J Orthop Trauma.* 2002;16:572.

Velhamos GC, Toutouzas KG. Vascular trauma and compartment syndromes. *Surg Clin North Am.* 2002;82:1.

Whitesides TE, Haney TC, Morimoto K, et al. Tissue pressure measurements as a determinant of the need for fasciotomy. *Clin Orthop Relat Res.* 1975;113:43–51.

43

Measurement of Compartment Pressures

Gregory J. Lopez and Maurizio A. Miglietta

Indications
- Suspected compartment syndrome
- Rising creatine phosphokinase (CPK) level without a source in the setting of trauma

Contraindications
- **Relative Contraindications**
  - Overlying skin cellulitis
  - Coagulopathy

Risks/Consent Issues
- Pain (site of needle insertion)
- Bleeding (local at needle puncture site)
- Infection (theoretical risk of iatrogenic infection)

Landmarks/Relevant Anatomy
- The forearm consists of three compartments (see Fig. 43.1). All compartments are entered one-third of the way from the elbow to the wrist with the arm at heart level and in supination (palm up). At this level, the posterior border of the ulna is easily palpated, just distal to the elbow.
  - The volar (palmar) compartment contains the wrist and finger flexors. Needle entry is medial to palmaris longus tendon, 1 to 2 cm deep.
  - The dorsal compartment contains the wrist and finger extensors. Needle entry is 1 to 2 cm lateral to the posterior ulna border, 1 to 2 cm deep.
  - The mobile wad contains the brachioradialis and radial flexors of the wrist. Needle insertion is 1 to 1.5 cm into the muscle, which laterally overlies the radius.
- The buttock contains three compartments: One containing the tensor fascia lata; one containing gluteus medius and minimus; and one containing the gluteus maximus.
  - Landmarks vary from person to person
  - In all cases, the needle should be at the point of maximal tenderness
- The thigh is composed of two compartments; the needle is easily passed into the point of maximal tenderness.
  - The anterior contains the quadriceps and femoral neurovascular bundle
  - The posterior contains the hamstring group and the sciatic nerve, which gives rise to the common tibial and common fibular nerve
- The leg contains four compartments (see Fig. 43.2). All compartments are entered one-third of the way from the knee to the ankle with the leg at heart level.
  - The anterior compartment contains the tibialis anterior, responsible primarily for dorsiflexion of the foot, and toe extensors; ***this compartment is most***

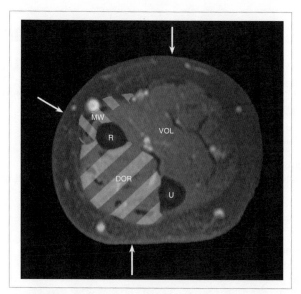

FIGURE 43.1: The three compartments of the forearm. R, radial bone; U, ulna bone; VOL, volar compartment; DOR, dorsal compartment; MW, mobile wad.

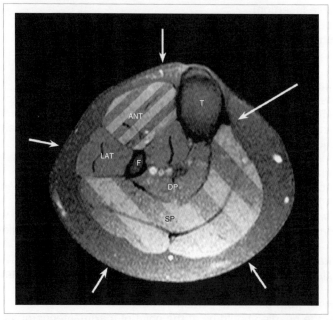

FIGURE 43.2: The four compartments of the leg. T, tibial bone; F, fibula bone; ANT, anterior compartment; LAT, lateral compartment; DP, deep posterior compartment; SP, superficial posterior compartment.

commonly affected by compartment syndrome. Needle entry is 1 cm lateral to the anterior border of the tibia 1 to 3 cm deep, while the patient is supine.

• The deep posterior compartment contains the tibialis posterior muscle (which inverts the foot) and the toe flexors. Needle entry is posterior to the medial border of the tibia, angled toward the posterior border of the fibula, 2 to 4 cm deep, with the patient supine.

- The superficial posterior compartment contains the plantar flexors of the foot—the soleus, gastrocnemius, and plantaris muscles; as well as the sural nerve. Needle entry is either side of the midline of the calf, 2 to 4 cm deep, with the patient prone.
- The lateral compartment is located anterolaterally and contains the foot everters as well as the fibular nerve. Needle entry is just anterior to the posterior border of the fibula, 1 to 1.5 cm deep, with the patient supine.

Technique

- Variety of tonometers is commercially available.
- Alternatively, measurements can be made using an arterial-line assembly.
  - Assemble your materials.
    - Arterial-line assembly, transducer, monitor, and stand
    - An 18-gauge side-port needle or slit catheter
  - Setup the arterial-line transducer and apparatus as would be for inserting an arterial line.
  - Attach the side-port needle or slit catheter to the arterial-line assembly and flush.
  - Zero the apparatus at the level of the compartment.
  - Select your entry site and cleanse it with 10% iodine solution or 2% chlorhexidine/70% ethyl alcohol (ChloraPrep). Allow to dry.
  - Administer local anesthesia and/or systemic analgesia as appropriate (avoid injection of muscle or fascia as this can affect measurements).
  - Insert the needle into your selected compartment, perpendicular to the skin.
    - For fractures, insert at level of the fracture (±5 cm)
    - Feel the "pop" as you enter the compartment through the deep fascia
  - Verify placement by gently compressing the compartment distal to the needle.
  - Record the *mean* pressure (allow needle to equilibrate).
  - Remove needle from the compartment, inspect and flush as needed.
  - Repeat the measurement of the same compartment.
  - Cover puncture site with a clean, dry dressing.
- Whitesides technique (in the absence of the above) may be used:
  - Assemble your materials.
    - A 20-mL syringe
    - Two IV extension tubing sets
    - Four-way stopcock
    - Sterile saline
    - Mercury manometer (dial-style or aneroid pressure gauges are not calibrated at low pressures and should not be used)
    - An 18-gauge needle or spinal needle
  - In a sterile manner, assemble the apparatus (see Fig. 43.3).
    - Attach the two IV extension tubing sets to the four-way stopcock.
    - Attach the 20-mL syringe to the remaining port on the four-way stopcock.
    - Attach the manometer to the female-end of the apparatus.
    - Attach the 18-gauge needle to the male-end of the apparatus.
    - On the four-way stopcock, set the manometer's port to the "off" position. Aspirate enough sterile saline to fill half of the first section of tubing.
    - Ensure that there are no air bubbles in the column as this will effect your measurement.
  - Prepare the site of needle insertion in sterile manner as described above
  - Insert the needle into the compartment of interest.
  - Set the four-way stopcock so that all three ports are open.

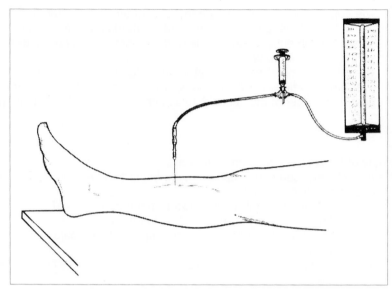

FIGURE 43.3: Schematic for a bedside compartment pressure measuring device. (From Simon RS, Brenner BE. *Emergency procedures and techniques*, 4th ed. Philadelphia: Lippincott Williams & Wilkins; 2002:293, with permission.)

- Zero the apparatus: The top of the column of saline must be at the same height as the needle.
- Slowly compress the syringe and observe the column of water in the IV tubing; the pressure at which the fluid begins to infuse is the pressure of the compartment.
- Remove needle from the compartment.
- Cover puncture site with a clean, dry dressing.

Complications
- Infection
- Local bleeding or hematoma

Common Pitfalls
- Needle is occluded by tissue plugs or blood clots
- Needle is up against an occluding structure, or placed in tendon, fascia, or the wrong compartment
- Failure to zero the apparatus
- Air bubbles in the column of saline

Pearls
- In one study, readings with a simple 18-gauge needle or spinal needle on an arterial-line assembly were 11.5 to 32 mm Hg above the compartment pressure, therefore their use is discouraged.
- If you suspect compartment syndrome, before measurement of pressures, your first action should be to release any extrinsic compression of the limb—bivalve casts, remove restrictive or circumferential dressings and place leg level. Do not elevate the leg above the heart as this may decrease perfusion.

▪ Owing to the potentially devastating complications of compartment syndrome and the low complication rate and ease of measurement, clinicians should have a low threshold for measurement of compartment pressures, especially in patients with altered mental status or who are unable to communicate.

▪ The compartment pressure used as an indication for fasciotomy varies from study to study. Additionally, measurements of compartment pressure using the Whitesides technique are notoriously inaccurate.

▪ Clinicians must take into account the *entire clinical picture* before ruling out compartment syndrome based on a ''low'' compartment pressure or proceeding to fasciotomy in an asymptomatic patient with elevated compartment pressures.

Suggested Readings

Boody AR, Wongworawat MD. Accuracy in the measurement of compartment pressures: A comparison of three commonly used methods. *J Bone Joint Surg Am.* 2005;87: 2415–2422.

Simon RS, Brenner BE. *Emergency procedures and techniques*, 4th ed. New York: Lippincott Williams & Wilkins; 2002:293.

Whitesides TE, Haney TC, Morimoto K, et al. Tissue pressure measurements as a determinant for the need of fasciotomy. *Clin Orthop Relat Res.* 1975;113:43–51.

44

Knee Arthrocentesis

Richard F. Petrik

Indications
- Used to provide evacuation of abnormal collections of fluid from the joint space for synovial fluid analysis
  - Septic arthritis
  - Crystal arthropathy
  - Hemarthrosis
  - Inflammatory process
- Used to diagnose occult fracture or ligamentous injury
- Used to decrease/relieve pressure in the joint to provide pain relief
- Used to inject methylene blue and test for joint capsule integrity when overlying laceration potentially extends into joint space
- Used to instill medication for treatment and pain relief

Contraindications
- **Absolute Contraindications**
  - Abscess/cellulitis in the tissue overlying the site to be punctured (often infectious arthritis can mimic an overlying soft tissue infection)
- **Relative Contraindications**
  - Bleeding diatheses or anticoagulant therapy
  - Prosthetic joint
  - Known bacteremia

Risks/Consent Issues
- Potential for introducing infection (sterile technique must be utilized)
- Procedure can cause pain (local anesthesia will be given)
- Needle puncture can cause localized bleeding
- Re-accumulation of fluid may occur
- Risk of injuring articular cartilage with needle tip

Landmarks
- **Parapatellar Approach**
  - Can use medial or lateral approach.

- Enter 1 cm from the edge of the patella along the superior one-third of the medial or lateral border.
- Direct the needle along the inferior surface of the patella and toward the intercondylar notch (see Fig. 44.1).

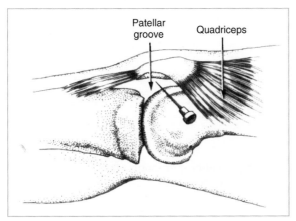

FIGURE 44.1: Medial parapatellar approach. (From Simon RR, Brenner BE. *Emergency procedures and techniques,* 4th ed. Philadelphia: Lippincott Williams & Wilkins; 2002:245.)

Technique
- **Patient Preparation**
  - Position knee fully extended or passively flexed 15 degrees with a towel roll behind popliteal region.
  - Make sure the patient relaxes his/her quadriceps as this will open up the joint space.
  - Confirm landmarks and, if needed, mark the needle insertion point.
  - Sterilize the area where the needle will be inserted with povidone-iodine solution or comparable skin antiseptic.
  - Wipe injection site with alcohol to avoid introduction of iodine into the synovium.
  - Drape the area with sterile towels.
- **Analgesia**
  - Use a small-bore (25-gauge) needle to raise a wheal of anesthetic.
  - Inject lidocaine with epinephrine at the site of puncture.
  - Anesthetize the subcutaneous tissue and a track toward the joint.
  - Avoid entering the joint space if synovial fluid analysis is desired.
- **Aspiration**
  - Using as large a needle as possible, preferably 18 gauge, advance slowly toward the joint space providing negative pressure on the syringe plunger at all times.
  - Angle the needle along the posterior surface of the patella toward the intercondylar notch until synovial fluid is aspirated.
  - Free flow of fluid confirms proper needle position.
  - Use caution and avoid trauma to bone and articular surfaces with needle tip.
  - Once the procedure is completed, withdraw the needle.
  - Apply pressure over the area of insertion for 30 seconds or until bleeding stops.

- Wipe off all excess povidone-iodine solution on the skin.
- Apply clean dressing.

Complications
- Iatrogenic infection
- Excessive pain during procedure
- Localized bleeding
- Re-accumulation of effusion
- Injury to articular cartilage if proper technique is not utilized

Common Pitfalls
- Improper use of sterile technique
- Use of inadequate local anesthesia
- Failure to appreciate the osseous anatomy and proper landmarks
- Failure to advance the needle far enough into the joint space

Pearls
- Send aspirated fluid for cell count with differential, gram stain and culture, and microscopic evaluation of crystals. See Arthrocentesis Appendix for a guideline of fluid analysis.
- Compressing the suprapatellar region with an elastic bandage or with the help of an assistant will "milk" the joint space and facilitate completion of aspiration.
- When aspirating the knee, if the first syringe becomes full, use extension tubing or a clamp on the hub of the needle to avoid moving it excessively when changing syringes.
- If the needle becomes clogged with debris, gently readjust the needle, ease up on the force of aspiration, or reinject a small amount of aspirated fluid.
- A clear fracture on x-ray may obviate the need for arthrocentesis and may require further imaging studies with consultation.
- Septic arthritis may cause skin changes similar to that of an overlying cellulitis. It is imperative that this distinction be made so that this clinical imitator is not seen as a relative contraindication to arthrocentesis, which is essential for the timely diagnosis of a septic joint.

Suggested Readings
Simon R, Brenner BE. *Emergency procedures and techniques*, 4th ed. Maryland: Williams & Wilkins; 2002.

45

Elbow Arthrocentesis

Joseph P. Underwood, III

Indications

- Used to provide evacuation of abnormal collections of fluid from the joint space for synovial fluid analysis
  - Septic arthritis
  - Crystal arthropathy
  - Hemarthrosis
  - Inflammatory process
- Used to diagnose occult fracture or ligamentous injury
- Used to decrease/relieve pressure in the joint to provide pain relief
- Used to inject methylene blue and test for joint capsule integrity when overlying laceration potentially extends into joint space
- Used to instill medication for treatment and pain relief

Contraindications

- **Absolute Contraindications**
  - Abscess/cellulitis in the tissues overlying the site to be punctured (often infectious arthritis can mimic an overlying soft tissue infection)
- **Relative Contraindications**
  - Bleeding diatheses or anticoagulant therapy
  - Known bacteremia

Risks/Consent Issues

- Potential for introducing infection (sterile technique must be utilized)
- Procedure can cause pain and discomfort (local anesthesia will be given)
- Needle puncture can cause localized bleeding
- Re-accumulation of fluid may occur
- Risk of injuring articular cartilage with needle tip

Landmarks

Arthrocentesis of the radiohumeral joint (elbow) is performed at the center of the triangle composed of the olecranon, head of the radius, and the lateral epicondyle of the humerus (see Fig. 45.1).

Technique

- **Patient Preparation**
  - Position patient on stretcher in supine position.
  - Place patient's affected arm on a procedure table.
  - With the elbow extended, palpate the depression between the radial head and the lateral epicondyle of the humerus. While still palpating, flex the elbow to

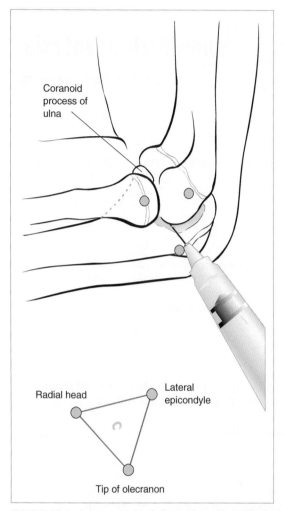

Coranoid
process of
ulna

Radial head

Lateral
epicondyle

Tip of olecranon

FIGURE 45.1: Arthrocentesis of elbow. (From Clark MC, Rothrock SG. Arthrocentesis. In: Henretig FM, King C, eds. *Textbook of pediatric emergency procedures*. Philadelphia: Williams & Wilkins; 1997:1070, with permission.)

90 degrees and pronate the forearm. Place the palm down flat on a procedure table. If helpful, mark the insertion point. If an effusion is present it should be easily palpable.
- Sterilize the area where the needle will be inserted with povidone-iodine solution or a comparable antiseptic.
- Wipe injection site with alcohol to avoid introduction of iodine into synovium.
- Drape the area with sterile towels.
- **Analgesia**
  - Use a 25-gauge needle to raise a wheal of anesthetic.
  - Inject lidocaine with epinephrine at the site of puncture.
  - Anesthetize the subcutaneous tissue and track toward the joint.
  - Avoid entering the joint space if synovial fluid analysis is desired.
- **Aspiration**
  - A 22-gauge needle is inserted from a lateral position distal to the lateral epicondyle and is directed medially. While advancing, gentle aspiration should be applied on the 10-mL syringe.

- The clinician should feel a slight reduction in resistance as the needle passes into the joint space and synovial fluid should flow easily.
- Once the procedure is completed, withdraw the needle.
- Apply pressure over the area of insertion for 30 seconds or until bleeding stops.
- Wipe off all excess povidone-iodine solution on the skin.
- Apply clean dressing.

Complications

- Iatrogenic infection
- Increased pain
- Localized bleeding
- Re-accumulation of effusion
- Injury to articular cartilage if proper technique not utilized

Common Pitfalls

- Improper use of sterile technique
- Use of inadequate local anesthesia
- Failure to appreciate the osseous anatomy and proper landmarks
- Failure to advance the needle far enough into the joint space

Pearls

- Send aspirated fluid for cell count with differential, gram stain and culture, and microscopic evaluation of crystals. See Arthrocentesis Appendix for a guideline of fluid analysis.
- Patients presenting after joint trauma must have plain radiographs to rule out underlying fracture. However, patients with unclear or equivocal radiographic findings should undergo arthrocentesis as this is highly sensitive for the diagnosis of fracture, especially in the case of radial head fractures.

Suggested Readings

May HL, ed. *Emergency medical procedures*. New York: John Wiley and Sons; 1984.

Roberts J, Hedges J. *Clinical procedures in emergency medicine*, 4th ed. Philadelphia: WB Saunders; 2004.

Schwartz G, ed. *Principles and practice of emergency medicine*, 3rd ed. Vol. 1. Pennsylvania: Lea & Febiger; 1992.

Simon R, Brenner BE. *Emergency procedures and techniques*, 4th ed. Maryland: Williams & Wilkins; 2002.

46

Ankle Arthrocentesis

Teresa M. Amato

Indications
- Used to provide evacuation of abnormal collections of fluid from the joint space for synovial fluid analysis
  - Septic arthritis
  - Crystal arthropathy
  - Hemarthrosis
  - Inflammatory process
- Used to diagnose occult fracture or ligamentous injury
- Used to decrease/relieve pressure in the joint to provide pain relief
- Used to inject methylene blue and test for joint capsule integrity when overlying laceration potentially extends into joint space
- Used to instill medication for treatment and pain relief

Contraindications
- **Absolute Contraindications**
  - Abscess/cellulitis in the tissues overlying the site to be punctured (often infectious arthritis can mimic an overlying soft tissue infection)
- **Relative Contraindications**
  - Bleeding diatheses or anticoagulant therapy
  - Known bacteremia

Risks/Consent Issues
- Potential for introducing infection (sterile technique must be utilized)
- Procedure can cause pain and discomfort (local anesthesia will be given)
- Needle puncture can cause localized bleeding
- Re-accumulation of fluid may occur
- Risk of injuring articular cartilage with needle tip

Landmarks
- Ankle arthrocentesis may be performed at either the tibiotalar joint (the medial approach) or the subtalar joint (the lateral approach) with the medial approach being the most common.
  - Medial approach: The malleolar sulcus is a small depression that is bordered by the medial malleolus medially and the anterior tibial tendon laterally. The tendon is easily identified by having the patient dorsiflex the foot. In addition, the extensor hallucis longus lies laterally to the anterior tibial tendon. This tendon may be easily identified by having the patient flex the big toe.

- Lateral approach: The lateral malleolus is easily palpable. The joint space lies just below the distal tip of the lateral malleolus (see Fig. 46.1).

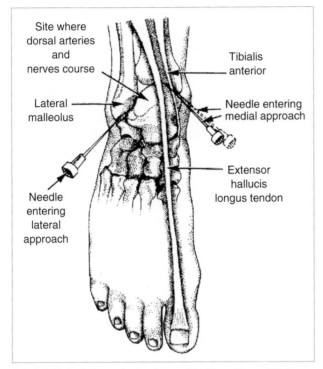

Site where dorsal arteries and nerves course

Tibialis anterior

Lateral malleolus

Needle entering medial approach

Needle entering lateral approach

Extensor hallucis longus tendon

FIGURE 46.1: Arthrocentesis of the ankle. (From Simon RR, Brenner BE. *Emergency techniques and procedures*, 4th Ed. Philadelphia: Lippincott Williams & Wilkins; 2002:246, with permission.)

Technique
- **Patient Preparation**
  - Confirm landmarks and, if needed, mark the needle insertion point.
  - Sterilize the area where the needle will be inserted with povidone-iodine solution or comparable skin antiseptic.
  - Wipe injection site with alcohol to avoid introduction of iodine into synovium.
  - Drape the area with sterile towels.
- **Analgesia**
  - Use a 25-gauge needle to raise a wheal of anesthetic.
  - Inject lidocaine without epinephrine at the site of puncture.
  - Anesthetize the subcutaneous tissue and track toward the joint.
  - Avoid entering the joint space if synovial fluid analysis is desired.
- **Aspiration**
  - Medial approach
    - The patient should be placed in a supine position, the knee extended, and the foot slightly plantar-flexed (after identifying the landmarks with dorsiflexion).
    - Alternatively, the patient can (if capable) sit on the side of a stretcher and hang his/her leg, placing the foot on a stool. This fixes the joint in a

stable position and avoids the posterior pooling of fluid in the joint that may occur when the patient is in the supine position.

▷ Insertion: Insert a 20- or 22-gauge needle just medial to the anterior tibial tendon directing it toward the anterior edge of the medial malleolus.

▷ Advance the needle 2 to 3 centimeters until the joint space is entered. While advancing, gentle aspiration should be applied on the 10-mL syringe.

○ Lateral approach

▷ The patient should be placed in a supine position; the foot should be perpendicular to the leg.

▷ Insertion: Insert a 20- or 22-gauge needle just below the tip of the lateral malleolus directing the needle medially toward the joint space.

▷ Advance the needle 2 to 3 centimeters until the joint space is entered. While advancing, gentle aspiration should be applied on the 10-mL syringe.

○ Free flow of fluid confirms proper needle position.

○ Once the procedure is completed, withdraw the needle.

○ Apply pressure over the area of insertion for 30 seconds or until bleeding stops.

○ Wipe off all excess povidone-iodine on the skin.

○ Apply clean dressing.

Complications

- Iatrogenic infection
- Increased pain
- Localized bleeding
- Re-accumulation of effusion
- Injury to articular cartilage if proper technique not utilized

Common Pitfalls

- Improper use of sterile technique
- Use of inadequate local anesthesia
- Failure to appreciate the osseous anatomy and proper landmarks
- Failure to advance the needle far enough into the joint space

Pearls

- Send aspirated fluid for cell count with differential, gram stain and culture, and microscopic evaluation of crystals. See Arthrocentesis Appendix for a guideline of fluid analysis.
- Septic arthritis may cause skin changes similar to that of an overlying cellulitis. It is imperative that this distinction be made so that this clinical imitator is not seen as a relative contraindication to arthrocentesis, which is essential for the timely diagnosis of a septic joint.

Suggested Readings

Cilip M, Chelluri L, Jastremski M, et al. *Emergency procedures*. Mexico: WB Saunders; 1992.

May HL, ed. *Emergency medical procedures*. New York: John Wiley and& Sons; 1984.

Schwartz G, ed. *Principles and practice of emergency medicine*, 3rd ed Vol. 1. Philadelphia: Lea & Febiger; 1992.

Simon RR, Brenner BE. *Emergency procedures and techniques*, 3rd ed. Maryland: Williams & Wilkins; 1994.

47

Shoulder Arthrocentesis

Caesar R. Djavaherian

Indications

- Used to provide evacuation of abnormal collections of fluid from the joint space for synovial fluid analysis
  - Septic arthritis
  - Crystal arthropathy
  - Hemarthrosis
  - Inflammatory process
- Used to diagnose occult fracture or ligamentous injury
- Used to decrease/relieve pressure in the joint to provide pain relief
- Used to inject methylene blue and test for joint capsule integrity when overlying laceration potentially extends into joint space
- Used to instill medication for treatment and pain relief

Contraindications

- **Absolute Contraindications**
  - Abscess/cellulitis in the tissue overlying the site to be punctured (often infectious arthritis can mimic an overlying soft tissue infection)
- **Relative Contraindications**
  - Known bacteremia
  - Bleeding diathesis or anticoagulant therapy
  - Prosthetic joint

Risks/Consent Issues

- Potential for introducing infection (sterile technique must be utilized).
- Procedure can cause pain and discomfort (local anesthesia will be given).
- Needle puncture can cause localized bleeding.
- Re-accumulation of fluid may occur.
- Risk of injuring articular cartilage with needle tip.

Landmarks

- **Anterior Approach**
  - Coracoid process and head of the humerus
- **Posterior Approach**
  - Posterolateral edge of the acromion

Technique

- **Patient Preparation**
  - Place the patient sitting upright with arm in slight external rotation.
  - Confirm landmarks and, if needed, mark the needle insertion point.

- Sterilize the area where the needle will be inserted with povidone-iodine solution or comparable skin antiseptic.
- Wipe injection site with alcohol to avoid introduction of iodine into synovium.
- Drape the area with sterile towels.

Analgesia
- Use a 25-gauge needle to raise a wheal of anesthetic.
- Inject lidocaine with epinephrine at the site of puncture.
- Anesthetize the subcutaneous tissue and a track toward the joint.
- Avoid entering the joint space if synovial fluid analysis is desired.

Aspiration
- Anterior approach
  - Insert an 18-guage needle attached to a 20-mL syringe just below and lateral to the coracoid process, medial to the head of the humerus.
  - Point the needle posterolaterally to avoid the joint capsule.
  - While advancing the needle, gentle aspiration on the syringe should be applied. The needle should be inserted 3 cm deep into this space or until fluid is aspirated (see Fig. 47.1)

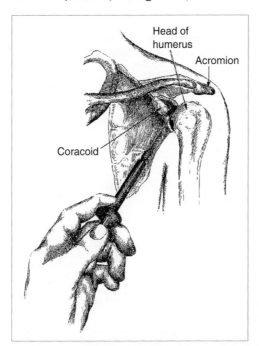

FIGURE 47.1: Anterior approach. (From Simon RR, Brenner BE. *Emergency procedures and techniques*, 4th ed. Philadelphia: Lippincott Williams & Wilkins; 2002:242, with permission.)

- Posterior approach
  - Insert an 18-guage needle attached to a 20-mL syringe 1 cm below and 1 cm medial to the posterolateral edge of the acromion.
  - Aim the needle anteriorly toward the coracoid process.
  - While advancing the needle, gentle aspiration on the syringe should be applied. The needle should be inserted 3 cm deep into this space or until fluid is aspirated (see Fig. 47.2)
- Once the procedure is completed, withdraw the needle.
- Apply pressure over the area of insertion for 30 seconds or until bleeding stops.

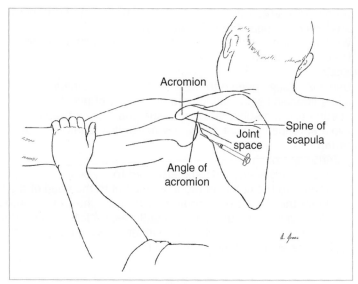

FIGURE 47.2: Posterior approach. (From Simon RR, Brenner BE. *Emergency procedures and techniques,* 4th ed. Philadelphia: Lippincott Williams & Wilkins; 2002:242.)

- Wipe off all excess povidone-iodine on the skin.
- Apply clean dressing.

Complications
- Iatrogenic infection
- Excessive pain during procedure
- Localized bleeding
- Re-accumulation of effusion
- Injury to articular cartilage if proper technique is not utilized

Common Pitfalls
- Improper sterile technique
- Use of inadequate local anesthesia
- Failure to appreciate the osseous anatomy and proper landmarks
- Failure to advance the needle far enough into the joint space

Pearls
- Send aspirated fluid for cell count with differential, Gram stain and culture, and microscopic evaluation of crystals. See Arthrocentesis Appendix for a guideline of fluid analysis.
- Septic arthritis may cause skin changes similar to that of an overlying cellulitis. It is imperative that this distinction be made so that this clinical imitator is not seen as a relative contraindication to arthrocentesis, which is essential to the timely diagnosis of a septic joint.
- Patients presenting after joint trauma must have plain radiographs taken to rule out underlying fracture.

Suggested Readings
Courtney P, Doherty M. Joint aspiration and injection. *Best Pract Res Clin Rheumatol.* 2005;19(3):345–369.

Li SF, Henderson J, Dickman E, et al. Laboratory tests in adults with monoarticular arthritis: Can they rule out a septic joint? *Acad Emerg Med.* 2004;11(3):276–280.

Lossos IS, Yossepowitch O, Kandel L. Septic arthritis of the glenohumeral joint. A report of 11 cases and review of the literature. *Medicine (Baltimore).* 1998;77(3):177–187.

Schaffer TC. Joint and soft-tissue arthrocentesis. *Prim Care.* 1993;20:757–770.

Simon R, Brenner BE. *Emergency procedures and techniques*, 4th ed. Maryland: Williams & Wilkins; 1994.

48

Interphalangeal Arthrocentesis

Hina Z. Ghory

Indications

- Used to provide evacuation of abnormal collections of fluid from the joint space for synovial fluid analysis
  - Septic arthritis
  - Crystal arthropathy
  - Hemarthrosis
  - Inflammatory process
- Used to diagnose occult fracture or ligamentous injury
- Used to decrease/relieve pressure in the joint to provide pain relief
- Used to inject methylene blue and test for joint capsule integrity when overlying laceration potentially extends into joint space
- Used to instill medication for treatment and pain relief

Contraindications

- **Absolute Contraindications**
  - Abscess/cellulitis in the tissues overlying the site to be punctured (often infectious arthritis can mimic an overlying soft tissue infection)
- **Relative Contraindications**
  - Bleeding diatheses or anticoagulant therapy
  - Prosthetic joint
  - Known bacteremia

Risks/Consent Issues

- Potential for introducing infection (sterile technique must be utilized)
- Procedure can cause pain and discomfort (local anesthesia will be given)
- Needle puncture can cause localized bleeding
- Re-accumulation of fluid may occur
- Risk of injuring articular cartilage with needle tip

Landmarks

- The landmarks for aspiration of the small joints of the upper and lower extremities are similar.
- The fibrous tendon sheaths, nerves, and vessels are located on the volar/plantar surface of the joint, so the dorsal approach should be used.
- Approach from either side of the extensor tendons.
- Remember: The undersurface of the extensor tendon is attached to the dorsal joint capsule surface.

Technique

- **Patient Preparation**
  - Confirm landmarks and, if needed, mark the needle insertion point.

- Sterilize the area where the needle will be inserted with povidone-iodine solution or comparable skin antiseptic.
- Wipe injection site with alcohol to avoid introduction of iodine into synovium.
- Drape the area with sterile towels.

Analgesia
- Use a 25-gauge needle to raise a wheal of anesthetic.
- Inject lidocaine without epinephrine at the site of puncture.
- Anesthetize the subcutaneous tissue and track toward the joint.
- Avoid entering the joint space if synovial fluid analysis is desired.

Aspiration
- Passively flex the interphalangeal joint 20 to 30 degrees, applying distal traction.
- Assuming that the "dorsal crease line" is an imaginary line connecting the dorsal points of the interphalangeal skin creases, place the needle in the dorsal crease line as shown in Figure 48.1.
- "Lifting up" the extensor tendon with your needle, insert the needle tip under the tendon (Fig. 48.1).
- For metacarpophalangeal/metatarsophalangeal joints, passively flex the joint and apply distal traction. Note the separation between the metacarpal/metatarsal and proximal phalanx. Place the needle lateral or medial to the extensor tendon into the fossa (see Fig. 48.2).
- In the case of the first metacarpophalangeal joint, insert the needle radial to the extensor pollicis longus tendon, and medially in the case of the first metatarsophalangeal joint (see Fig. 48.3).
- Free flow of fluid confirms proper needle position.
- Once the procedure is completed, withdraw the needle.
- Apply pressure over the area of insertion for 30 seconds or until bleeding stops.
- Wipe off all excess povidone-iodine on the skin.
- Apply clean dressing.

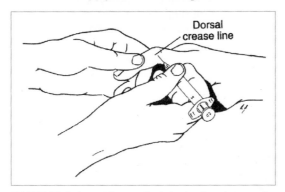

Dorsal crease line

FIGURE 48.1: Insert the needle tip in the dorsal crease line at the joint. (From Simon RR, Brenner BE. *Emergency procedures and techniques,* 4th ed. Philadelphia: Lippincott Williams & Wilkins; 2002:238. with permission.)

Complications
- Iatrogenic infection
- Excessive pain during procedure
- Localized bleeding
- Re-accumulation of effusion
- Injury to articular cartilage if proper technique is not utilized

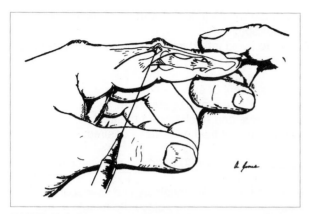

FIGURE 48.2: Distract the joint and "lift up" the extensor tendon with the needle tip. (From Simon, R. and Brenner, B. Emergency procedures and techniques, 4th ed. Maryland: Williams and Wilkins; 2002. With permission.)

Common Pitfalls

- Improper use of sterile technique
- Use of inadequate local anesthesia
- Failure to appreciate the osseous anatomy and proper landmarks
- Failure to advance the needle far enough into the joint space

Pearls

- Send aspirated fluid for cell count with differential, Gram stain and culture, and microscopic evaluation of crystals. See Arthrocentesis Appendix for a guideline of fluid analysis.
- Septic arthritis may cause skin changes similar to that of an overlying cellulitis. It is imperative that this distinction be made so that this clinical imitator is not seen as a relative contraindication to arthrocentesis, which is essential for the timely diagnosis of a septic joint.

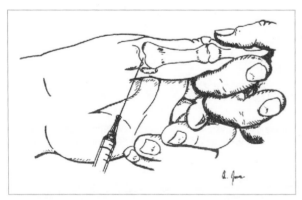

FIGURE 48.3: Arthrocentesis of the metacarpophalangeal joint of the thumb. (From Simon RR, Brenner BE. *Emergency procedures and techniques,* 4th ed. Philadelphia: Lippincott Williams & Wilkins; 2002:238. with permission.)

Suggested Readings

Jastremski MS, Dumas M, Penalaver L. *Emergency procedures*. Mexico: WB Saunders; 1992.

Lee GKW, Lau CS. Intraarticular injection of steroid. *Hong Kong Practitioner*. 1997;19:482–488.

May HL, ed. *Emergency medical procedures*. New York: John Wiley and Sons; 1984.

Marx JA, Hockberger RS, Walls RM, et al. eds. *Rosen's emergency medicine: Concepts and clinical practice*, Vol 2. 5th ed. Mosby; 2002.

Schwartz GR, Cayten CG, Mangelsen MA, et al. eds. *Principles and practice of emergency medicine*, Vol. 1. 3rd ed. Philadelphia: Lea & Febiger; 1992.

Simon R, Brenner BE. *Emergency procedures and techniques*, 4th ed. Philadelphia: Lippincott Williams & Wilkins; 2002:238.

49 Wrist (Radiocarpal) Arthrocentesis

Sadie Johnson

Indications

- Used to provide evacuation of abnormal collections of fluid from the joint space for synovial fluid analysis
  - Septic arthritis
  - Crystal arthropathy
  - Hemarthrosis
  - Inflammatory process
- Used to diagnose occult fracture or ligamentous injury
- Used to decrease/relieve pressure in the joint to provide pain relief
- Used to inject methylene blue and test for joint capsule integrity when overlying laceration potentially extends into joint space
- Used to instill medication for treatment and pain relief

Contraindications

- **Absolute Contraindications**
  - Abscess/cellulitis in the tissues overlying the site to be punctured (often infectious arthritis can mimic an overlying soft tissue infection)
- **Relative Contraindications**
  - Known bacteremia
  - Bleeding diatheses or anticoagulant therapy

Risks/Consent Issues

- Potential for introducing infection (sterile technique must be utilized)
- Procedure can cause pain and discomfort (local anesthesia will be given)
- Needle puncture can cause localized bleeding
- Re-accumulation of fluid may occur
- Risk of injuring articular cartilage with needle tip

Landmarks

- **Dorsal Approach**
  - For the radiocarpal approach, place the wrist in 20 degree flexion and extend the thumb.
  - Palpate the dorsal radial tubercle (Lister tubercle) and the extensor pollicis longus tendon as it courses over the distal radius.
  - Palpate the depression that is distal to the tubercle and on the ulnar side of the extensor carpi radialis brevis tendon.
- **Ulnocarpal Approach**
  - Flex the wrist 20 degrees and palpate the depression between the ulnar styloid process and pisiform bone.
  - This approach may be problematic because multiple tendons travel through this region.

Technique
- **Patient Preparation**
  - Confirm landmarks and, if needed, mark the needle insertion point.
  - Sterilize the area where the needle will be inserted with povidone-iodine solution or comparable skin antiseptic.
  - Wipe injection site with alcohol to avoid introduction of iodine solution into the synovium.
  - Drape the area with sterile towels.
  - Place the wrist in neutral, relaxed position.
  - Apply gentle traction and ulnar deviation to the hand to open the joint space.
- **Analgesia**
  - Use a 25-gauge needle to raise a wheal of anesthetic.
  - Inject lidocaine with epinephrine at the site of puncture.
  - Anesthetize the subcutaneous tissue and a track toward the joint.
  - Avoid entering the joint space if synovial fluid analysis is desired.
- **Aspiration**
  - Use a 22-gauge needle attached to a 5- or 10-mL syringe.
  - For the radiocarpal approach, direct the needle just distal to the border of the distal radius.
  - Insert the needle in the depression on the ulnar side of the extensor carpi radialis brevis tendon and between the distal radius and lunate bone (see Fig. 49.1).
  - For the ulnocarpal approach direct the needle between the distal border of the ulnar styloid process and the pisiformis bone (see Fig. 49.2).
  - Provide negative pressure on the syringe plunger as the needle is inserted in the joint cavity.
  - Easy aspiration of fluid confirms proper needle position.
  - Use caution and avoid trauma to bone, tendons, and articular surfaces with needle tip.
  - Once the procedure is completed, withdraw the needle.
  - Apply pressure over the area of insertion for 30 seconds or until bleeding stops.
  - Wipe off all excess povidone-iodine on the skin.
  - Apply clean dressing.

Complications
- Iatrogenic infection
- Increased pain
- Localized bleeding
- Re-accumulation of effusion
- Injury to articular cartilage if proper technique not utilized

Common Pitfalls
- Improper use of sterile technique
- Use of inadequate local anesthesia
- Failure to appreciate the osseous anatomy and landmarks
- Failure to advance the needle far enough into the joint space

Pearls
- When using the radiocarpal approach, avoid the anatomic snuff box that contains the radial artery and superficial radial nerve.

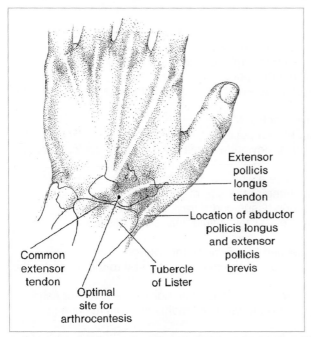

FIGURE 49.1: Radiocarpal arthrocentesis. (From Simon RR, Brenner BE. *Emergency procedures and techniques,* 4th ed. Philadelphia: Lippincott Williams & Wilkins; 2002:239. with permission.)

- The ulnocarpal approach to this joint should be avoided whenever possible to avoid injury to tendons traveling into the hand.
- Send aspirated fluid for cell count with differential, Gram stain and culture, and microscopic evaluation of crystals. See Arthrocentesis Appendix for a guideline of fluid analysis.
- Septic arthritis may cause skin changes similar to that of an overlying cellulitis. It is imperative that this distinction be made so that this clinical imitator is not seen as a relative contraindication to arthrocentesis, which is essential to the timely diagnosis of a septic joint.
- Patients presenting after joint trauma must have plain radiographs taken to rule out underlying fracture.

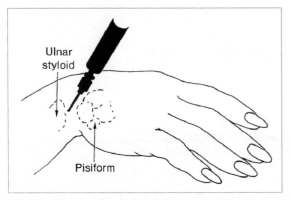

FIGURE 49.2: Ulnocarpal joint arthrocentesis. (From Simon RR, Brenner BE. *Emergency procedures and techniques,* 4th ed. Philadelphia: Lippincott Williams & Wilkins; 2002:240. with permission.)

Suggested Readings

Harris ED Jr, Budd RC, Firestein GS, et al. eds. *Kelley's textbook of rheumatology*, 7th ed. Philadelphia: WB Saunders; 2004.

Marx JA, Hockberger RS, Walls RM, et al. eds. *Rosen's emergency medicine: Concepts and clinical practice*, Vol. 2. 5th ed. Mosby; 2002.

Schwartz GR, Cayten CG, Mangelsen MA, et al. eds. *Principles and practice of emergency medicine*, Vol. 1. 3rd ed. Philadelphia: Lea & Febiger; 1992.

Simon R, Brenner BE. *Emergency procedures and techniques*, 4th ed. Maryland: Williams & Wilkins; 2002.

50 Arthrocentesis Appendix: Joint Fluid Analysis

Wallace A. Carter

Synovial fluid test	Laboratory tube
Gram stain and culture	Sterile tube or specific culture medium
Cell count and differential	EDTA: lavender top tube
Crystals	Heparin: green top tube
Chemistries (e.g., glucose, ANA, anti-Lyme Ab, RF)	SST: gold top tube or Plain: red top tube

EDTA, ethylenediaminetetra-acetic acid; ANA, antinuclear antibody; RF, rheumatoid factor; SST, serum separator tube.

- **Normal Fluid**
  - An ultradiasylate of plasma with protein and hyaluronic acid
  - Clear to straw colored
  - Viscosity of oil
- **Crystals**
  - Gout
    - Monosodium urate (MSU) crystals
    - Negative birefringence
    - Needle shaped
  - Pseudogout
    - Calcium pyrophosphate dihydrate (CPPD) crystals
    - Weak positive birefringence
    - Rhomboid and/or polymorphic shaped
  - Rarely, crystal arthritis and septic arthritis can occur concomitantly.
- **Septic Arthritis**
  - Leukocyte counts as low as 5,000 have been associated with early septic joints.
  - Most septic joints have a white cell count greater than 50,000, with more than 75% polymorphonuclear leukocytes (see Table 50.1).

Pearls

- If only a small sample is obtained, it is most important to send for Gram stain and culture to rule out infectious arthritis.
- One to 2 mL is enough for Gram stain, culture, and wet prep for crystals.
- Mucin clot and string test are physical tests of viscosity and inflammation, which are less reliable than laboratory analyses and are therefore not widely used.
- Although leukocyte count and differential will generally distinguish noninflammatory, inflammatory, and septic arthritides, leukocyte counts as low as 5,000 have been associated with early septic joints.
- Patients with **sickle cell disease** who are being evaluated for the possibility of joint infection are at increased risk for Salmonella species being the causative organism. Patients who are active **intravenous drug abusers** are at risk for Pseudomonas species being the causative organism.

TABLE 50.1: Synovial fluid analyses

Diagnosis	Appearance	WBC/mm^3	PMN%	Glucose (vs. serum level)
Normal	Clear	<200	<25	Same
DJD	Clear	<4,000	<25	Same
Trauma	Colored	<4,000	<25	Same
Crystalline (MSU/CPPD)	Turbid	2,000–50,000	>75	Lower
SLE, RA, IBD, CTD	Turbid	2,000–50,000	50–75	Lower
Septic	Purulent	5,000–>100,000	>75	Very low

WBC, white blood cell; PMN, polymorphonuclear leukocyte; DJD, degenerative joint disease; MSU, monosodium urate; CPPD, calcium pyrophosphate dihydrate; SLE, systemic lupus erythematosus; RA, rheumatoid arthritis; IBD, inflammatory bowel disease; CTD, connective tissue disease.

- Patients with negative cultures and synovial fluid suspicious for inflammatory arthritis should be evaluated for **Lyme disease** especially if they have a potential exposure within 1 year and a history of asymmetric, recurrent, and remitting joint pains.

Section Editor: Moira Davenport

51 Shoulder Dislocation and Reduction

Robert J. Preston and David J. Berkoff

Indications
- History and clinical examination consistent with shoulder dislocation
  - Anterior dislocations (>90%)
    - Occurs following excessive abduction and external rotation of the arm or, rarely, a blow to the posterior shoulder.
    - Prominent humeral head anteriorly and a shallow depression below the acromion may be observed.
  - Posterior dislocations (~5%)
    - Occurs following excessive adduction and internal rotation on a flexed arm, a fall on an outstretched hand, or a direct blow to the anterior shoulder.
    - Patient may hold and maintain the limb in a state of internal rotation and adduction.
  - Inferior dislocations (luxatio erecta)
    - Arm will typically be held fixed in an overhead position as the humeral head lays immobilized inferior to the glenoid fossa.
- Radiographs demonstrate glenohumeral dislocation

Contraindications
- An associated fracture
  - Orthopedic consultation is recommended
- An associated neurologic deficit
  - Closed reduction may still be attempted but multiple forceful attempts should be avoided

Risks/Consent Issues
- Recurrent dislocation
  - An age-dependent phenomenon depending on age at time of first dislocation. Rates range from 65% to 90% for those younger than 20, 60% to 70% for ages 20 to 40, and 2% to 4% if older than 40.
- Risks associated with conscious sedation
- Neurovascular injury during relocation
- Fracture during relocation

Landmarks

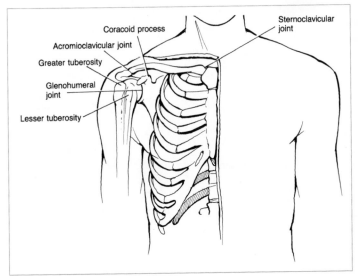

FIGURE 51.1: The essential anatomy of the shoulder. (From Schaider J, Simon RR. Shoulder injuries. In: Wolfson AB, ed. *Harwood-Nuss' clinical practice of emergency medicine*, 4th ed. Philadelphia: Lippincott Williams & Wilkins; 2005:1033, with permission.)

Technique
- **Physical Examination**
  - Inspect the shoulder joint by comparing both the affected and unaffected extremity.
  - Perform a thorough neurovascular examination.
    - Damaged axillary nerve results in a sensory deficit over the deltoid (the so-called sergeant's-stripe pattern) or an impaired deltoid contraction.
    - All major nerves to the arm should be assessed as ulnar and radial nerve lesions have also been reported.
- **Radiographs**
  - Should be obtained before procedure if there is a concern for a fracture or to definitively determine the position/type of the dislocation.
  - Plain films should typically be obtained in the anteroposterior (AP), scapular Y, and axillary lateral view.
  - In anterior dislocations, the humeral head is anterior in the axillary lateral view, and anterior to the center of Y in the trans-scapular view.
  - In posterior dislocations, a partial vacancy of the glenoid fossa (vacant glenoid sign) and >6 mm space between the glenoid rim and humeral head (positive rim sign) on the AP view are diagnostic. The humeral head is posterior on axillary lateral view and posterior to center Y on trans-scapular view.
- **Sedation, Analgesia, and Muscle Relaxation**
  - Current best practice involves the use of procedural sedation and analgesia before reduction.
  - Intra-articular lidocaine is also useful to reduce pain associated with reduction.
    - Fill a 20-mL syringe with 1% lidocaine and attach a 1.5 in. 20-gauge needle.

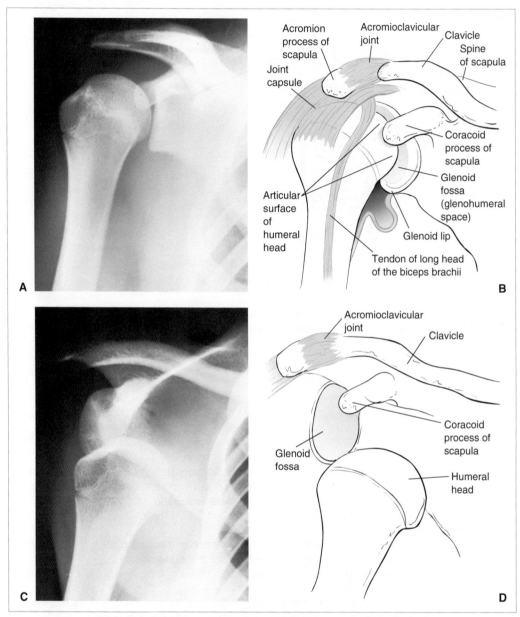

FIGURE 51.2: **A, B:** Normal shoulder joint. **C, D:** Anterior dislocation of the shoulder. (From Young GM. Reduction of common joint dislocations and subluxations. In: Henretig FM, King C, eds. *Textbook of pediatric emergency procedures*. Philadelphia: Williams & Wilkins; 1997:1083, with permission.)

    ▷ Prepare the shoulder with povidone-iodine solution.
    ▷ Insert the needle 2 cm inferiorly and directly lateral to the acromion, in the lateral sulcus left by the absent humeral head.
    ▷ Withdraw to ensure you are not in a blood vessel and then inject 15 to 20 mL of lidocaine into the joint space.

  ■ **Shoulder Reduction**
     ° For all methods of shoulder reduction, the guiding principle should be a gradual and gentle application of technique.

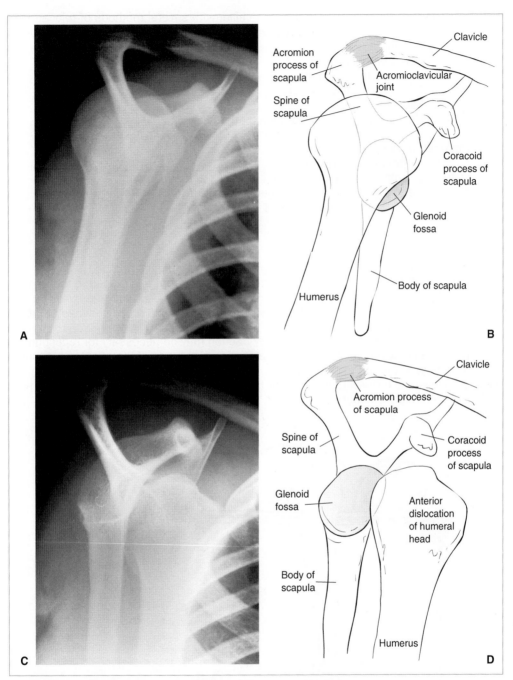

FIGURE 51.3: Scapular Y view of the shoulder. **A, B:** Normal. **C, D:** Anterior dislocation. (From Young GM. Reduction of common joint dislocations and subluxations. In: Henretig FM, King C, eds. *Textbook of pediatric emergency procedures.* Philadelphia: Williams & Wilkins; 1997:1085, with permission.)

- The treating physician should be familiar with several methods of relocation because no technique is 100% effective. Following techniques are described in this chapter:
  - ▶ Stimson maneuver
  - ▶ Scapular manipulation
  - ▶ Traction–countertraction
  - ▶ Milch technique
  - ▶ Hennepin or external rotation method
  - ▶ Posterior dislocation reduction

- **Postreduction Care**
  - Obtain postreduction x-rays.
  - Check postreduction neurovascular status and document the findings.
  - Sling and swath or apply shoulder immobilizer for 2 to 3 weeks.
  - Arrange orthopedic follow-up in 1 to 2 weeks.

Stimson Maneuver

- Patient is positioned prone with dislocated arm overhanging the bed.
- Weight of 5 to 15 lbs (initially supported by the surgeon) is strapped to the wrist of the affected extremity.
- Gradually, traction is exerted on the shoulder by slow and steady release of the surgeon's support.
- Up to 30 minutes of sustained, steady traction may be necessary for reduction.
- Reduction may be facilitated by delicate external rotation of the affected extremity.
- Advantages: Can be performed by the lone practitioner without assistance.
- Disadvantages: Often requires more time and materials (weights and straps) than may be readily available.

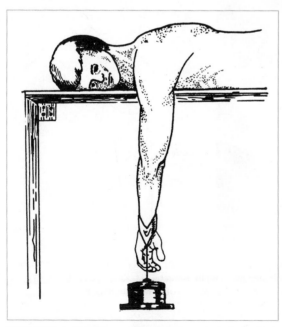

FIGURE 51.4: The Stimson technique for reducing an anterior shoulder dislocation. (From Simon RR, Brenner BE. *Emergency procedures and techniques*, 4th ed. Philadelphia: Lippincott Williams & Wilkins; 2002:279, with permission.)

Scapular Manipulation
- Place the patient in either a prone or seated position.
- Palpate the inferior tip of the scapula. Manipulate the scapula by pushing the scapular tip medially with one hand and push the superior scapula laterally with the other hand.
- An assistant should exert gentle traction on the injured extremity (alternatively weights can be used). Simultaneous external rotation of the humerus may also aid in the relocation effort.
- Advantages: Easy to perform with a high degree of safety, efficacy, and patient tolerance.
- Disadvantages: Requires two people.

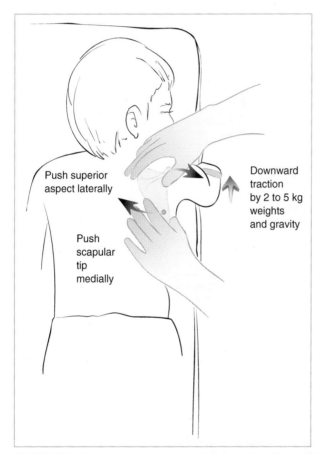

Push superior aspect laterally

Push scapular tip medially

Downward traction by 2 to 5 kg weights and gravity

FIGURE 51.5: Reduction by scapular manipulation. (From Young GM. Reduction of common joint dislocations and subluxations. In: Henretig FM, King C, eds. *Textbook of pediatric emergency procedures*. Philadelphia: Williams & Wilkins; 1997:1086, with permission.)

Traction–Countertraction Method
- Position the patient supine with a sheet wrapped around the upper torso and under the axilla of the injured extremity. Have an assistant holds the sheet to apply countertraction.
- Apply gentle traction to the injured, extended extremity.

- Consider placing a second sheet around the flexed elbow of the patient and tying it around your back. Then lean back while holding the patient's forearm and elbow (above and below the sheet) to apply gently traction.
- The practice of placing a foot in the axilla of the patient to gain leverage for traction (the so-called Hippocratic technique) should be avoided.
- Advantages: A popular method in the emergency department where familiarity has resulted in reportedly high success rates.
- Disadvantages: Requires two people and may take several minutes of slow gentle traction to be efficacious.

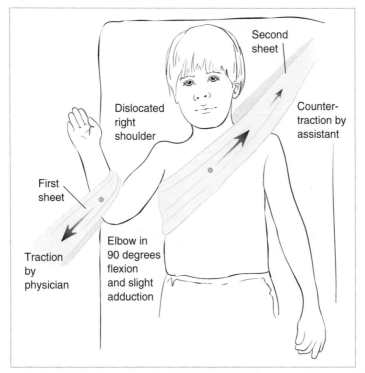

FIGURE 51.6: Reduction by traction/counter-traction. (From Young GM. Reduction of common joint dislocations and subluxations. In: Henretig FM, King C, eds. *Textbook of pediatric emergency procedures.* Philadelphia: Williams & Wilkins; 1997:1086, with permission.)

Milch Technique
- This technique has been likened to harvesting an apple from a tree.
- It may take several minutes to complete, taking special care to avoid sudden jerky movements.
- Place the patient supine with the injured shoulder at the bed edge.
- Abduct the injured arm and bring the palmar aspect of the hand up toward the head slowly and gently; patients tolerate this motion better than expected.
- Apply gentle traction and external rotation.
- Stubborn reductions may be facilitated by pressure being applied to the humeral head upward, in the direction of the glenoid fossa.
- Advantage: High patient tolerance and few reported side effects.
- Disadvantages: Requirement for patient cooperation is relatively high compared to other techniques.

Hennepin/External Rotation Method

- Place patient in the supine position with the arm adducted at side.
- With the elbow flexed to 90 degrees and supported by the surgeon, externally rotate the arm.
- Typically, reduction will occur before the arm has reached the coronal plane, but gentle elevation of the humeral head can be used to complete the relocation.
- Advantages: Shoulder muscles permit relocation with minimal manipulation and analgesia.
- Disadvantages: Success may be limited to those in whom frequent dislocation/relocation cycles occur.

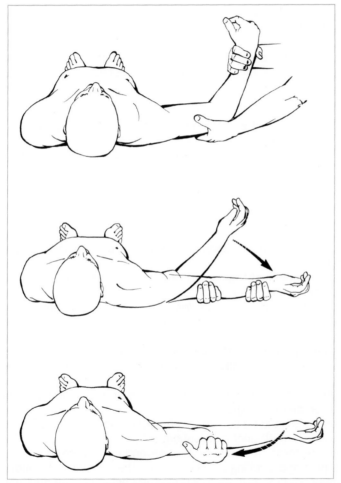

FIGURE 51.7: Hennepin technique for anterior shoulder dislocation reduction. (From Schaider J, Simon RR. Shoulder injuries. In: Wolfson AB, ed. *Harwood-Nuss' clinical practice of emergency medicine*, 4th ed. Philadelphia: Lippincott Williams & Wilkins; 2005:1037, with permission.)

Posterior Dislocation Reduction

- With the patient lying supine, place axial traction on the humerus.
- The assistant should apply gentle anterior pressure at the posterior humeral head.

- Slow internal and external rotation in addition to gentle traction will facilitate reduction.
- Advantages: Well known technique for posterior relocation.
- Dislocation: Success rate not uniformly high, particularly in cases of delayed presentation.

Complications
- Orthopedic
  - Fracture of the greater tuberosity, glenoid rim (Bankart lesion), humeral head (Hill-Sachs deformity) or humeral neck
  - Rotator cuff tear
  - Residual shoulder stiffness
  - Recurrent dislocation
- Neurovascular
  - Brachial plexus injury (especially axillary nerve palsies)
  - Laceration or thrombosis of vascular structures (especially axillary artery)

Common Pitfalls
- Not documenting pre- and postreduction neurovascular status appropriately in the patient record
- Failing to provide sufficient muscle relaxation and analgesia before reduction attempts
- Using aggressive force and being impatient rather than applying gentle maneuvers and constant traction

Pearls
- An audible "clunk" is often heard upon successful relocation, and fasciculation of the deltoid muscle may occur.
- The ability to place the palm of the injured extremity on the contralateral shoulder is often indicative of relocation success.
- Older patients should be immobilized for *less* time than younger patients, and should be followed up *sooner* (5 to 7 days) due to the risk of developing frozen shoulder.
- Nerve injuries generally have a good prognosis, but the patient should be informed of the findings and the need for follow-up. Symptoms may take many months to resolve.
- Posterior dislocations are often missed due to either an incomplete physical examination or incomplete radiographs.
- Posterior dislocations should be considered following the "3 Es": epileptic seizure, electric shock, or ethanol intoxication.
- Rotator cuff tears are easier to evaluate after several days when there is resolution of the pain and swelling associated with the original dislocation.
- Hill-Sachs deformity—a groove in the posterolateral aspect of the humeral head suggestive of recurrent dislocations—may be visible on radiographs before and after reduction.

Suggested Readings
Roberts JR, Hedges JR. *Clinical procedures in emergency medicine*, 4th ed. Philadelphia: WB Saunders; 2004:949–960.
Simon RR Brenner BE. *Emergency procedures and techniques*, 4th ed. Philadelphia: Lippincott Williams & Wilkins; 2002:276–280.

52

Knee Dislocation and Reduction

James E. Rodriguez and Maureen Gang

Indications

- Clinical suspicion of knee dislocation with neurovascular compromise (see Fig. 52.1)

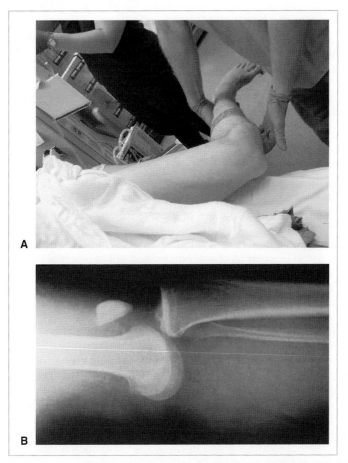

A

B

FIGURE 52.1: Clinical suspicion of knee dislocation with neurovascular compromise. (From Silverberg M. Knee dislocations. In: Greenberg MI, ed. *Greenberg's text-atlas of emergency medicine.* Philadelphia: Lippincott Williams & Wilkins; 2005:522, with permission).

- Radiographic evidence of anterior, posterior, lateral, medial, or rotary knee dislocation
    - Anteroposterior (AP) and lateral plain films usually show knee dislocations

Contraindications
- Multiple unsuccessful reduction attempts with adequate sedation
    - Repeated attempts at reduction may further traumatize tissues and increase the likelihood of neurologic/vascular damage
    - Irreducible knee dislocations are time sensitive orthopedic emergencies that should be brought to the operating room as quickly as possible
- Relative contraindications
    - "Dimple sign" of the skin of the anteromedial knee
        - Associated with posterolateral knee dislocation with entrapment of tissues within the joint space and extrusion of the medial femoral condyle from the joint capsule

Risks/Consent Issues
- Knee reduction is a limb-saving procedure and as such it may be performed even if informed consent cannot be attained.
- Procedural sedation may be complicated by loss of airway reflexes, respiratory arrest, and potential allergic/adverse reaction.
- Reduction attempts may result in injury to connective tissues, associated fractures, vascular structures, or neurologic anatomy as well as iatrogenic fractures.

Technique
- **Preprocedural Preparation**
    - Assess the patient as per Advanced Trauma Life Support (ATLS) protocols and perform resuscitation and treatment of life-threatening injuries before attempting knee reduction.
    - Neurovascular examination is critical!
        - Consider using Doppler to check pulses and ankle-brachial index (ABI).
            - ABI is the systolic blood pressures (attained by Doppler acoustics) of the distal injured extremity, divided by the same measure from an uninjured upper extremity.
            - ABI ratio of <0.9 is suspicious for arterial damage.
        - Document presence and character of the posterior tibial and dorsal pedal pulses bilaterally.
        - Document presence and character of popliteal pulse, bruit, thrill, and/or hematoma.
        - Neurologic examination with emphasis on the condition of common peroneal and posterior tibial branches of the sciatic nerve (see "Pearls" section for further details).
    - Attain expeditious plain films of knee if possible.
    - Administer tetanus prophylaxis and intravenous antibiotics if indicated.
    - Consent patient for conscious (or "moderate") sedation.
- **Knee Reduction**
    - The first practitioner grasps the distal femur to hold its position.
    - A second practitioner grasps the ankle/distal tibia.
    - Gentle and persistent axial traction is applied by the second practitioner, while the first practitioner maintains countertraction (see Fig. 52.2).
    - Application of axial traction for 1 minute will often cause complete reduction.

- If reduction has not been achieved after 1 minute, continue with the additional maneuver.

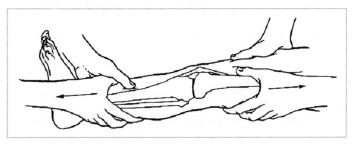

FIGURE 52.2: Gentle and persistent axial traction is applied by the second practitioner, while the first practitioner maintains counter traction. (From Gough JE, Rodriguez LE. Knee injuries. In: Wolfson AB, ed. *Harwood-Nuss' clinical practice of emergency medicine*, 4th ed. Philadelphia: Lippincott Williams & Wilkins; 2005:1089, with permission.)

- **ANTERIOR** dislocation: A third practitioner grasps the posterior aspect of the distal femur and applies gentle, persistent anterior force while axial traction/countertraction is maintained.
- **POSTERIOR** dislocation: Now the second practitioner (grasping the proximal tibia) also grasps the posterior aspect of the proximal tibia and applies gentle, persistent anterior force to the proximal tibia while axial traction/countertraction is maintained.
- **MEDIAL, LATERAL,** or **ROTATORY** dislocation: The second practitioner (grasping the proximal tibia and applying axial traction) also applies gentle, persistent force on the proximal tibia in the direction **opposite** to that of the dislocation while axial traction/countertraction is maintained (see Fig. 52.3).

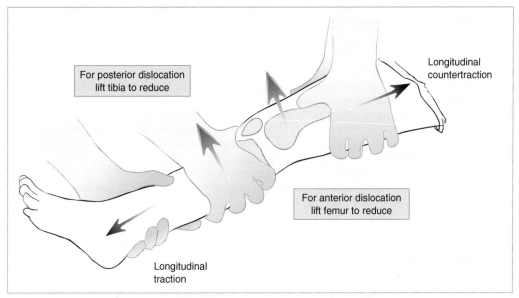

FIGURE 52.3: Technique for reduction of knee joint dislocation. (From Young GM. Reduction of common joint dislocations and subluxations. In: Henretig FM, King C, eds. *Textbook of pediatric emergency procedures*. Philadelphia: Williams & Wilkins; 1997:1098, with permission.)

- **Post Reduction**
  - Perform and document a second complete physical examination with emphasis on any changes to the neurologic and vascular status.
  - Stabilize the reduced knee
    - Apply a long leg posterior splint with the knee in 15 to 20 degree of flexion.
    - An extension knee immobilizer is less optimal but may be used instead of a splint.
    - Circumferential casting or occlusive dressings should be avoided.
  - Obtain postreduction radiographs.
  - Emergent arteriography and/or surgical intervention should be seriously considered if:
    - There was any evidence of ischemia or vascular compromise either before or after the reduction, including the ABI results.
    - The reduction could not be attained or is incomplete.
  - If emergent arteriography and/or surgery are not pursued, the patient must be admitted and receive close monitoring and serial neurologic and vascular reassessments every 1 to 2 hours.

Complications
- Popliteal vessel disruption
- Deep vein thrombosis
- Compartment syndrome, occurs 24 to 48 hours after the injury
- Pseudoaneurysms, occurs hours to months after the injury
- Arterial thrombosis
- Injury to the peroneal or tibial nerves
- Skin necrosis of the knee
- Damage to the articular surfaces, osteoarthritis, and loss of knee function
- Multiple simultaneous ligament sprains/ruptures

Common Pitfalls
- Failure to consider vascular injury despite a normal clinical examination
- Attempting reduction with inadequate procedural sedation
- Significant delay in reduction in order to attain radiographs
  - While radiographs can be helpful to characterize the dislocation and reveal associated fractures, they are not needed before reduction can be attempted if neurovascular compromise is suspected.
- Assuming the obvious knee dislocation is the only injury
  - Most knee dislocations are due to high energy trauma and are associated with other occult injuries.

Pearls
- Closed reduction should always be attempted with emergent priority if the injured extremity has clinical evidence of ischemia.
  - While subsequent emergent operative intervention is always indicated in a dislocated knee with distal ischemia, expeditious preoperative reduction may restore blood flow and improve the ultimate outcome.

- Ischemia left uncorrected for more then 6 to 8 hours is associated with subsequent loss of the limb.
- The dimple sign is a characteristic puckering of the skin along the anteromedial knee.
  - Dimple sign is associated with posterolateral knee dislocation with entrapment of tissues within the joint space and extrusion of the medial femoral condyle from the joint capsule.
  - Dislocations with a dimple sign are usually impossible to reduce nonoperatively.
  - Such dislocations are associated with skin necrosis and peroneal nerve injury.
  - Consult orthopedic service.
- Common peroneal nerve injury is the most common neurologic complication associated with knee dislocation.
  - Some peroneal deficit with 20% to 30% of knee dislocations
  - This injury is more common with posterolateral knee dislocations
  - Peroneal nerve function may be tested by checking the strength of ankle dorsiflexion and the sensation of the dorsum of the foot
- Posterior tibial nerve dysfunction is also associated with knee dislocation.
  - Tibial nerve function may be tested by checking the strength of ankle plantar-flexion and the sensation of the plantar side of the foot.

Suggested Readings

Antosia RE, Robert E, Lyn E, et al. *Rosen's emergency medicine: Concepts and clinical practice*, 5th ed. St Louis: Mosby; 2002:689–692.

Fanelli GC, Daniel FD, Edison CJ, et al. *DeLee and Drez's orthopaedic sports medicine*, 2nd ed. Copyright © 2003 Philadelphia: WB Saunders; 2003:2111–2200. An Imprint of Elsevier.

Gough JE, Rodriguez LE. *Harwood—Nuss' clinical practice of emergency medicine*, 4th ed. Philadelphia: Lippincott Williams & Wilkins; 2005:1084–1089.

Hollis JD, Daley BJ. 10-Year review of knee dislocations: Is arteriography always necessary. *J Trauma Inj Infect Crit Care.* 2005;59(3):672–676.

Levy BA, Zlowodzki MP, Graves M, et al. Screening for extremity arterial injury with the arterial injury with the arterial pressure index. *Am J Emerg Med.* 2005; 23(5):689–695.

Mills WJ, Barei DP, McNair P. The value of the ankle–brachial index for diagnosing arterial injury after knee dislocation: A prospective study. *J.Trauma Inj Infect Crit Care.* 2004;56(6):1261–1265.

Niall DM, Nutton RW, Keating JF. Palsy of the common peroneal nerve after traumatic dislocation of the knee. British Editorial Society of Bone and Joint Surgery. *J Bone Joint Surg.* 2005;87-B(5):664–667.

Nystrom M, Samimi S, Ha'Eri GB. Two cases of irreducible knee dislocations occurring simultaneously in two patients and a review of the literature. *Clin Orthop Relat Res.* 1992;277:197.

Reckling FW, Peltier LF. Acute knee dislocations and their complications. *Clin Orthop Relat Res.* 2004;422:135–141.

Robert DM, Stallard TC. Emergency department evaluation and treatment of knee and leg injuries. *Emerg Med Clin North Am.* 2000;15:67–84.

Silverberg M. Greenberg's text atlas of emergency medicine: A visual guide to diagnosis and treatment. *Knee dislocations*, Chapters 15–64. Philadelphia: Lippincott Williams & Wilkins; 2005:522.

Simon RR, Brenner BE. *Emergency procedures and techniques*, 4th ed. Philadelphia: Lippincott Williams & Wilkins; 2002:284.

Ulfberg J, McNamara R, Roberts: Clinical procedures in emergency medicine. In: *Management of common dislocations*, Chapters 50, 4th ed. Philadelphia: WB Saunders; 2004:977–998.

53 Patellar Dislocation and Reduction

Maria Vasilyadis, Moira Davenport, and Jeffrey Manko

Indications
- Clinical suspicion of patellar dislocation
  - The knee is at 20 to 30 degrees of flexion
  - Most dislocations occur laterally
    - Other types include superior, medial, and intra-articular
- Dislocated patella on x-ray

Contraindications
- Fracture
- Effusion

Landmarks
- Abnormal excursion of extensor mechanism over the femoral condyles often results in dislocation
- Patellar dislocations most commonly occur laterally, due to a weakened medial retinaculum and loss of lateral trochlear groove

Technique
- Patellar dislocations frequently relocate spontaneously before the patient seeks treatment.
- **IV Sedation and Muscle Relaxation**
  - Often the procedure may be accomplished without use of sedation or muscle relaxation.
  - Current best practice involves the use of procedural sedation and analgesia before reduction.
- **Reduction Procedure**
  - Reduction is performed by manually subluxing the patella, usually medially given the lateral nature of the dislocation, while extending the extremity.
    - A palpable relocation should be felt and confirmed by relief of the patient's symptoms.
  - Reduction may be difficult due to the medial patellar facet being locked on to the lateral femoral condyle.
    - In these cases, apply downward pressure to the lateral patella which creates the external rotational force needed to unlock the facet (see Fig. 53.2).
- **Post Procedure**
  - Postreduction films should include an anteroposterior, lateral, and sunrise (Merchants) patellar view to evaluate for any fractures or osteochondral avulsion fragments which may need arthroscopic removal at a later time.

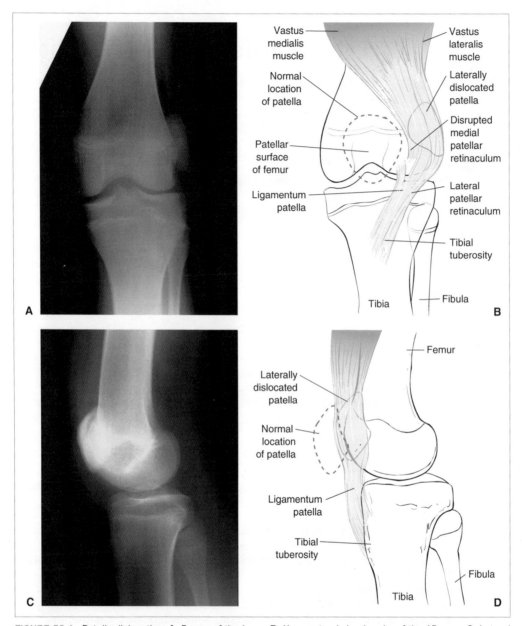

FIGURE 53.1: Patella dislocation. **A:** P x-ray of the knee. **B:** Key anatomic landmarks of the AP x-ray. **C:** Lateral x-ray of the knee. **D:** Key anatomic landmarks of the lateral x-ray. (From Young GM. Reduction of common joint dislocations and subluxations. In: Henretig FM, King C, eds. *Textbook of pediatric emergency procedures.* Philadelphia: Williams & Wilkins; 1997:1089, with permission.)

- Immobilization in full leg extension for 3 to 6 weeks is warranted, preferably in a commercially available knee immobilizer or a Jones-type compression dressing.
- Patients should be instructed to elevate the extremity and apply ice to the area to reduce swelling.
- Provide and prescribe appropriate analgesia for pain.
- Crutches maybe used as an aid for weight bearing as tolerated.

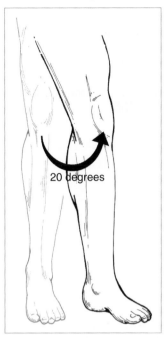

20 degrees

FIGURE 53.2: Apprehension test.

- Orthopedic follow-up should be given within 2 weeks of event.
- Patients may be instructed to do straight-leg raises to strengthen the quadriceps muscle; however, this should be deferred until the patient is seen by an orthopedic surgeon and proper physical therapy regimens are arranged.
- Patellar-stabilizing braces may be worn at a later time.

Complications
- Pain
- Inability to relocate, requiring surgical treatment
- Moderate rate of recurrence

Common Pitfalls
- Confusing a knee dislocation as a patellar dislocation
  - Knee dislocations are true orthopedic emergencies due to the high incidence of popliteal artery injury
- Not assessing for patellar dislocations in multitrauma patients
- Improper follow-up

Pearls
- Reduction can often be accomplished without sedation and analgesia.
- Patients often present to physicians after dislocation has spontaneously relocated.

Suggested Readings

Henretig F, King C. *Textbook of pediatric emergency procedures.* Williams & Wilkins; 1997:1088–1091.

Roberts JR, Hedges JR. *Clinical procedures in emergency medicine*, 4th ed. WB Saunders; 2004:982–983.

Simon RR, Brenner BE. *Emergency procedures and techniques*, 4th ed. Philadelphia: Lippincott Williams & Wilkins; 2002;285–286.

54 Elbow Dislocation and Reduction

Anand K. Swaminathan and Elizabeth M. Borock

Indications

- Clinical suspicion of acute anterior, posterior, lateral, medial, or divergent dislocation with neurovascular compromise
  - The clinical presentation depends on the type of dislocation.
  - Suspected dislocation is clinically confirmed by disruption of the relationship between the tip of the olecranon and the distal epicondyles of the humerus in comparison with the unaffected elbow.
- Radiographic evidence of anterior, posterior, lateral, medial, or divergent dislocation

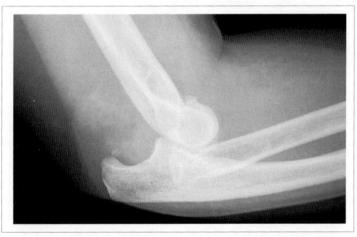

FIGURE 54.1: Posterior dislocation of the olecranon. (From Campbell C. Elbow dislocation. In: Greenberg MI, ed. *Greenberg's text-atlas of emergency medicine*. Philadelphia: Lippincott Williams & Wilkins; 2005:492, with permission.)

Contraindications

- Multiple failed reduction attempts with adequate sedation should prompt consultation with orthopedic surgeon
- Irreducible elbow dislocations may require operative management

Risks/Consent Issues

- Procedural sedation may be associated with loss of airway reflexes and respiratory arrest
- Soft tissue injury may occur with reduction attempts
- Fractures and neurovascular injury may occur with reduction attempts

Landmarks

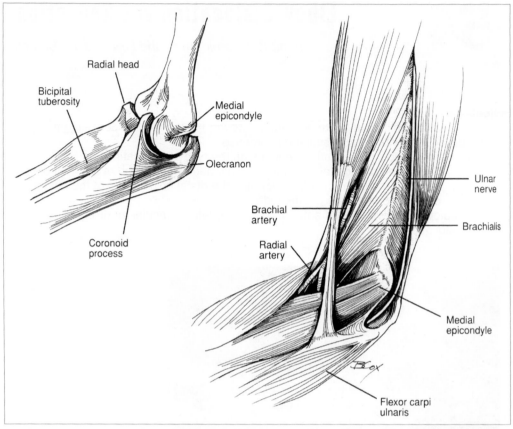

FIGURE 54.2: Elbow anatomy. (From McCue FC III, Sweeney T, Urch S. The elbow, wrist, and hand. In: Perrin DH, ed. *The injured athlete,* 3rd ed. Philadelphia: Lippincott Williams & Wilkins; 1999, with permission.)

Technique
- Perform a complete neurovascular check before any reduction attempt.
- Obtain radiographs of the affected joint and consider radiographs of one joint above and below the injury (shoulder and wrist).
  - Complex dislocations (those with associated fractures) may require consultation with orthopedic surgery.
- Anesthesia/analgesia: Consider parenteral analgesics. Reduction may also be attempted with injection of local anesthetic alone into the elbow joint.
- Reduction technique is determined by the type of dislocation.

Technique: Posterior Dislocation
- Eighty percent of all elbow dislocations
- Mechanism of injury: Most commonly caused by a fall on an outstretched hand with the arm in extension.
- Clinical Presentation: Shortened forearm that is held in flexion with a prominent olecranon posteriorly. In addition, a defect may be palpable above the olecranon.

- Associated injuries are as follows:
  - Numerous fractures including radial head and coronoid process are common.
  - Neurologic symptoms accompany approximately 15% to 22% of dislocations.
    - ▶ Ulnar nerve injury is most common followed by median nerve injury.
    - ▶ Radial nerve injury commonly occurs when the dislocation is complicated by radial head fracture.
    - ▶ Traction leading to stretch injury, local swelling, and entrapment during reduction are common causes of nerve injury.
  - Brachial artery injury occurs in 5% to 13% of posterior dislocations.
- **Reduction Techniques**
  - Traditional traction method
    - ▶ Place patient in supine position.
    - ▶ An assistant stabilizes the humerus by wrapping both hands around arm just distal to axilla.
    - ▶ The physician grasps the wrist with one hand and places the other hand just above the antecubital fossa with the thumb on the olecranon.
    - ▶ The physician applies slow, steady in-line traction while the assistant applies steady countertraction.
    - ▶ The elbow is held in slight flexion and the wrist is held in supination as traction is applied.
    - ▶ Reduction is accompanied by a "clunk" that is heard or felt.

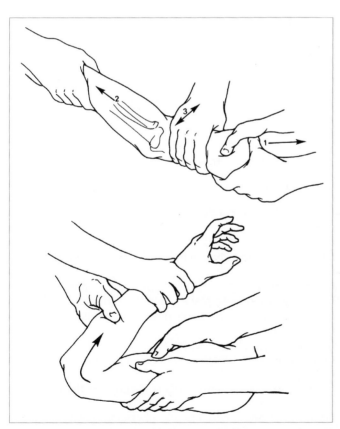

FIGURE 54.3: Technique for reduction of posterior dislocation of the elbow. (From Perron AD. Elbow injuries. In: Wolfson AB. *Harwood-Nuss' clinical practice of emergency medicine,* 4th ed. Philadelphia: Lippincott Williams & Wilkins; 2005:1046, with permission.)

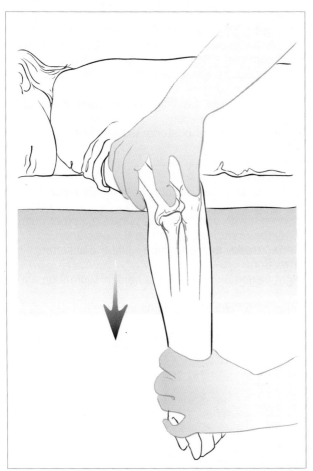

FIGURE 54.4: Technique for reduction of elbow joint dislocation. (From Young GM. Reduction of common joint dislocations and subluxations. In: Henretig FM, King C, eds. *Textbook of pediatric emergency procedures.* Philadelphia: Williams & Wilkins; 1997:1097, with permission.)

> Alternatively, the forearm may be gently flexed in an effort to reduce the joint.
- Seated position
  > Patient is seated in a high backed chair with arm hanging over the back of the chair in a flexed position.
  > The physician applies traction by gently pulling down on the patient's hand while guiding the olecranon into place using the other hand.
  > The physician may also elect to simply apply downward pressure onto the olecranon to reduce the elbow.
  > Reduction is once again signaled by a "clunk."
  > This method has the advantage of requiring only a single physician.
- Prone technique
  > Patient is positioned prone with the arm hanging flexed over the edge of the stretcher.
  > Traction is applied to the forearm, either by the physician or with weights.
  > Forward and downward pressure that is applied to the olecranon with the physician's thumbs will facilitate reduction.
  > Assistant applying gentle countertraction on the humerus may also help.

Technique: Anterior Dislocation
- Ten percent to 15% of elbow dislocations
- Mechanism: Direct posterior trauma to the olecranon with the elbow in flexed position.
- Clinical presentation: The upper arm is shortened and the forearm appears elongated. Arm is held with the elbow fully extended and the forearm supinated. There is anterior tenting of the proximal forearm and prominence of the distal humerus posteriorly.
- Associated injuries are:
  - These injuries require a large amount of force and are often open.
  - Brachial artery injury is common in open dislocations.
  - Ulnar nerve injury is uncommon.
- Reduction technique—for closed dislocations only
  - Patient is positioned supine on stretcher.
  - The assistant encircles humerus with both hands and applies countertraction.
  - The physician grasps the wrist with one hand and applies in-line traction while the second hand is positioned at the proximal forearm, and applies downward pressure.
  - Reduction is signaled by an audible or tactile "clunk."

Technique: Medial/Lateral Dislocation
- Epidemiology: Very rare
- Mechanism: Fall on outstretched hand with arm in extension with an additional vector force which displaces the radius/ulna medially or laterally
- Reduction technique
  - Same as posterior reduction technique
  - Arm should be placed in slight extension

Post Reduction Care
- Ensure stability after reduction by gentle range of motion.
- Perform a complete neurovascular check.
- Immobilize the elbow in 90 degree flexion with a long-arm posterior splint.
- Obtain postreduction radiographs to confirm reduction and to check for associated injuries.

Complications
- Delayed vascular compromise
  - May result from reduction attempts or continued soft tissue swelling.
  - Attempt to loosen splint, if already in place.
  - Consider arteriogram, surgical consultation.
- Median or ulnar nerve injury
- Inability to properly range elbow
  - Often caused by entrapped medial epicondyle fracture fragment.
  - Requires surgical intervention.
- Anterior dislocations have a high rate of associated vascular injury.
  - Emergent orthopedic consultation is required for any open anterior dislocation as well as any anterior dislocation with suspected vascular compromise.
- Myositis ossificans may occur when significant hemarthroses accompanies dislocation.

Common Pitfalls

▪ Use of inadequate anesthesia or analgesia
▪ Failure to check neurovascular status before, or after reduction attempts
▪ Failure to recognize associated injury within the elbow joint (i.e., fractures)
▪ Failure to assess one joint distal and one joint proximal to the injury

Pearls

▪ Always examine the prereduction films (if obtained) before attempting reduction. Always examine postreduction films.
▪ If available, have a colleague help you with countertraction.
▪ If one technique fails to reduce the joint, try a different technique.
▪ Treat open dislocations like open fractures—tetanus, antibiotics, early orthopedic consultation.

Suggested Readings

Geideerman JM. *Humerus and elbow–Rosen's emergency medicine concepts and clinical practice*, 6th ed. Mosby; 2006:647–670.

Hildebrand KA, Patterson SD, King GJW. Acute elbow dislocations: Simple and complex. *Orthop Clin North Am*. 1999;30(1):63–79.

Kumar A, Ahmed M. Closed reduction of posterior dislocation of the elbow: A simple technique. *J Orthop Trauma*. 1999;13(1):58–59.

Mehta JA, Bain GI. Elbow dislocations in adults and children. *Clin Sports Med*. 2004;23:609–627.

Platz A, Heinzelmann M, Ertel W, et al. Posterior elbow dislocation with associated vascular injury after blunt trauma. *J Trauma*. 1999;46(5):948–950.

Rasool MN. Dislocations of the elbow in children. *J Bone Joint Surg [Br]*. 2004; 86-B(7):1050–1058.

Silverberg M. *Greenberg's text atlas of emergency medicine: A visual guide to diagnosis and treatment*. Lippincott Williams & Wilkins;2005:492–493.

Simon RR, Brenner BE. *Emergency procedures and techniques*, 4th ed. Philadelphia: Lippincott Williams & Wilkins; 2002:281.

Ufberg JW, McNamara RM. *Management of common dislocations–Roberts and Hedges clinical procedures in emergency medicine*, 4th ed.WB Saunders; 2004:964–969.

55 Hip Dislocation and Reduction

Tania V. Mariani and Rama B. Rao

Indications
- Clinical suspicion of hip dislocation
  - Hip pain with obvious deformity in the setting of a motor vehicle crash, pedestrian struck by a vehicle, falls, or sports-related injuries
- Radiographic evidence of hip dislocation

Contraindications
- Associated femoral neck fracture
- Coexistent fracture in dislocated extremity

Risks/Consent Issues
- Inadvertently converting a dislocation to a fracture-dislocation
  - Especially in the elderly with osteoporotic bones
- Oversedation may lead to inability to protect the airway and subsequent aspiration

Landmarks
- **Posterior Hip Dislocation**
  - Mechanism of injury—femoral head is forced out of the acetabulum and rests posteriorly
  - Extremity position—shortened, adducted, and internally rotated

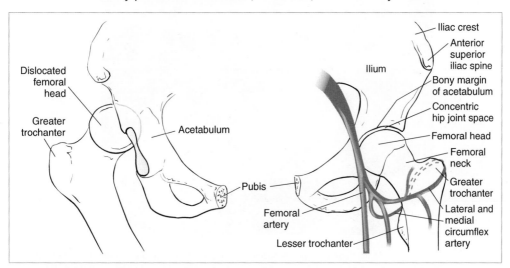

FIGURE 55.1: Normal (left) and dislocated (right) hip. (From Young GM. Reduction of common joint dislocations and subluxations. In: Henretig FM, King C, eds. *Textbook of pediatric emergency procedures*. Philadelphia: Williams & Wilkins; 1997:1093, with permission.)

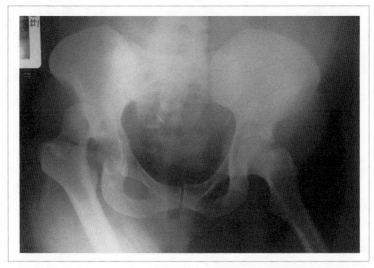

FIGURE 55.2: Anteroposterior pelvis radiograph of a posterior hip dislocation of the right hip. (From Tornetta Paul III. Hip dislocations and fractures of the femoral head. In: Bucholz RW, Heckman JD, Court-Brown C, eds. *Rockwood and green's fractures in adults,* Vol. 2, 6th ed. Philadelphia: Lippincott Williams & Wilkins; 2006:1718, with permission.)

Anterior Hip Dislocation
- Mechanism—forced abduction with the hip in a flexed position or forced hyperextension of the hip
- Extremity position—abducted and externally rotated

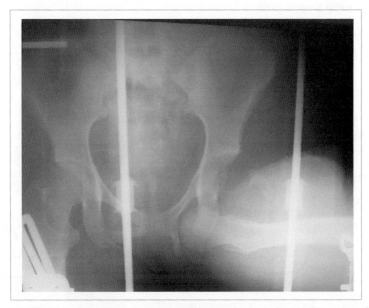

FIGURE 55.3: Anteroposterior pelvis radiograph of an anterior hip dislocation of the left hip. (From Tornetta Paul III. Hip dislocations and fractures of the femoral head. In: Bucholz RW, Heckman JD, Court-Brown C, eds. *Rockwood and green's fractures in adults*, Vol. 2, 6th ed. Philadelphia: Lippincott Williams & Wilkins; 2006:1720, with permission.)

Technique

- **Preprocedure**
  - Radiographs
    - ▷ Should be obtained preprocedure only if there is a concern for a fracture or to determine the position of the dislocation

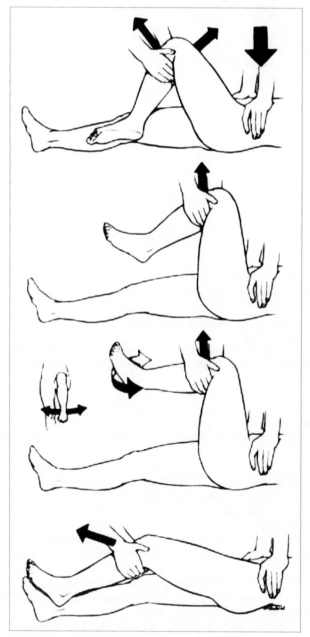

FIGURE 55.4: Allis maneuver for reduction of posterior hip dislocation. (From Tornetta Paul III. Hip dislocations and fractures of the femoral head. In: Bucholz RW, Heckman JD, Court-Brown C, eds. *Rockwood and green's fractures in adults*, Vol 2, 6th ed. Philadelphia: Lippincott Williams & Wilkins; 2006:1730, with permission.)

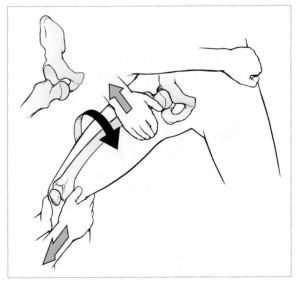

FIGURE 55.5: Modified Allis maneuver for reduction of anterior hip dislocation. (From Tornetta Paul III. Hip dislocations and fractures of the femoral head. In: Bucholz RW, Heckman JD, Court-Brown C, eds. *Rockwood and green's fractures in adults*, Vol 2, 6th ed. Philadelphia: Lippincott Williams & Wilkins; 2006:1730, with permission.)

- IV sedation and muscle relaxation
  - Current best practice involves the use of procedural sedation and analgesia before reduction.

■ **Posterior Dislocation Reduction: Allis Maneuver**
- Patient is placed supine.
- Downward stabilization of the pelvis is performed by an assistant.
- With the knee flexed, apply in-line traction with gentle flexion of the hip to 90 degrees.
- Perform gentle internal-to-external rotation as the hip is flexed.
- Once reduction is achieved, legs are immobilized in slight abduction through the placement of pillows between the knees.
- Repeat physical examination to ensure neurovascular integrity of the affected extremity.
- The reduced hip should be tested for stability by gently placing it through full range of motion to test if the hip will dislocate again.
- Reduction is confirmed by repeat radiographs.

■ **Anterior Dislocation Reduction**
- Patient is placed supine.
- Downward stabilization of the pelvis is performed by an assistant.
- In-line traction is applied as the hip is simultaneously flexed and internally rotated.
- Once the head clears the rim of the acetabulum, the hip is abducted.
- Once reduction is achieved, legs are immobilized in slight abduction through the placement of pillows between the knees.
- A repeat physical examination should be performed to ensure neurovascular integrity of the affected extremity.
- The reduced hip should be tested for stability by gently placing it through full range of motion to test if the hip will dislocate again.
- Reduction is confirmed by repeat radiographs.

Complications
- Sciatic nerve injury
- Avascular necrosis of the femoral head
- Converting a dislocation to a fracture/dislocation
- Traumatic arthritis
- Joint instability

Common Pitfalls
- Use of inadequate sedation
- Inadequate pain control
- Inadequate force for traction
- Delay in reduction

Pearls
- Posterior hip dislocations constitute 80% to 90% of hip dislocations.
- Orthopedic consultation should be obtained for hip dislocation in the presence of a fracture.
- Stabilization of the pelvis by an assistant greatly improves the ease of reduction.
- Traction should be applied inferior to the knee in line with the deformity.
- If evidence of neurovascular injury exists, the dislocation should be treated as an emergency and should be reduced immediately.
- Avascular necrosis of the femoral head is a major concern in hip dislocations; to minimize the risk, reduction should be performed as soon as possible.
- Reduction of prosthetic hip dislocations should be left to the orthopedic consultant secondary to risks of loosening components of the prosthesis, fracture of the surrounding bone, or movement of the acetabular capsule.

Suggested Readings

Green DP, DeLee JC. *Fractures and dislocations of the hip—fractures in adults*, Vol 2. Philadelphia: JB Lippincott Co; 1991.

Marx J, Hockberger R, Walls R. *Rosen's emergency medicine: Concepts and clinical practice*, 6th ed. Mosby; 2006:756–759.

Roberts JR, Hedges JR. *Clinical procedures in emergency medicine*, 4th ed. WB Saunders; 2004:975–981.

Tintinalli JE, Kelen GD, Stapczynski JS. *Emergency medicine: A comprehensive study guide*, 6th ed. McGraw-Hill; 2004:1723–1725.

56 Ankle Dislocation and Reduction

Cassandra Jo Haddox and Mara S. Aloi

Indications
- Dislocated Ankle Joint
    - Demonstrated on plain film radiographs
    - Clinically dislocated with neurovascular compromise

Contraindications
- Open dislocations without neurovascular compromise may be better managed in the operating room with prior cleaning before reduction
- After one or two unsuccessful attempts at reduction, orthopedic consultation should be considered

Risk/Consent Issues
- Neurovascular damage may result from reduction attempt
- Closed reduction may be unsuccessful and operative repair may be required
- Risks of IV analgesia/sedation
- Risks of regional anesthesia

Landmarks
- The ankle joint is a modified saddle joint that comprises the distal fibula, tibia, and the talus bone of the foot.
- Is a stable joint with strong ligamentous support.
- Dislocations are a result of great forces applied to the ankle and are often associated with fractures; pure dislocations are uncommon.

Technique
- **Preprocedure Examination**
    - Search for other injuries, especially if high-energy mechanism.
    - Check neurovascular status of the foot.
    - Get prereduction radiographs of dislocation (anteroposterior [AP], lateral, mortise views).
        - If there is neurovascular compromise, perform reduction before radiograph.
    - Try to ascertain the mechanism of injury.
- **Analgesia and Sedation**
    - Conscious (or ''moderate'') sedation
    - Regional analgesia
        - Bier block
        - Hematoma block
- **Procedure:** Technique depends on type of dislocation

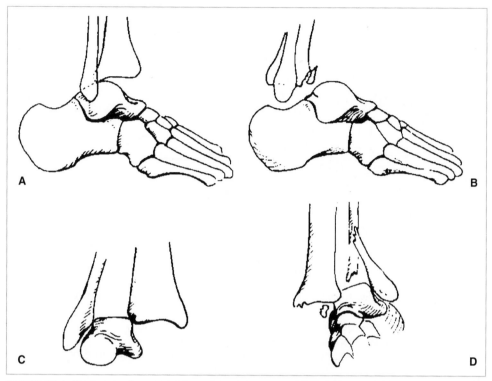

FIGURE 56.1: Four types of ankle dislocations. **A:** Posterior. **B:** Anterior. **C:** Superior. **D:** Lateral. (From Simon RR, Brenner BE. *Emergency procedures and techniques*, 4th ed. Philadelphia: Lippincott Williams & Wilkins; 2002:285, with permission.)

Posterior Dislocation
- Usually result of forced plantar flexion or a strong forward force applied to the posterior tibia
- Most are associated with a fracture of one or more malleoli
- Presents typically with the ankle held in plantar flexion with foot shortened in appearance and resistant to dorsiflexion
- Technique
  - Patient is placed in supine position and the knee is flexed to 45 degrees to relax the Achilles tendon.
  - If two people are available this can be done by an assistant, or the patient's knee can hang over the end of the bed.
  - Assistant also provides countertraction over the calf.
  - Physician places one hand on the heel and the other on the forefoot.
  - Plantar flex the foot while pulling it forward and applying downward traction. Assistant provides downward pressure on the lower leg.

Anterior Dislocation
- Usually result of forced dorsiflexion of the foot or a blow to the tibia directed posteriorly while the foot is fixed
- Dorsalis pedis pulse may be lost secondary to pressure from the talus
- Most common cause is deceleration injuries as seen in motor vehicle accidents
- Also associated with malleolar fractures or a fracture of the anterior lip of the tibia

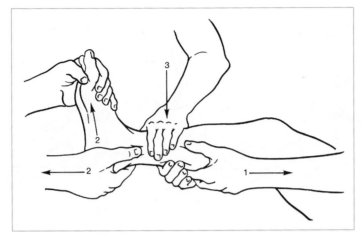

FIGURE 56.2: Technique of reduction of posterior dislocation of the ankle. (From Shah K. Ankle and foot injuries. In: Wolfson AB, ed. *Harwood-Nuss' clinical practice of emergency medicine*, 4th ed. Philadelphia: Lippincott Williams & Wilkins; 2005:1097, with permission.)

- Presents typically with foot held in dorsiflexion with elongated appearance
- Technique
  - Establish same patient setup as in posterior dislocation.
  - Assistant provides countertraction over the calf.
  - Physician places one hand on the heel and the other on the forefoot.
  - Slightly dorsiflex the foot to free the talus.
  - Straight longitudinal traction is applied while the foot is pushed directly backward.
  - Assistant provides upward pressure on the back of the lower leg.

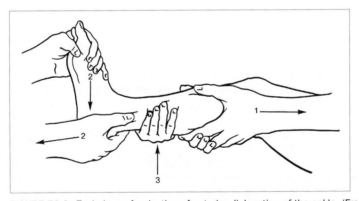

FIGURE 56.3: Technique of reduction of anterior dislocation of the ankle. (From Shah K. Ankle and foot injuries. In: Wolfson AB, ed. *Harwood-Nuss' clinical practice of emergency medicine*, 4th ed. Philadelphia: Lippincott Williams & Wilkins; 2005:1097, with permission.)

Superior Dislocation

- Uncommon
- Usually result of significant axial force resulting in diastasis of the tibiofibular joint (talus driven upward into the mortise)
- Commonly results from a person landing on his feet from a significant height

- Emergency consultation with an orthopedist required for open reduction and internal fixation
- Evaluate carefully for a concomitant spine injury
- Technique
  - Splint, then call for an emergent consultation with an orthopedist.

Lateral Dislocation

- Most common ankle dislocation seen in the emergency department (ED)
- Usually result of marked inversion of the foot
- Always associated with malleolar fractures or distal fibula fracture
- Less commonly associated with rupture of the deltoid ligament
- Presents with foot laterally displaced with the skin very taut over the medial aspect of the ankle joint
- Technique
  - Place one hand on the heel and the other on the forefoot.
  - Apply longitudinal traction to the foot.
  - While assistant applies countertraction to the leg, gently manipulate the foot medially. Usually produces a palpable thud.
  - Orthopedic consultation is generally required.

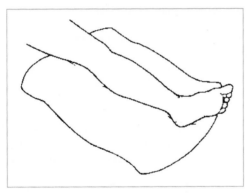

FIGURE 56.4: The typical position of a lateral ankle dislocation. (From Simon RR, Koenigsjnecht SJ: Emergency Orthopedics: The Extremities. New York: McGraw-Hill, 524, 2000, with permission.)

Postreduction Care

- Recheck neurovascular status and document the findings.
- Order postreduction radiographs.
- Adequate immobilization is required for comfort and to prevent repeat dislocation.
  - Ankle is splinted at 90 degrees with a long-leg posterior splint.
- Follow-up for orthopedic consultation is required within 48 to 72 hours for closed fractures without neurovascular compromise.
- Open injuries or fracture dislocations with neurovascular compromise require emergent orthopedic consultation.
- Recommendations for follow-up care are dependent on the injury and its severity. Necessity to admit to the hospital must be determined in consultation with an orthopedic surgeon.
- Patient should not bear weight on that extremity for approximately 6 weeks.

Complications
- Nonunion or malunion
- Synostosis—union of two or more bones to form one bone
- Entrapment of the tibialis posterior tendon or of a fracture fragment
- Cartilaginous injury
- Osteochondral fractures of the talar dome
- Joint stiffness and decreased range of motion
- Arterial injury (anterior and posterior tibial, peroneal)
- Avascular necrosis of the talus
- Compartment syndrome (rare)

Common Pitfalls
- Inadequate analgesia and muscle relaxation
- Failure to assess vascular integrity immediately
  - Delaying reduction for x-rays
- Failure to check neurovascular status after reduction attempts

Pearls
- Knowledge of the anatomy and forces which caused the injury aid in choosing proper reduction maneuver.
- Use adequate doses of analgesic agents and muscle relaxants.
- Proceed in a slow and gentle manner.
- Contact an orthopedist if multiple attempts in reduction are needed.

Suggested Readings

Banks AS, Downey MS, Martin DE, et al. *McGlamry's comprehensive textbook of foot and ankle surgery*, 3rd ed. Philadelphia: Lippincott Williams & Wilkins; 2001.

Connolly JF. *The management of fractures and dislocations: An atlas*, 3rd ed. Philadelphia: WB Saunders; 1981.

Coughlin MJ, Mann RA. *Surgery of the foot and ankle*, 7th ed. New York: Mosby; 1999.

Hedges JR, Roberts JR. *Clinical procedures in emergency medicine*, 4th ed. Philadelphia: WB Saunders; 2004.

Koenigsknecht SJ, Simon RR. *Emergency orthopedics: The extremities*, 4th ed. New York: McGraw-Hill; 2001.

Shah K. Ankle and foot injuries. In: *The clinical practice of emergency medicine*, 4th ed. Philadelphia: Lippincott Williams & Wilkins; 2005.

Simon RR, Brenner BE. *Emergency procedures and techniques*, 4th ed. Philadelphia: Lippincott Williams & Wilkins; 2002:284–285.

57

Digit Dislocation and Reduction

Taylor J. Kallas and David J. Berkoff

Indications
- Clinical suspicion of digit dislocation
  - Obvious deformity of the joint
  - History of trauma to joint
- Radiographic evidence of dislocation

Contraindications
- Any fracture associated with the dislocation
- Thumb dislocation
  - Owing to entrapment of the volar plate, it will be difficult to reduce this joint without operative intervention

Landmarks
- Nerves run on lateral surface of digits at the 2, 4, 8, and 10 o'clock positions
- Flexor tendons run on volar surface of digit
- Extensor tendons run on dorsal surface of digit
- Collateral ligaments maintain stability on lateral surface of joints (see Fig. 57.1)

Risks/Consent Issues
- Patients with failed closed reduction will usually need open reduction
  - When failing after two attempts under sufficient anesthesia, suspect a complex dislocation
- Many patients will have persistent pain and/or swelling after reduction
- Risk of causing further damage during reduction

Technique
- **Anesthesia**
  - Before attempting any digit reduction, a digital block is recommended for anesthesia.
  - See Chapter 41 for various techniques.
- **Finger Dislocations**
  - Proximal interphalangeal (PIP) joint dislocations
    - Dorsal PIP dislocations
      - Reduced by hyperextending the joint and gently adding longitudinal traction followed by dorsal pressure on the base of the middle phalanx while moving the digit back into flexion.
      - After reduction is accomplished, the finger should be tested for stability in flexion, extension, and lateral motion.

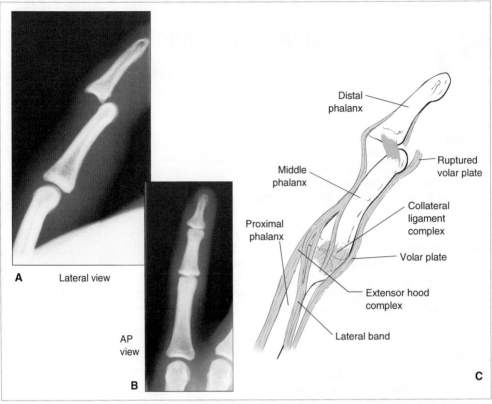

FIGURE 57.1: Radiographic (A, B) and schematic (C) representation of an interphalangeal joint dislocation. AP, anteroposterior. (From Young GM. Reduction of common joint dislocations and subluxations. In: Henretig FM, King C, eds. *Textbook of pediatric emergency procedures.* Philadelphia: Williams & Wilkins; 1997:1080, with permission.)

- Once the joint is determined to be stable, the finger should be splinted in 20 to 30 degrees of flexion for 3 weeks. Another option is wrapping the joint with a self-adherent wrap (e.g., Coban) and buddy taping the finger for 3 to 6 weeks.
- Referral to a hand surgeon is recommended, especially for those with significant articular fractures.
- Volar PIP dislocations
  - Is much less common than dorsal dislocations.
  - Reduction is performed by hyperflexing the finger then using gentle longitudinal traction.
  - The PIP should be splinted in full extension for 3 weeks and patient should be referred to a hand surgeon for follow-up.
  - Volar dislocations are often complicated by injury to the central slip of the extensor tendons. This is important because if these injuries are improperly splinted, a boutonniere deformity may develop. These injuries should be splinted in full extension for a minimum of 6 weeks.
  - Owing to the complications associated with these dislocations, referral to a hand surgeon is required.
- Lateral PIP dislocations
  - Easily reduced by gentle extension in the direction of the injury and longitudinal traction.

♦ After reduction the digit may be buddy taped or splinted.
♦ Referral to hand surgeon is recommended (see Fig. 57.2).

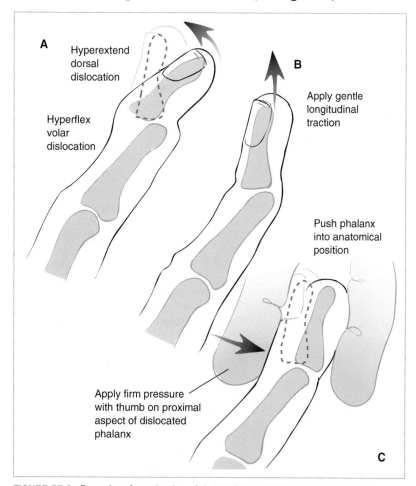

FIGURE 57.2: Procedure for reduction of dorsal distal interphalangeal (DIP) joint dislocation. (From Young GM. Reduction of common joint dislocations and subluxations. In: Henretig FM, King C, eds. *Textbook of pediatric emergency procedures*. Philadelphia: Williams & Wilkins, 1997:1080, with permission.)

○ Distal interphalangeal (DIP) joint dislocations
  ▷ Most commonly are dorsal dislocations.
  ▷ Reduce using the same techniques described in dorsal PIP dislocations.
  ▷ Range of motion may be partially intact in a DIP injury.
  ▷ Do not confuse with a mallet finger injury.
○ Metacarpal phalangeal (MCP) joint dislocations (see Fig. 57.3)
  ▷ Volar dislocations are infrequent and will nearly always require open reduction.
  ▷ Dorsal MCP dislocations are most common.
    ♦ May be either simple or complex.
    ♦ Complex dislocations occur when the volar plate becomes trapped in the joint and these usually require open reduction.
    ♦ Closed reduction of simple dorsal dislocation is accomplished by first placing the wrist into flexion to relax flexor tendons. Next step is to

hyperextend the joint and then apply pressure at base of proximal phalanx while bringing the back into flexion.

- Longitudinal traction should be avoided in these injuries as it may convert a simple dislocation into a complex one.
- Splint with the MCP joint in 30 degrees of flexion.

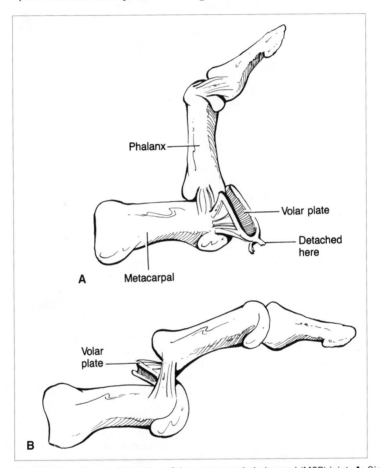

FIGURE 57.3: Dorsal dislocation of the metacarpal phalangeal (MCP) joint. **A:** Simple dorsal dislocation. **B:** Complex dorsal dislocation; note entrapment of the volar plate. (From Jackimczyk K, Shepherd SM, Blackburn P. Hand injuries. In: Wolfson AB, ed. *Harwood-Nuss' clinical practice of emergency medicine*, 4th ed. Philadelphia: Lippincott Williams & Wilkins; 2005:1064, with permission.)

Toe Dislocations
- Metatarsal phalangeal (MTP) joint dislocations
  - Dislocation of the MTP joint is nearly always a dorsal dislocation due to a hyperextension injury
  - May be simple or complex as with MCP joint dislocations
  - Reduction is accomplished by first plantar flexing the ankle to relax the flexor tendons. Next step is to hyperextend the joint along with gentle longitudinal traction and applying pressure at the base of proximal phalanx while bringing the digit back into flexion.
  - Toe should then be placed in a dorsal splint and patient should be referred for orthopedic follow-up.

- Interphalangeal joint dislocations
  - ▶ Dislocation of interphalangeal (IP) joint is usually due to an injury that provides an axial load in the toe.
  - ▶ These dislocations may be reduced as in the hand by applying longitudinal traction, recreating the injury, and placing pressure at the base of the dislocated phalanx.
  - ▶ Toes are usually buddy taped after reduction for 10 to 14 days for lesser toes and for 3 weeks for first toe IP dislocations.
  - ▶ Patients should be referred for orthopedic follow-up.

Precautions

- Prereduction x-rays are recommended. It is important to include a true lateral film of the injured digit; otherwise it is possible to miss a fracture.
- Joint stability should be assessed after all successful reductions.
- Follow-up with a hand surgeon should be ensured for all patients after reduction.
- If reduction is accomplished in the field before evaluation, a careful history should be taken to try ensure that the injury was not a volar dislocation so that the appropriate splinting method may be applied to avoid boutonniere deformity.

Pearls

- Adequate anesthesia, usually with a digital block, and cooperation of patient maximizes potential for successful reduction.
- Pre- and postreduction films are necessary to determine extent of injury, and proper alignment of joint.
- Referral to hand surgeon is recommended in all patients with dislocations of the fingers due to the long-term disability associated with these injuries.
- Reductions of first MCP dislocations (thumb) are likely to be difficult or impossible if sesamoids are intact.

Suggested Readings

Henretig F, King C. *Textbook of pediatric emergency procedures*. Williams & Wilkins; 1997:1080–1081.

Simon RR, Brenner BE. *Emergency procedures and techniques*, 4th ed. Philadelphia: Lippincott Williams & Wilkins; 2002:282.

Wolfson AB, Linden CH, Shepherd SM, et al. *Harwood-Nuss' clinical practice of emergency medicine*, 4th ed. Philadelphia: Lippincott Williams & Wilkins; 2005: 1064–1066.

Section Editor: Sanjey Gupta

58

Perianal Abscess: Incision and Drainage

Brian Chung and Todd Mastrovitch

Definition
- Resulting from infection of soft tissue surrounding the rectum, which is caused by obstruction of anal crypts and ducts. Untreated abscesses can lead to life-threatening sepsis.

Classification of Anorectal Abscesses
- Perianal: Superficial subcutaneous abscess located at the anal orifice
- Ischiorectal: Located deep to external anal sphincter
- Intersphincteric: Located between internal and external anal sphincters
- Supralevator: Located superior to levator ani muscle, adjacent to rectum (see Fig. 58.1)

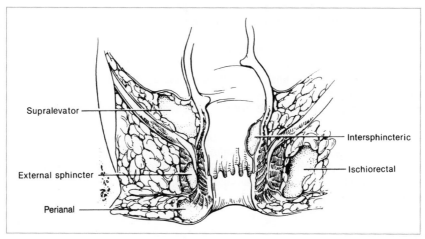

FIGURE 58.1: Anorectal abscesses. (From Coates WC. Perianal, rectal, and anal diseases. In: Wolfson AB, ed. *Harwood-Nuss' clinical practice of emergency medicine,* 4th ed. Philadelphia: Lippincott Williams & Wilkins; 2005:409, with permission.)

Indications/Contraindications
- Only perianal abscesses without fistulae in ano should be treated in the emergency department (ED) or clinic setting. All other perirectal or perianal abscesses with fistula should be drained in the operating room.

Risks/Consent Issues

- Procedure can cause pain (local anesthesia will be given)
- Local bleeding and hematoma formation

Technique

- Consider mild oral sedative or anxiolytic for the patient before procedure.
- Place patient in the prone position.
- Separate buttocks with adhesive tape to the lateral aspect of the hip (see Fig. 58.2).

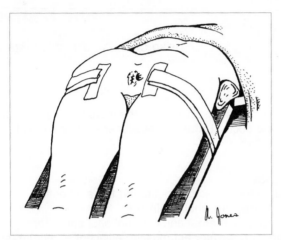

FIGURE 58.2: When excising a thrombosed external hemorrhoid or performing incision and drainage of an anal abscess, separate the buttocks by using 3-in. adhesive tape, as shown, to provide optimal exposure. (From Simon RR, Brenner BE. *Emergency procedures and techniques*, 4th ed. Philadelphia: Lippincott Williams & Wilkins; 2002:33, with permission.)

- Infiltrate area around the abscess with up to 5 mg/kg of 1% lidocaine with epinephrine (1:100,000).
- Using a no.11 blade, a linear or elliptical incision is made over the most fluctuant part of the abscess.
- Express as much as possible from the abscess with gentle squeezing pressure (see Fig. 58.3).
- Explore abscess with a hemostat to break loculations.
- Irrigate the abscess with normal saline (see Fig. 58.4).
- Pack cavity lightly with sterile packing material to allow incision to stay open, thereby allowing continuous drainage.
- Dress wound for patient comfort.

Complications

- Fistula formation
- Systemic infection

Common Pitfalls

- Use of inadequate local anesthesia
- Making the initial skin incision too small
- Failure to adequately break loculations
- Overpacking the wound will not allow for proper drainage and healing

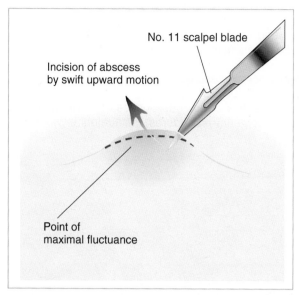

No. 11 scalpel blade

Incision of abscess
by swift upward motion

Point of
maximal fluctuance

FIGURE 58.3: Linear incision of a cutaneous abscess. (From Young GM. Incision and drainage of a cutaneous abscess. In: Henretig FM, King C, eds. *Textbook of pediatric emergency procedures.* Philadelphia: Williams & Wilkins; 1997:1202, with permission.)

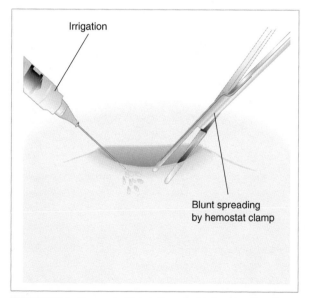

Irrigation

Blunt spreading
by hemostat clamp

FIGURE 58.4: Removal of loculations and irrigation of an abscess. (From Young GM. Incision and drainage of a cutaneous abscess. In: Henretig FM, King C, eds. *Textbook of pediatric emergency procedures.* Philadelphia: Williams & Wilkins; 1997:1203, with permission.)

Pearls

- Antibiotics are generally not required unless overlying cellulitis is present.
- If adequate analgesia cannot be achieved, consider incision and drainage in the operating room (OR) with general anesthesia.
- Packing is to be replaced at 48-hour intervals until infection has cleared.
- Advise the patient to take sitz bath daily for comfort until healing is complete.

Suggested Readings

Coates WC. Perianal, rectal, and anal diseases. In: Wolfson AB, ed. *Harwood-Nuss' clinical practice of emergency medicine*, 4th ed. Philadelphia: Lippincott Williams & Wilkins; 2005:409.

Simon RR, Brenner BE. *Emergency procedures and techniques*, 4th ed. Philadelphia: Lippincott Williams & Wilkins; 2002:33.

Young GM. Incision and drainage of a cutaneous abscess. In: Henretig FM, King C, eds. *Textbook of pediatric emergency procedures*. Philadelphia: Williams & Wilkins; 1997:1203.

59 Paronychia: Incision and Drainage

Alison E. Suarez and Audrey Paul

Definition
- A localized infection around the area of the nail root limited to the area above the nail and beneath the cuticle (perionychium).

Indications
- Localized infection with failure of spontaneous drainage

Contraindications
- Herpetic whitlow (common mimic)
- Coagulopathy

Technique
- Soak eponychium (cuticle).
- Depending on patient age and size of paronychia, consider digital block under sterile setting (see Chapter 41).
- Hold a no. 11 blade or sharp end of a large-bore needle parallel to the nail and insert it through the nail fold until pus is obtained.
- For large paronychia, elevate the nail fold skin and insert small piece of packing gauze to ensure continuous drainage for 24 hours.
- Following removal of packing, soak finger in warm water to promote healing.

Complications
- Osteomyelitis
- Abscess
- Extension of infection
- Destruction of nail matrix, compromising nail growth

Common Pitfalls
- Failure to incise and drain infection, leading to above stated complications
- Failure to recognize herpetic whitlow in which incision and drainage is contraindicated and may cause viremia or bacterial infection

Pearls
- Treat with antibiotics (first-generation cephalosporin) if overlying cellulitis is present.
- Actual skin incision or removal of the nail is rarely required.

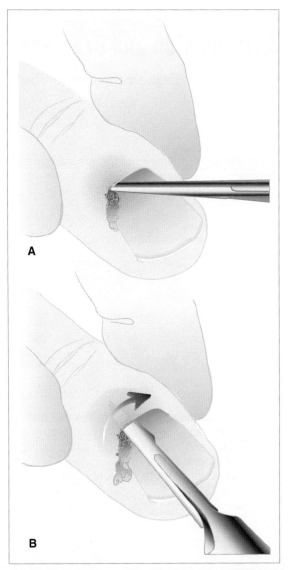

FIGURE 59.1: Drainage of the paronychia. (From Henretig FM. Incision and drainage of a paronychia. In: Henretig FM, King C, eds. *Textbook of pediatric emergency procedures*. Philadelphia: Williams & Wilkins; 1997:1207, with permission.)

- Drainage can sometimes occur on simple lifting of the nail fold skin with sterile needle allowing the pus to drain.
- Chronic infection is most likely due to Candida.
- Chronic paronychias that do not respond to conservative therapy need to be evaluated for possible malignancy.

60 Felon: Incision and Drainage

Alison E. Suarez and Audrey Paul

Definition
- An infection or abscess occurring in the pulp of the volar surface of the distal phalanx

Indications
- Fluctuance of the distal pulp with pain increased upon application of pressure
- Failure of resolution of infection after conservative therapy

Contraindications
- Herpetic whitlow (common mimic)
- Infection extending proximal to distal interphalangeal (DIP) joint
- Coagulopathy

Risks/Consent Issues
- Procedure can cause pain (local anesthesia will be given)
- Local bleeding or hematoma formation
- Infection (sterile technique will be utilized)

Technique
- Immobilize the involved digit.
- Perform digital block under sterile setting (see Chapter 41).
- Apply tourniquet for hemostasis.
- Types of incision:
  - Vertical incision—most favored for definite
  - Lateral J-shaped incision—avoid the digital nerve by making the incision just below the nail
- Make incision at area of maximal fluctuance.
- Disrupt loculations GENTLY using curved hemostat.
- Irrigate wound with sterile saline using 18-gauge catheter.
- GENTLY pack with gauze, which is removed in 24 to 48 hours.
- Apply nonadhesive dressing.
- Splint the involved finger.
- Encourage elevation to minimize pain.

Complications
- Digital nerve injury
- Osteomyelitis
- Painful neuroma

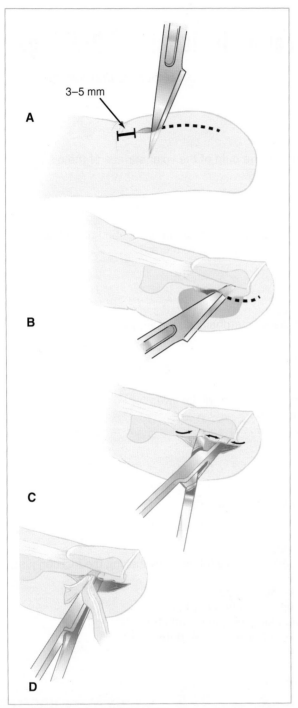

3–5 mm

A

B

C

D

FIGURE 60.1: **A:** Longitudinal incision on the palmar surface of the distal finger. **B:** J-shaped lateral incision of a felon. **C:** Disruption of loculations within a felon. **D:** Wick placement. (From Bethel CA. Incision and drainage of a felon. In: Henretig FM, King C, eds. *Textbook of pediatric emergency procedures*. Philadelphia: Williams & Wilkins; 1997:1214, with permission.)

- Flexor tenosynovitis
- Skin necrosis
- Septic arthritis
- Fingertip deformity

Common Pitfalls
- Incision and drainage of herpetic whitlow
- Use of conservative treatment in cases where incision and drainage are necessary
- Incision that crosses crease of DIP joint resulting in finger contracture and deformity

Pearls
- Proper technique of drainage has been controversial. The vertical incision carried out over the center of the abscess is associated with the lowest rate of complications.
- Use of a fish-mouth incision is associated with a high rate of complications including instability of the finger pad and anesthesia.
- Swelling due to a felon will not typically cross the DIP joint.
- Conscious sedation may be needed if pain is not controlled with digital block.
- If incision and drainage is made over the area of maximal fluctuance, packing may not be required.
- Always administer antistaphylococcal/antistreptococcal antibiotic coverage.
- Ensure close follow-up with a hand surgeon.
- Consider admission for the diabetic or immunocompromised patient.

Suggested Readings
Clark D. Common acute hand infections. *Am Fam Physician*. 2003;68:2167–2176.

Henretig F, King C, eds. *Textbook of pediatric procedures*. Lippincott Williams & Wilkins; 1997.

Jebson PJ. Infections of the fingertip. Paronychias and felons. *Hand Clin*. 1998;14: 547–555.

Rockwell P. Acute and chronic paronychia. *Am Fam Physician*. 2001;63:1113–1116.

Simon R. *Emergency procedures and techniques*, 4th ed. Lippincott Williams & Wilkins; 2002.

Wolfson AB, ed. *Harwood-Nuss' clinical practice of emergency medicine*, 4th ed. Lippincott Williams & Wilkins; 2005.

61

Subungual Hematoma

Peter A. Binkley and David Barlas

Indications

- Trephination: To create a fistula through the nail to the hematoma
  - Used for the decompression, drainage, and pain relief of simple subungual hematomas
- Nail removal and nail bed laceration repair
  - Used for large hematomas that cannot be managed adequately with trephination or elevation of the nail
  - Used for nail bed lacerations
  - Used for partial nail avulsion or subluxation when the nail is unstable or when there is nail fold disruption

Contraindications

- Significant crush injuries or missing/destroyed nail matrix warrant specialty consultation

Risks/Consent Issues

- Procedure can cause pain (local anesthesia will be given for nail bed repairs)
- Local bleeding
- Infection can develop after any wound repair (sterile technique will be utilized)

Landmarks

- Typical subungual hematomas are on the sterile matrix under the nail
- Germinal matrix: Region where new nail is formed
  - This area should not be injured during trephination and repair
  - Injury to this area should be documented and referred to a specialist to ensure optimal cosmetic outcome

Technique

- Obtain x-ray of digit if bone fracture is a consideration.
- **Trephination**
  - The goal is to form a hole of sufficient size through the nail to drain the hematoma.
  - An 18-gauge needle, scalpel, heated paper clip, disposable electrocautery device, or drill may be utilized.
  - If using a needle or scalpel, apply gentle pressure with the tip of the instrument perpendicular to the surface of the nail, twisting the instrument until blood is released.
  - A heated paper clip creates a wider hole but may tattoo the nail bed.

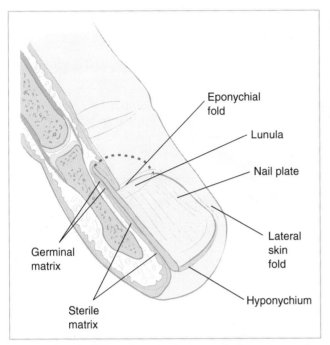

FIGURE 61.1: Anatomy of the finger and nail bed. (From Eberlein R. Hand and finger injuries. In: Henretig FM, King C, eds. *Textbook of pediatric emergency procedures*. Philadelphia: Williams & Wilkins, 1997:1048, with permission.)

- Electrocautery or drilling is quickly performed and effective.
- Instructions upon discharge are to soak the finger in warm water twice a day for 7 days to allow the blood to continue to drain.
- **Nail Bed Laceration Repair**
  - Perform digital block under sterile setting (see Chapter 41).
  - Gather needed materials: Iris scissors, hemostats, and suture set with fine absorbable sutures (5-0 to 7-0 chromic or Vicryl).
  - Apply tourniquet for hemostasis.
  - Remove the nail from the nail bed matrix.
    - Insert closed Iris scissors along the underside of the nail horizontally.
    - Gently spread the scissors and advance in repeated movements, gradually progressing to the nail root and separating the entire nail from the nail bed.
    - Once the nail is free from the nail bed and eponychium, it is grasped with hemostats and gently pulled using longitudinal traction freeing the nail.
  - Repair the nail bed laceration.
    - Using fine absorbable sutures, suture the laceration with interrupted stitches.
    - Significantly destroyed nail beds or germinal matrix involvement should prompt hand surgeon consultation.
    - Rinse and reinsert the nail in the anatomic position.
    - If necessary, secure the nail with a 5-0 suture stitch.
    - If the nail is damaged or not available, gently pack petroleum gauze between the nail matrix and eponychium.
  - Splint the finger.

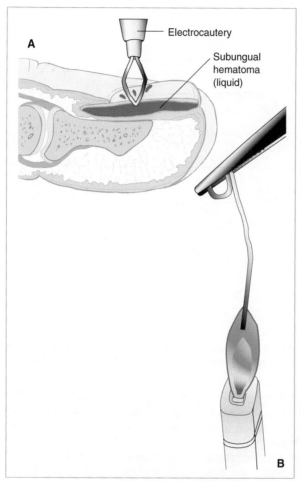

FIGURE 61.2: Nail trephination. (From Eberlein R. Hand and finger injuries. In: Henretig FM, King C, eds. *Textbook of pediatric emergency procedures*. Philadelphia: Williams & Wilkins, 1997:1051, with permission.)

- Discharge instructions are to maintain elevation of digit and to return for wound check in 2 days.
- The replaced nail should be left in place for 2 to 3 weeks.

Complications
- Infection
- Poor cosmetic outcome
    - Split nail
    - Adhesions between cuticle and nail matrix

Common Pitfalls
- Failure to obtain x-ray and diagnose fracture
- Failure to recognize and treat nail bed laceration

Pearls

- Advise patient that there is no guarantee of the final cosmetic outcome.
- Always suspect tuft fracture with significant nail bed lacerations.
- Oral antibiotics are indicated when patients have a concurrent fracture since this technically constitutes an open fracture; osteomyelitis of the distal phalanx after tuft fracture and subungual hematoma is very uncommon.

62

Wound Closure and Suture Techniques

Anthony Berger and Brenda L. Liu

Indications

- Goals are to optimize wound strength, reduce inflammation, avoid infection, and minimize scar formation
  - Time to wound cleaning is the most important factor
  - To preserve viable tissue and restore continuity and function of tissue

Contraindications

- Heavily contaminated wounds
- Presentation time for primary closure is after 12 hours for standard lacerations.
- Presentation time for primary closure is after 24 hours for lacerations of the face or other highly vascular areas.
- Wounds under high tension should not be closed by skin adhesives alone.
- Any animal or human bite and most puncture wounds should not be closed acutely.

Risk/Consent Issues

- Cleaning of and repair of wounds cause pain.
  - Local anesthetics are indicated for all wound repairs in conscious, alert patients.
- Infection is always a risk in wound repair.
- Wound repair always results in some scarring and can affect cosmetic appearance permanently.
- Tendon, nerve, and vascular injury can occur at time of initial injury or at time of repair.
- Risk of retained foreign body exists despite best methods of foreign body identification and removal, such as local exploration, radiographs, ultrasonography, and irrigation.
  - Adequate exploration for foreign bodies must be performed and documented.

Technique

- **Patient and Wound Preparation**
  - Position the patient to prevent falling or fainting during wound repair.
  - Practice universal precautions.
  - Prepare the surrounding skin with povidone-iodine solution and cover with sterile drapes before manipulation of any kind.
- **Local anesthesia:** Lidocaine (1% or 2%) with or without epinephrine
  - Epinephrine is contraindicated in areas of high risk for ischemia, such as fingers, ears, nose, toes, and penis.
  - Use small gauge needle (25 or 27 gauge) to directly inject into subcutaneous tissue within the laceration.
  - To decrease pain, inject through the wound and not through the skin.

- Use adequate amount for anesthesia but avoid high volumes that will lead to significant tissue distortion, possible cosmetic embarrassment, or systemic toxicity.
  - Maximum dose: 3 to 5 mg/kg 1% lidocaine, 7 mg/kg 1% lidocaine with epinephrine
- Consider regional blocks for repairs in cosmetically important areas (face, hands, etc.) to avoid distortion of tissue.
- **Wound cleansing:** Copious amounts of sterile water or sterile saline via high-power irrigation with a large syringe and splatter shield or an 18-gauge catheter.
- **Wound Exploration**
  - After cleansing, the true depth of the wound is appreciated.
  - Look for deeper tissue involvement and explore the wound.
  - If tendon or vascular structures are visualized, inspect through full range of motion and test for state of function.
- **Radiography and/or sonography:** If the possibility of underlying fracture and/or foreign body exists, image the affected area and document.
- **Select Method of Repair**
  - Dermabond
  - Staples
  - Sutures

Dermabond (Liquid Adhesive)
- Indicated for simple wounds under low tension
- **Advantages**
  - Ease of use, speed, and safety
  - No return visit necessary (sloughs off in 5 to 10 days and serves as own dressing)
  - Much less painful
- **Disadvantages**
  - Moderate closure strength—cannot be used on joints or areas with high tension
  - Cannot be used in hairy areas
- Caution when using around eyes to prevent accidental runoff into eyes
- Equivalent tensile strength at 7 days when compared to sutures
- **Procedure**
  - Clean the wound.
  - Approximate wound edges with forceps or fingers.
  - Apply three to four layers along the wound length or perpendicularly to it (as strips).
  - Maintain manual support for 60 seconds.

Staples
- Indicated for superficial scalp lacerations, linear lacerations on extremities, scalp or trunk, and wounds under low tension.
- **Advantages**
  - Ease of use, speed, and safety
  - Easily removed and excellent tensile strength
- **Disadvantages**
  - Less refined closure
  - Possible greater scarring
  - Uncomfortable removal

TABLE 62.1: Suture size and location

Size	Superficial (nonabsorbable)	Deep (absorbable)
2-0	Suture chest tube	
3-0	Foot	Chest, abdomen, back
4-0	Scalp, chest, abdomen, foot, extremity	Scalp, extremity, foot
5-0	Scalp, brow, mouth, chest, abdomen, hand	Brow, nose, lip, face, hand
6-0	Ear, lid, brow, face, mouth, nose	

- No significant differences found with infection, healing, or patient acceptance when compared to suturing.
- **Procedure**
  - Anesthetize and clean wound (debride as necessary).
  - Cover with sterile drapes.
  - If necessary, close deep fascia with absorbable sutures.
  - Evert wound edges before placing staple, if possible utilizing the services of an assistant with forceps. Do not press too hard.
  - Allow the staple crossbar to sit 1 to 2 mm above wound edge.
  - Place enough staples to adequately appose tissue edges.

Sutures
- **General Rules**
  - Deep stitches require 3-0 or 4-0 absorbable sutures.
  - Skin closure requires 4-0 or 5-0 nonabsorbable sutures.
  - Face, lips, eyelid wounds: Consider 6-0 sutures.
  - High skin tension areas: Consider 3-0 or 4-0 sutures.
  - Always select the smallest size that will hold the skin edges together.
- **Nonabsorbable Sutures**
  - **Silk:** Has the best knot security, the best tie ability, the least tensile strength, and causes significant tissue reactivity. Used in intraoral mucosa.
  - **Ethilon:** Has good knot security, good tensile strength, minimal tissue reactivity, and good tie ability. Best suited suture material for typical wound closure.
  - **Prolene:** Poorest knot security, best tensile strength, least tissue reactivity, and fair tie ability.
- **Absorbable Sutures**
  - **Vicryl:** Good knot security, good tensile strength, minimal tissue reactivity, best tie ability, 30-day suture duration. Used for deep repair to reduce wound tension.
  - **Surgical and chromic gut:** Fair knot security, fair tensile strength, greatest tissue reactivity, poor tie ability, 5- to 7-day suture duration. Used for intraoral wounds.
- **Procedure**
  - Anesthetize and clean wound (debride as necessary).
  - Prepare the skin with povidone-iodine or chlorhexidine solution
  - Minimize trauma by handling skin with toothed forceps and by using small sutures.
  - Relieve tension by undermining with a scissor and by using layered sutures.

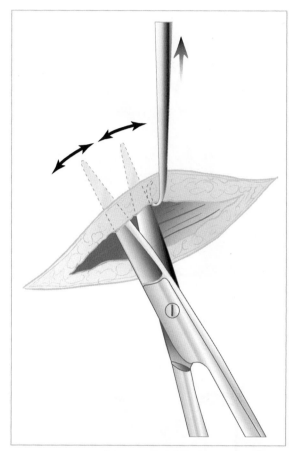

FIGURE 62.1: Undermining a wound reduces the degree of tension present after the repair. (From McNamara R, Loiselle J. Laceration repair. In: Henretig FM, King C, eds. *Textbook of pediatric emergency procedures*. Philadelphia: Williams & Wilkins; 1997:1152, with permission.)

- **Subcutaneous layer closure**
  - ▷ Reapproximate fascia as needed.
  - ▷ Close the subcutaneous layer in sections, starting in the middle and then bisecting adjacent sections until adequate tension has been relieved from the skin edges.
  - ▷ Insert the suture at the bottom of the layer and draw it through to just beneath the dermis on the same side of the wound.
  - ▷ Re-enter beneath the dermis on the adjacent side and draw through to the bottom of the subcutaneous (SQ) layer.
  - ▷ Tie the knot such that it remains at the bottom of the wound, thereby preventing a palpable knot near the skin surface.
- **Interrupted stitch**
  - ▷ Most commonly used stitch. If one fails, the rest will maintain closure.
  - ▷ Insert the needle at 90 degrees to the skin surface and include sufficient SQ tissue in the bite and carry the suture through to the opposite side.
  - ▷ Generally, the distance between sutures should equal the distance from the wound to the needle insertion site for each stitch.
  - ▷ The stitch depth should be greater than its width to produce eversion of wound edges.

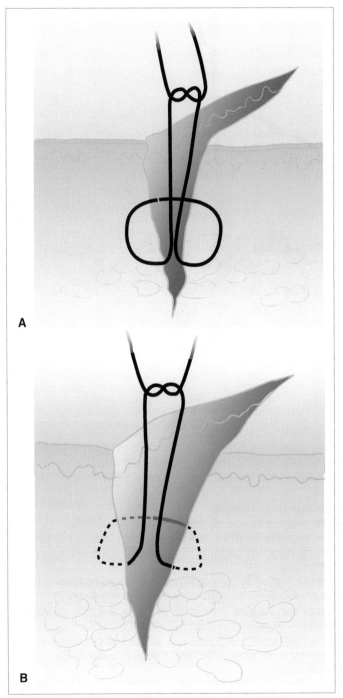

FIGURE 62.2: **A:** The buried subcutaneous suture. **B:** The horizontal dermal stitch. (From McNamara R, Loiselle J. Laceration repair. In: Henretig FM, King C, eds. *Textbook of pediatric emergency procedures*. Philadelphia: Williams & Wilkins; 1997:1155, with permission.)

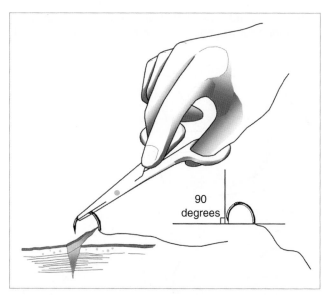

FIGURE 62.3: Interrupted stitch. Courtesy of Anthony Berger.

▷ Tying the knot requires an initial double loop around the needle driver, and then only one loop for the next three to four ties, alternating directions with each one for a strong durable knot.

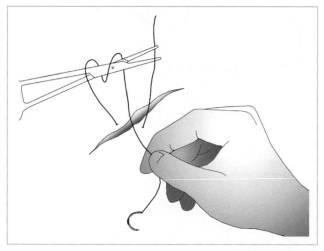

FIGURE 62.4: First tie of an interrupted stitch. Courtesy of Anthony Berger.

- **Mattress stitch**
    - ▷ Variation of the interrupted stitch, which can be vertical or horizontal
    - ▷ Used when approximation of wound edges requires more tensile strength
    - ▷ Vertical mattress stitch
        - ◆ The first stitch is made by passing the needle more widely separated from the wound edges and deeper into the wound than usual.
        - ◆ The needle is then passed back through the epidermis and lower dermis taking a small bite of the skin from both sides and approximating the edges.

◆   Tie the suture as an initial double loop around the needle driver, then one loop for the next three to four ties, alternating directions with each throw.

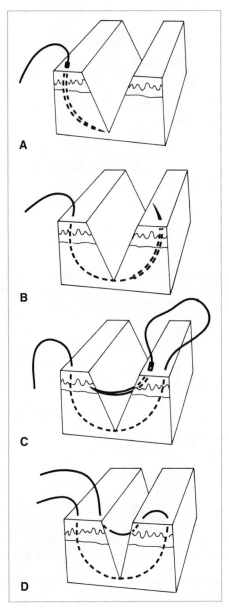

A

B

C

D

FIGURE 62.5: Vertical mattress stitch. (From Simon RR, Brenner BE. *Emergency procedures and techniques,* 4th ed. Philadelphia: Lippincott Williams & Wilkins; 2002:379, with permission.)

▶   Horizontal mattress stitch
    ◆   The first stitch is made 0.5 to 1 cm away from the wound edge.
    ◆   Pass the needle through the opposite side.
    ◆   Then enter the skin perpendicularly to the last motion and exit on the other side of the wound.

◆ Tie the suture as an initial double loop around the needle driver, then one loop for the next three to four ties, alternating directions with each throw.

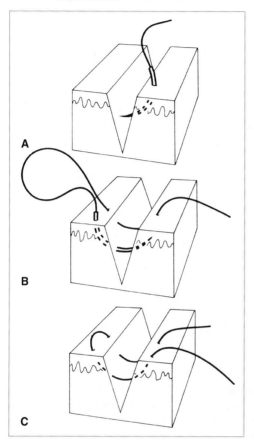

FIGURE 62.6: Horizontal mattress stitch. **A:** Pass the needle 0.5 to 1 cm away from wound edge deeply into the wound. **B:** Then pass the needle through the opposite side so it reenters the wound parallel to the initial suture. **C:** Enter the skin perpendicularly to provide some eversion of the wound edges, and enter and exit both the wound and skin at the same depth; otherwise, "buckling" and irregularities occur in the wound margin. (From Simon RR, Brenner BE. *Emergency procedures and techniques,* 4th ed. Philadelphia: Lippincott Williams & Wilkins; 2002:381, with permission.)

Continuous or "running" stitch
  ▶ Used for linear wounds that require minimal debridement.
  ▶ Advantages include speed of repair, strength, and minimal knot tying.
  ▶ Disadvantages
      ◆ One break in the stitch will cause the entire repair to unravel
      ◆ Sutures with differing tensions along the wound
  ▶ Technique
      ◆ Begin with a single suture that is tied to anchor the rest of the suture.
      ◆ Do not cut the stitch.
      ◆ Pass the needle perpendicular to the skin edge (the same distance and depth as interrupted stitches) continuously, until the edge of the wound is reached.
      ◆ After each pass, pull the suture thread to keep the wound closed.

◆ Close the running stitch by leaving a loop on one end of the wound that can be tied to the remaining suture thread as you would in a simple interrupted stitch (see Fig. 62.7).

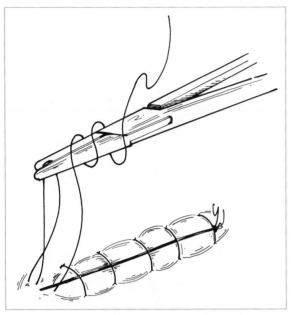

FIGURE 62.7: Running stitch. Courtesy of Anthony Berger.

Follow-up and Suture/Staple Removal

▪ Patients should be instructed to have a wound check in 2 days if wound is at high risk for infection or if patient is at high risk, such as a diabetic or immunocompromised patient.
▪ Consider antibiotics for patients with high-risk wounds.
  ◦ Antibiotic selection varies by institution and region and should be chosen on the basis of likely pathogen.
▪ The proper removal time of sutures/staples should be conveyed to the patient because it affects wound closure and cosmetics.

Area	Length of time (days)
Face	3–5
Scalp	7–9
Chest	8–10
Back	10–14
Forearm	10–14
Fingers and hand	8–10
Lower extremity	8–12
Foot	10–12
Overlying joint	14

▪ Tetanus immunization should be updated if required
  ◦ In general, if greater than 5 years since last tetanus shot, give Td booster

- Patients should be instructed to return if signs of symptoms of infection occur
  - Increasing pain, redness, or warmth
  - Fever
  - Purulent drainage

Complications
- **Infection**
  - Incidence of wound infection (assuming proper irrigation and sterile technique) is still 2% to 3%
  - Lowest incidence of infection—scalp, face, neck, trunk
  - Higher incidence of infection—extremities, especially hands and feet and in large, complex lacerations
- **Cosmesis**
  - Keloid formation
  - Larger suture material causes more scarring
  - Poor alignment (i.e., vermillion border) leads to poor cosmetic result

Pearls
- Obtain complete medical history with attention to complicating risk factors (e.g., human immunodeficiency virus/acquired immunodeficiency syndrome [HIV/AIDS], diabetes).
- Always inquire about patient's tetanus status.
- When suturing, adhere to the principles of minimizing trauma to tissues, relieving tension by undermining, using deep sutures, and realigning skin edges accurately.
- The Golden Period: The maximum time after injury that a wound may be safely closed without significant risk of infection is not a fixed number of hours.

Suggested Readings
Roberts JR, Hedges JR. *Clinical procedures in emergency medicine*, 4th ed. WB Saunders; 2004.

Simon RR, Brenner BE. *Emergency procedures and techniques*, 4th ed. Philadelphia: Lippincott Williams & Wilkins; 2002:335–395.

Singer AJ, Hollander JE. *Lacerations and acute wounds an evidence-based guide*. FA Davis Co; 2003.

63

Foreign Body Removal: Ticks, Rings and Fish Hooks

William C. Manson and Heidi E. Ladner

Indications
- Indicated only if location of foreign body (FB) is certain
- Removal may be done in 30 minutes or less

Relative Contraindications
- Involvement of joint—orthopedic consultation may be required
- Coagulopathies or bleeding diathesis
- Allergy to anesthetic
- Chronic medical problems that delay healing, such as diabetes, uremia, or immunocompromised state
- Involvement of abdomen/pelvis/thorax
- Near major vascular structures that are difficult to visualize
- Uncooperative, difficult, or intoxicated patient
- FB not localized

Risks/Consent Issues
- Procedure can cause pain (local anesthesia will be given)
- Local bleeding
- Whenever the skin is broken, there is potential for introducing infection (sterile technique will be utilized)
- Risk of injuring local neurovascular structures
- Scar at site of FB removal
- Patient must be informed that all FBs may not be removed
- Retained wood FBs always develop an inflammatory response, but retained bullets rarely produce inflammation
- Certain FBs may carry bacterial contamination, such as dirt, pieces of clothing, and shoe soles

Technique
- **Localize the FB**
  - Get multiple projections of plain x-ray using a soft tissue technique (e.g., under-penetrated film); to locate radiopaque FBs, place a marker (i.e., needle) on the skin surface at the wound entrance before the x-ray procedure.
  - Although glass and metal are easily located with plain films, ultrasonographic localization may be required for wood and thorns.
  - All intraorbital and intracranial FBs must be imaged by computed tomography (CT).
  - If a patient has a previously explored wound demonstrating signs of infection, poor wound healing, or persistent pain, consider doing a CT.
- **Patient Preparation**
  - Sterilize and drape the area from where FB will be removed.
  - Anesthetize area either via local infiltration or appropriate nerve block.

General Removal Techniques
- Enlarge the entrance to wound with an adequate skin incision.
- Spread the soft tissue with hemostats, avoiding use of fingers.
  - ▶ Hemostats can help find glass in a wound by creating a clicking sound when tapped against glass.
- If visualization is inadequate, consider excision of small block of tissue, only if no significant neurovascular structures are involved.
- When searching for a thorn or needle, consider an elliptical incision, undermine the skin in all directions, and then compress the sides, expelling the FB.
- Closure of the wound after thorough irrigation is indicated unless exploring a contaminated wound.

Tick Removal
- Nonmechanical means of tick removal is not recommended (i.e., drowning the tick in petroleum jelly), because it may cause the tick to regurgitate, increasing infection risk.

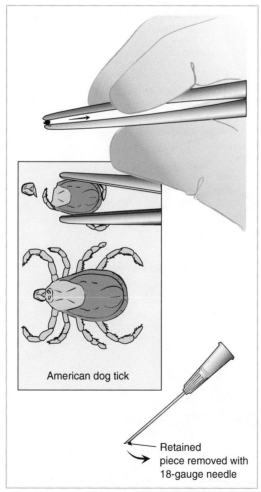

American dog tick

Retained piece removed with 18-gauge needle

FIGURE 63.1: Tick removal. (From Bond GR. Evenomation management and tick removal. In: Henretig FM, King C, eds. *Textbook of pediatric emergency procedures*. Philadelphia: Williams & Wilkins; 1997:1328, with permission.)

- Mechanical removal
  - Using the tip of forceps, grab the tick as close as possible to the patient's skin, and apply steady traction.
  - Ensure that all mouth parts are removed. Use an 18-gauge needle to remove retained pieces.
  - Thoroughly cleanse the area with soap and water.
- In patients at high risk of Lyme disease, consider administration of 200 mg of doxycycline in a single dose (or amoxicillin in pediatrics) (see Fig. 63.1).

Ring Removal
- Initial attempt at ring removal should be with soap and water.
- **String-Wrap Method**
  - Consider a digital block to reduce pain and minimize swelling.
  - With 25+ in. of string, umbilical tape, or suture, pass the tip between the ring and finger.
  - Using the distal end of the string, wrap clockwise (proximal to distal), including the proximal interphalangeal (PIP) and distal finger, ensuring compression.
  - Do not leave gaps between the wraps of string.

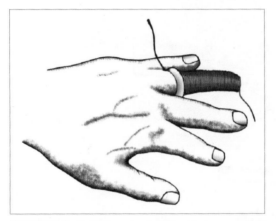

FIGURE 63.2: Ring removal using the string-wrap method.

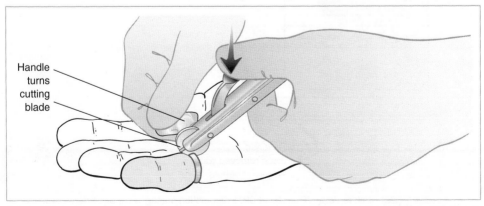

Handle turns cutting blade

FIGURE 63.3: Ring cutter method of ring removal. (From Fuchs SM. Ring removal. In: Henretig FM, King C, eds. *Textbook of pediatric emergency procedures*. Philadelphia: Williams & Wilkins; 1997:1231, with permission.)

- Unwrap the string from the proximal end, slowly forcing the ring over the PIP and distal finger, unraveling the ring with the string.
- If this technique fails, consider using a ring cutter.
- **Ring Cutters**
  - Reassure the patient that the ring cutter will not cut the finger.
  - Turn the ring such that the thinnest portion is on the palmar side of the finger.
  - Gently slide the ring cutter guard under the ring (this will likely cause some pain due to swelling of the distal finger).
  - Grasp the ring cutter handle firmly such that the cutting wheel is against the ring.
  - Turn the wheel until the ring is cut.
  - Pull off the ring with hemostats or clamps; alternatively, make another cut in the ring.

Fish Hook Removal

- Determine if fish hook is single, multiple, or trebled, and also note the number and location of the barbs.
- Administer 1% lidocaine locally.
- Advance the hook through the anesthetized skin.
- Clip off the barb, and remove the rest of the hook in a retrograde manner.

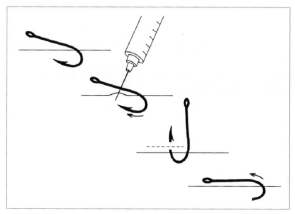

FIGURE 63.4: Hook removal.

Complications

- Bleeding
- Infection
- Scarring
- Pain
- Nerve damage
- Incomplete removal
- Retained FBs such as wood always lead to inflammation
- Rarely, retained FBs containing lead may lead to systemic lead poisoning

Common Pitfalls

- Failing to consider possibility of retained FBs with simple lacerations
- Inadequate number of views on plain film

- Making the initial skin incision too small
- Making the skin incision lateral to the plane of the FB
- Tick: Leaving remnants of the mouth parts in the skin
- Failing to use adequate anesthesia, either local or a regional block
- Failing to address tetanus immunization status

Pearls
- Always inform patient that the FB may not be located.
- Always inform patient about the possibility of a retained FB.
- Always start with multiple views on plain film to localize FB. If unsuccessful, consider ultrasonography or CT scan.
- Make skin incisions along skin folds or Kraissel lines to minimize scars.
- When removing thorns or needles, consider making an elliptical incision and undermining the wound.
- Before attempting ring removal, wrap the finger with a tight bandage from distal to proximal to exsanguinate the digit and reduce swelling.
- Always ensure adequate local anesthesia. If insufficient, consider a digital or regional block.
- DO NOT guarantee the patient that no FB remains in the soft tissue.

Suggested Readings
Roberts JR, Hedges JR. *Clinical procedures in emergency medicine*, 4th ed. WB Saunders; 2004;703–705, 711–713.

Simon RR, Brenner BE. *Emergency procedures and techniques*, 4th ed. Philadelphia: Lippincott Williams & Wilkens; 2002;419–422.

64

Escharotomy and Burn Care

Steven Shuchat and Jeffrey P. Green

Indications
- Used to decompress accumulated edema under tight, unyielding eschar following full-thickness burn (classic and modern classifications of burns are given in Table 64.1)
- Circumferential extremity burn with evidence of neurovascular compromise:
  - Cyanosis
  - Deep tissue pain
  - Progressive paresthesia
  - Decreased or absent pulses
  - Elevated compartment pressure
  - Decreased arterial flow on Doppler ultrasonography
  - Pulse oximetry <95% of affected extremity (without systemic hypoxia)
- Thoracic burn with evidence of respiratory compromise due to eschar
- Circumferential neck burn
- Abdominal burn with evidence of increased intra-abdominal pressure (usually estimated by bladder pressure)
- Circumferential penile burn

Contraindications
- No evidence of tissue hypoperfusion on physical examination
- Normal findings on arterial Doppler ultrasonography
- Adequate respiration despite eschar
- No evidence of increased intra-abdominal pressure

Risk/Consent Issues
- Often difficult to obtain consent from major burn victims; escharotomy is a life-saving procedure and should be performed even if informed consent from the patient cannot be obtained
- Procedure can cause pain (local and systemic analgesia will be provided)
- Risk of bleeding (minimized with proper technique)
- Whenever the skin is broken, there is potential for introducing infection (sterile technique will be utilized)

Landmarks
Escharotomy sites are depicted in Figure 64.1.

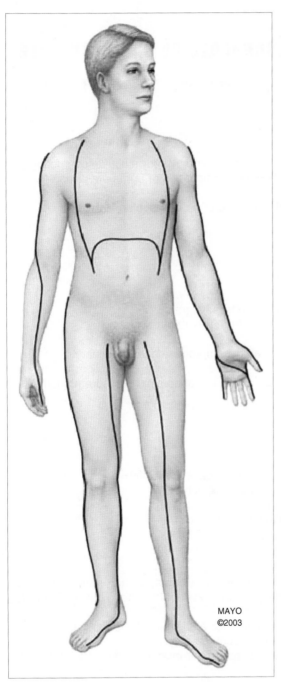

MAYO
©2003

FIGURE 64.1: Escharotomy sites. (From Haro LH, Miller S, Decker WW. Burns. In: Wolfson AB, ed. *Harwood-Nuss' clinical practice of emergency medicine,* 4th ed. Philadelphia: Lippincott Williams & Wilkins; 2005:1106, with permission.)

TABLE 64.1: Burn depth classification

Classic classification	Modern classification	Burn depth	Appearance	Healing
First degree	Superficial	Epidermis only	Painful, dry, red Blanch with pressure	3–6 days No scarring
Second degree	Superficial partial thickness	Epidermis and superficial dermis	Red, weeping, usually blister Blanch with pressure	7–21 days Scarring unusual
	Deep partial thickness	Epidermis and deep dermis	Usually blister, waxy, and dry, white to red color Nonblanching	Greater than 21 days Scarring severe
Third degree	Full thickness	Extends through and destroys dermis	Waxy-white to charred black, dry, inelastic skin Nonblanching	No spontaneous healing Severe scarring with contractures

Technique

- Follow guidelines in "General Burn Management" section.
- Escharotomy
  - Do not delay procedure for transfer to Burn Center.
  - Make incision to subcutaneous level so that eschar is released, preferably with Bovie cautery device to minimize bleeding.
  - Thoracic escharotomy
    - Make longitudinal incisions along each midclavicular line from 2 cm below the clavicle to the tenth rib; connect with two transverse incisions across the chest, forming a square.
  - Extremity eschar
    - Make incision to subcutaneous layer only.
    - Cut through the entire length of the burn eschar.

General Burn Management

- First ensure Airway, Breathing and Circulation (ABCs) and administer supplemental oxygen
- Strongly consider endotracheal intubation if:
  - Burns to the face and neck are present
  - Soot in and around the mouth and nose
  - Hoarseness, stridor, wheezing, or development of acute coughing
  - Carbonaceous sputum
- Give IV fluids for resuscitation (for moderate to major burns)
  - Use Parkland formula: Ringers lactate 4 mL × weight (kg) × % of total body surface area (TBSA) burned (excluding superficial burns).
    - Give 1/2 of total volume over the first 8 hours from time of burn injury.
    - Give second 1/2 of total volume over the following 16 hours.
    - Titrate to maintain blood pressure and urine output of at least 1 mL/kg/hour.
    - Continue maintenance fluids in addition.
  - Place urinary catheter to monitor adequate resuscitation.

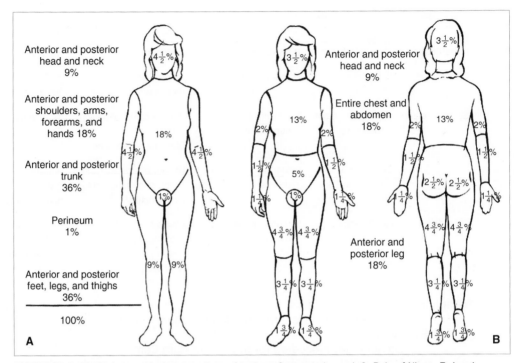

FIGURE 64.2: Methods to evaluate percentage of body surface area burned. **A:** Rule of Nines. **B:** Lund and Browder chart. (From Haro LH, Miller S, Decker WW. Burns. In: Wolfson AB, ed. *Harwood-Nuss' clinical practice of emergency medicine,* 4th ed. Philadelphia: Lippincott Williams & Wilkins; 2005:1103, with permission.)

- Provide pain management with frequent pain assessment
  - Acetaminophen and nonsteroidal anti-inflammatory drugs (NSAIDS) ± opioids for superficial burns
  - Opioids are necessary for partial-to-full thickness burns
- Administer tetanus prophylaxis
- Wound care, if not delaying transfer to burn unit:
  - Use sterile technique.
  - Clean with mild soap and tap water.
  - Debride sloughed or necrotic skin; avoid extensive debridement.
  - Remove ruptured blisters.
    - Intact blister management is controversial; it is recommended to unroof cloudy blisters or those where rupture is imminent (e.g., over joints).
  - Superficial burns do not need dressings; application of aloe vera cream is sufficient.
  - Deeper burns require chemoprophylaxis to prevent infection:
    - Apply silver sulfadiazine (Silvadene) to a thickness of 1/16th of an inch on burns other than the face where bacitracin is preferred.
    - Over the silver sulfadiazine, place three layers of gauze: first, a nonadherent gauze, ideally with a nonpetroleum-based lubricant. Then, a fluffed gauze layer capable of absorbing exudates. Finally, place an outer wrap with elastic gauze with enough pressure to keep the dressing in place.
      - Wrap all fingers and toes individually to prevent maceration and adherence.

    ◆   *Caveat:* If transferring to a nearby burn unit, covering wounds with sterile moist dressings is appropriate.

Disposition

- Patients with superficial burns may be safely discharged home
- For burns beyond superficial, apply American Burn Association Minimal Criteria for Transfer to Burn Center:
  - Partial-thickness and full-thickness burns: Greater than or equal to 10% TBSA in patients younger than 10 years or older than 50 years
  - Greater than or equal to 20% TBSA in other age-groups
  - Full-thickness burns: Greater than or equal to 5% TBSA in all age-groups
  - Circumferential burns of the extremities or chest
  - Partial- and full-thickness burns involving the face, eyes, ears, hands, feet, genitalia, perineum, or joints
  - Electrical burns, including lightning injuries
  - Chemical burns with threat of functional or cosmetic impairment
  - Inhalation injury in association with burns
  - Patients with burns having associated trauma or preexisting illness, such as acquired immunodeficiency syndrome (AIDS), diabetes, cancer, alcoholism
  - Children with burns seen in hospitals not having qualified personnel or equipment
  - Patients who will require special social or emotional care or long-term rehabilitation
- Patients with burns not being referred to Burn Center, but needing admission:
  - If there is suspicion of child abuse
  - Patients unable to care for wounds at home

Complications of Escharotomy

- Hemorrhage from superficial veins
- Infection
- Damage to underlying structures
- Complications of poorly done procedure
- Muscle necrosis
- Nerve injury, such as foot drop

Common Pitfalls

- Underestimating the extent of the burn; often burns will not fully declare their penetration for 24 to 72 hours
- Failure to frequently reevaluate airway patency
- Failure to consider concomitant carbon monoxide or cyanide exposure
- Failure to use Bovie cautery for escharotomy

Pearls

- More than one million thermal burns occur annually.
- Obtain carboxyhemoglobin level to evaluate for carbon monoxide poisoning for closed space burns.
- Suspect cyanide poisoning for burns involving wool, silk, nylon, and polyurethane found in furniture or paper.

- Never apply silver sulfadiazine to the face because it can cause skin discoloration.
- Always give tetanus prophylaxis.
- Individually wrap toes and fingers.
- For sulfa allergic patients, bacitracin is appropriate for initial burn infection prophylaxis.
- Escharotomy should not be delayed for transfer to Burn Center.

Suggested Readings

American College of Surgeons. *Resources for optimal care of the injured patient*, Chapter 14. Committee on Trauma, American College of Surgeons; 1999.

Simon RR, Brenner BE. *Emergency procedures and techniques*, 4th ed. Philadelphia: Lippincott Williams & Wilkins; 2002:395–397.

Wolfson AB. *Harwood-Nuss' clinical practice of emergency medicine*, 4th ed. Philadelphia: Lippincott Williams & Wilkins; 2005:1101–1107.

Section Editor: Jay Lemery

65

Epistaxis

James Hsiao

Indications

- ■ **Cauterization**
  - ● Active bleeding from an anterior source, when the source can be visualized
- ■ **Anterior nasal packing**
  - ● Active bleeding from an anterior source, when the source cannot be visualized
  - ● Cauterization fails
- ■ **Posterior nasal packing or balloon tamponade**
  - ● Anterior source cannot be identified AND
    - ▶ Bleeding from both nares OR
    - ▶ Blood is draining into the posterior pharynx
  - ● Anterior packing of both nares fails to control bleeding

Contraindications

- ■ None

Risks/Consent Issues

- ■ Procedure can cause pain or discomfort
- ■ Risk of infection, septal damage, and ulceration
- ■ Risk of balloon migration and airway obstruction with posterior packing

Landmarks

- ■ The type of procedure used depends on the source of bleeding. The source can be identified by direct visualization, or with use of a nasal speculum (described in more detail in the "Technique" section).
- ■ Nosebleeds are most commonly anterior (80% to 90%), originating from the Kiesselbach plexus in the septum.
- ■ Posterior nosebleeds originate from branches of the sphenopalatine artery in the posterior nasal cavity or nasopharynx. A posterior source is likely when an anterior source cannot be identified, when bleeding is from both nares, or when blood is draining into the posterior pharynx.

Technique

- ■ **Patient Preparation**
  - ● Ask the patient to lean forward and apply manual pressure to both nares for 10 to 20 minutes.

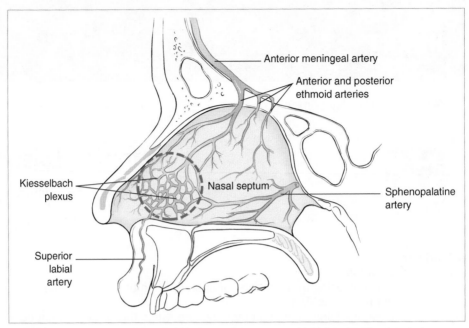

FIGURE 65.1: Anatomy of nasal septum. (From Kost SI, Post JC. Management of epistaxis. In: Henretig FM, King C, eds. *Textbook of pediatric emergency procedures*. Philadelphia: Williams & Wilkins; 1997:663, with permission.)

- If bleeding continues, ask the patient to blow his or her nose, which decreases the effects of local fibrinolysis and removes clots.
- Apply a topical anesthetic and vasoconstrictor.
  - Soak strips of cotton or gauze in 4% lidocaine and topical epinephrine (1:10,000) or 4% topical cocaine. Place in the nasal cavity for 15 to 20 minutes.
  - Alternatively, a topical anesthetic with a decongestant (2% lidocaine and 4% phenylephrine mixed 1:1) or oxymetazoline hydrochloride (Afrin) nasal spray may be used.
- Because patients may be apprehensive, and because packing may be uncomfortable, opiates may be given before the examination (strongly recommended in cases of posterior packing).
- Insert a nasal speculum and spread the nares vertically. Suction all remaining clots and blood. This permits visualization of most anterior sources.

Cauterization

- If an anterior source is visualized, cauterization should be attempted. To be effective, cautery should be performed after bleeding is controlled.
- Chemical cauterization can be performed using silver nitrate sticks. Apply the tip of a silver nitrate stick to the bleeding site for at least 20 seconds or until a gray eschar forms.
- If bleeding is vigorous, electrocauterization can be used. Apply the device to the bleeding site for 20 seconds or until a gray eschar forms.

Anterior Packing

- If the source of an anterior bleed cannot be identified, or if bleeding persists despite cauterization, an anterior pack can be placed.
- A Merocel nasal tampon can be used. Lubricate the tip with lidocaine or a topical antibiotic and insert the device along the floor of the nasal cavity.

Expansion and tamponade of the bleed will occur with 10 to 20 mL of saline insertion.

- Xeroform gauze ¹/₂-in. wide (dispensed in 72-in. strip) can also be used. Using forceps, grab 4 to 5 in. of gauze and advance into the nasal cavity as far as possible, then grasp another 4 to 5 in. and layer on top. Continue to layer in an accordion manner until the nose is tightly packed (see Fig. 65.2).

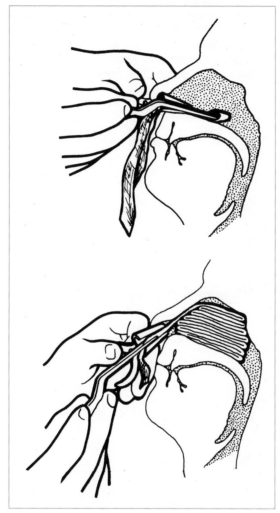

FIGURE 65.2: Anterior nasal packing. (From Simon RR, Brenner BE. *Emergency procedures and techniques,* 4th ed. Philadelphia: Lippincott Williams & Wilkins; 2002:313, with permission.)

- If bleeding persists despite initial packing, the contralateral naris can be packed. If bleeding still persists, it is likely coming from a posterior source.
- Instructions if nasal packing is successful are:
  - Packing should be left in for 3 to 5 days.
  - Antibiotics (penicillins or first-generation cephalosporins) should be prescribed for the duration.
  - Avoid nasal manipulation and nose blowing, as well as vasodilating actions such as physical exertion, spicy foods, and alcohol.
  - Follow-up with ENT specialist.

Posterior Packing

- Rolled gauze method

  - Prepare 3 × 3-in. or 2 × 2-in. gauze rolled and bound tightly around the middle with umbilical tape or silk (no. 0) tie. Ten inches of umbilical tape/silk tie should be left on each end.

  - Lubricate a rubber catheter with lidocaine or a topical antibiotic and feed it through the nose, pulling it through the mouth.

  - Tie the rolled gauze to the catheter, and pull the gauze back into the mouth by pulling on the catheter.

  - Once the pack lodges in the posterior portion of the nose, secure the tape anteriorly by tying it around a piece of gauze.

  - Apply an anterior pack to the same side, because bleeding may resume anterior to the posterior pack.

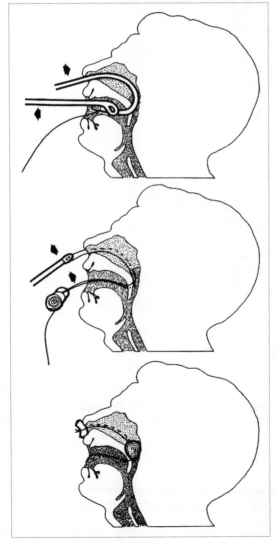

FIGURE 65.3: Posterior nasal packing. (From Simon RR, Brenner BE. *Emergency procedures and techniques,* 4th ed. Philadelphia: Lippincott Williams & Wilkins; 2002:314, with permission.)

- Epistat device (balloon tamponade)
  - ▶ Composed of anterior and posterior balloons.
  - ▶ Lubricate the catheter and advanced it along the floor of the nasal cavity.
  - ▶ Inflate the posterior balloon with 7 to 10 mL of saline and then pull forward until it lodges in the posterior portion of the nose.
  - ▶ Inflate the anterior balloon with 15 to 30 mL of saline.
  - ▶ Apply an anterior pack to the same side.
- Foley catheter
  - ▶ Catheter size (10- to 16-French) should be approximately the diameter of the external nares.
  - ▶ Check the balloon for an air leak.
  - ▶ Cut catheter tip distal to the balloon to prevent irritation of the posterior pharynx.
  - ▶ Lubricate the catheter and advanced it along the floor of the nasal cavity until it reaches the nasopharynx.
  - ▶ Inflate the balloon with 15 mL of saline and then pull forward until it lodges in the posterior portion of the nose.
  - ▶ Apply an anterior pack to the same side.

Note: Because of possible multiple complications with posterior packing (see following text), these patients should be admitted with involvement of ENT specialist.

Complications

See Figure 65.4 for algorithm for management of epistaxis.
- Infection (sinusitis, otitis media, abscess formation)
- Septal hematoma, ulceration, or perforation
- External nasal deformity
- Vasovagal episode
- Aspiration
- Balloon migration and airway obstruction with posterior packing
- Hypoxia and hypoventilation with posterior packing

Common Pitfalls

- Nasal packing, especially posterior, can be particularly uncomfortable for the patient. Consider giving opiates before the procedure.
- Because of the risks associated with posterior packing, admit all patients who require posterior packing.
- For patients discharged with anterior nasal packs, start oral antibiotics for the duration of the packing to prevent infection.
- Attempts at nasal packing may slow down but not completely stop the nasal hemorrhage. If bleeding persists, consult ENT specialist.

Pearls

- When bleeding from both nares, or when bleeding persists despite anterior packing on both sides, the source is likely posterior.
- Before attempting nasal packing, remember to apply manual pressure and topical anesthetics and vasoconstrictors—this may control the bleeding and obviate the need for packing.
- When applying a posterior pack, make sure to place an anterior pack on the same side, because bleeding may resume or persist anterior to the posterior pack.

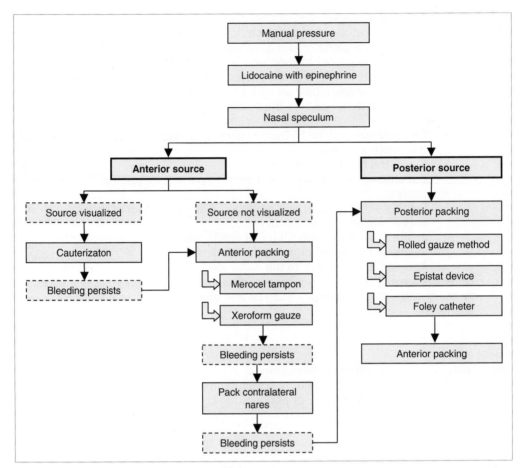

FIGURE 65.4: Algorithm for management of epistaxis.

Suggested Readings

Alter, H. *Approach to the patient with epistaxis*. UpToDate (web site). http://www .utdol.com. Accessed Aug 8, 2006.

Rosen P. *Atlas of emergency procedures*. St. Louis: Mosby; 2001:194–197.

Evans, Jeffrey. *Epistaxis*. Emedicine.com (web site). http://www.emedicine.com. Accessed Aug 8, 2006.

Kost S, Post C. Management of epistaxis. In: Henretig F, King C, eds. *Textbook of pediatric emergency procedures*. Baltimore: Williams & Wilkins; 1997:663–673.

Nosebleed (epistaxis). PatientPlus (web site). http://www.patient.co.uk. Accessed Aug 8, 2006.

Simon RR, Brenner BE. *Emergency procedures and techniques*, 4th ed. Lippincott Williams & Wilkins; 2002:309–316.

66

Eye Foreign Body Removal

Satchit Balsari

Indications
- All external foreign bodies (FBs) in the eye must be removed
- Patient usually complains of pain, redness, increased tearing, or FB sensation in the eye.

Contraindications
- Always check for intraocular FBs by conducting a meticulous examination and maintaining a high index of suspicion, especially when the mechanism of injury includes flying particles or projectiles.

Landmarks

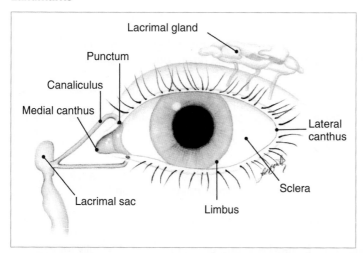

FIGURE 66.1: Periorbital structures. (From Knoop KJ, Dennis WR. Eye Trauma. In: Wolfson AB, ed. *Harwood-Nuss' clinical practice of emergency medicine.* 4th ed. Philadelphia: Lippincott Williams & Wilkins, 2005:946, with permission.)

Technique
- **Patient Preparation**
  - Place 0.5% tetracaine or 0.5% proparacaine drops in the eye (may use in both eyes to reduce the blink reflex).
  - In case of intense blepharospasm, administer an ipsilateral facial block.
- **Inspection**
  - Examine the conjunctiva and cornea carefully. Do not stop looking for FBs if one is found (there may be more!)

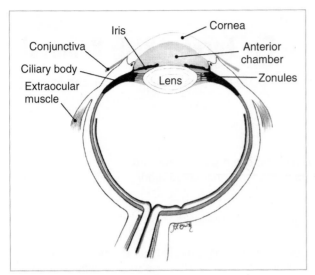

FIGURE 66.2: Cross section of the eye. (From Knoop KJ, Dennis WR. Eye Trauma. In: Wolfson AB, ed. *Harwood-Nuss' clinical practice of emergency medicine,* 4th ed. Philadelphia: Lippincott Williams & Wilkins; 2005:946, with permission.)

- Look behind both eyelids.
  - Pull down the lower eyelid and ask the patient to look up.
  - Evert the upper lid.
    - Use a cotton-tipped applicator or similar device as a fulcrum to evert the lid by pulling on the eyelashes down, out, and back.
- **Fluorescein Stain**
  - Gently touch the fluorescein strip to the lower eyelid conjunctiva and ask the patient to blink two to three times. Wipe away the excess.
  - Inspect the cornea for abrasions (fluorescein, when taken up by the alkaline Bowman membrane, will fluoresce). Patients with corneal abrasions may have FB sensation in the absence of a retained FB.
- **Slit Lamp Inspection**
  - Examine the fluorescein-stained cornea under the blue light of a slit lamp.
  - Vertical linear lesions on the cornea should raise suspicion for a FB under the eyelids.
  - If you see a FB extending through the full thickness of the cornea, consult an ophthalmologist.
  - Signs of an intraocular FB may be subtle or absent. Look carefully for the following:
    - Irregular pupil
    - Shallow anterior chamber
    - Collapsed iris
    - Positive Seidel test (extrusion of fluorescent material from the cornea)
    - Hyphema
    - Lens opacification
    - Decreased intraocular pressure
- **Foreign Body Visible**
  - Swab
    - If easily visualized, remove the particle with a moist sterile cotton-tipped applicator or nasopharyngeal swab.

- Irrigation
  - ▷ FB may be flushed out when the eye is irrigated gently with a stream from an Angiocath connected to a syringe containing saline.
  - ▷ If more copious irrigation is required, consider commercial devices such as the Morgan lens.
- Embedded FB
  - ▷ Cornea can be gently scraped with a small 25- or 27-gauge needle, attached to a syringe for stability (under the slit lamp).
  - ▷ Place hand on the patient's cheek bone for increased stability, and hold needle tip *tangential* to the globe surface.
  - ▷ Pick out and manipulate FB under slit lamp magnification.
  - ▷ Rust rings formed by the oxidation of iron-containing FBs may be removed along with the FB, with repeated picking. Note that rust rings can also be safely removed in 24 to 48 hours in the ophthalmologist's office as well.
  - ▷ Do not pick or burr in the visual axis—consult an ophthalmologist!
- **Aftercare**
  - May consider topical antibiotics
  - Patching not recommended
  - Topical anesthetics are not recommended for use at home (corneal toxicity, impairs corneal wound healing)

Complications
- Incomplete removal
- Second FB (patient may not have persistent FB sensation, due to anesthesia)
- Conjunctivitis
- Corneal epithelial injury
- Globe perforation (patch, protect, and call ophthalmology consult service)

Common Pitfalls
- Failing to evert the eyelid to look for a FB
- Become familiar with the slit lamp at your institution! Do not be intimidated.

Pearls
- If you suspect that an embedded or penetrated FB exists, obtain a computed tomography (CT) of the orbits. Avoid magnetic resonance imaging (MRI) if object is metallic or unknown.
- If deep corneal defects are present, fluorescein may enter the anterior chamber and be seen as "flare," different from the flare reaction of iritis.

67

Lateral Canthotomy

Dean Jared Straff

Indications

Retrobulbar hemorrhage is an ocular emergency that is most commonly a result of direct trauma to the eye, recent retrobulbar anesthesia, or eyelid surgery. If untreated, orbital compartment syndrome develops with resultant optic nerve ischemia and irreversible vision loss in as little as 90 to 120 minutes.

- **Primary Indications**
  - Retrobulbar hemorrhage with the following:
    - Acute loss of visual acuity
    - Increased intraocular pressure
    - Severe proptosis
    - Diffuse subconjunctival hemorrhage
    - Marked periorbital edema
  - An unconscious or uncooperative patient with an intraocular pressure greater than 40 mm Hg
- **Secondary Indications**
  - Suspected retrobulbar hemorrhage with the following:
    - Associated afferent pupillary defect
    - Ophthalmoplegia
    - Resistance to retropulsion
    - Cherry-red macula
    - Optic nerve head pallor
    - Severe eye pain

Contraindications

- Suspected ruptured globe

Landmarks

- The lateral canthal tendon is a combined tendon-ligament that provides structural fixation of the lids (tarsal plates) and orbicularis oculi muscle to the inner aspect of the bony lateral orbital wall (zygoma) just posterior to the orbital rim.
- The tendon has an inferior and superior crux.
- The point at which the tendon attaches is called *Whitnall tubercle*.
- Eisler pocket, a small pocket of orbital fat, lies anterior to the lateral canthal tendon.
- Upon cutting the inferior crux of the lateral canthal tendon, the lower lid loses its structural fixation to the lateral orbital wall and becomes lax, releasing the increased intraocular pressure from the eye.

Technique

- Positioning is critical. The patient must be in the supine position and has to be able to cooperate throughout the procedure. Unexpected head movement may lead

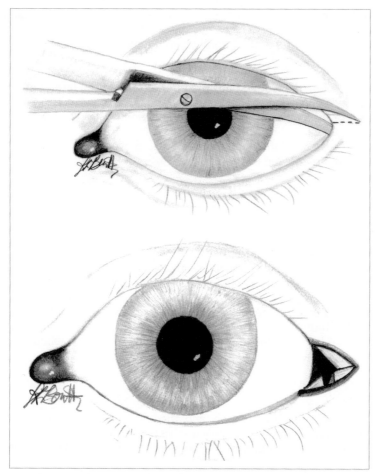

FIGURE 67.1: Lateral canthotomy and cantholysis. The inferior arm of the lateral canthal tendon has been incised to release the globe. (From Knoop KJ, Dennis WR. Eye trauma. In: Wolfson AB, ed. *Harwood-Nuss' clinical practice of emergency medicine,* 4th ed. Philadelphia: Lippincott Williams & Wilkins; 2005:952, with permission.)

to iatrogenic globe injury. Depending on the clinical scenario, the patient may need to be restrained, undergo conscious sedation, or even be intubated and paralyzed.

- The lateral canthus should be prepped and draped in a sterile manner.
- Irrigate the eye with normal saline to remove surrounding debris.
- **Anesthetize** the lateral canthus with approximately 1 mL of 1% or 2% lidocaine with epinephrine to obtain both local anesthesia and hemostasis.
- A **straight clamp** is placed horizontally across the lateral canthus (the skin of the lateral corner of the eye) for 1 to 2 minutes to compress tissues and achieve hemostasis.
- Release the clamp, leaving an impression for where the incision is to be made.
- Use a pair of forceps to pick up the skin around the lateral orbit.
- **Use scissors and cut** a 1 to 2 cm horizontal incision in the tissue starting at the lateral corner of the eye and extending laterally. This will open the skin, orbicularis muscle, orbital septum, palpebral conjunctiva, and exposes the Eisler pocket of fat.

- **Retract the lid down** and away from the lateral orbit, separating the conjunctiva and the skin.
- Palpate the inferior portion of the lateral canthal tendon by using your finger or the tip of the scissors.
- With the scissors pointed inferoposteriorly toward the lateral orbital rim (pointing away from the globe), dissect and **cut the inferior crux of the lateral canthal tendon**. This critical incision is approximately 1 to 2 cm in depth and length.
- If this procedure is insufficient, dissect superiorly and cut the superior crux of the lateral canthal tendon.
- Releasing the pressure of the hematoma will help prevent further visual loss or restore vision to the affected eye.

Complications
- Iatrogenic globe injury
- Excessive bleeding
- Local infection or abscess formation
- Fibrosis may develop limiting extraocular motility
- Improper direction of scissors superiorly may lead to injury to the levator aponeurosis, resulting in ptosis
- The lacrimal gland and lacrimal artery also lie superiorly; care must be taken to avoid these structures
- Loss of adequate lower lid suspension and ectropion (can be repaired at a later date by the ophthalmologist)

Common Pitfalls
- Failure to adequately position, sedate, and anesthetize the patient.
- It is extremely important to immediately test visual acuity post procedure. If vision fails to improve, operative orbital decompression or hematoma evacuation is required.

Pearls
- Despite high intraorbital pressures, only a small amount of blood is usually expressed from the hematoma upon completion of the emergent orbital decompression.
- Almost immediately after a successful procedure, there will be a noticeable improvement of extraocular muscle movements and visual acuity, resolution of afferent pupillary defect, decrease in intraocular pressure, and resolution of the severe eye pain.
- Formal intraocular pressure testing with instruments such as a Tono-Pen is contraindicated in patients with suspected ruptured globe injury.
- If it is unclear whether there is retrobulbar hemorrhage or another ocular process occurring, an emergent computed tomography (CT) scan of the orbits may be helpful to clarify the diagnosis. However, imaging may delay treatment and result in permanent vision loss.
- Always call an emergent ophthalmology consult when this procedure is performed.
- Retrobulbar hemorrhage can also occur spontaneously. It has been reported to occur in people with hemophilia, von Willebrand disease, disseminated intravascular coagulation, leukemia, hypertension, atherosclerosis, straining, venous anomalies, and intraorbital aneurysm of the ophthalmic artery.

Suggested Readings

McInnes G, Howes DW. Lateral canthotomy and cantholysis: A simple, vision saving procedure. *Can J Emerg Med*. 2002;4(1):49–52.

Roberts JR, Hedges JR, eds. *Clinical procedures in emergency medicine*, 4th ed. Portland, Ore: WB Saunders; 2004:1275.

Rosen P, Barkin R. *Emergency medicine: Concepts and clinical practice*. St Louis: Mosby; 2002:910.

Titinalli JE, Kelen GD, Strapczynski JS. *Emergency medicine: A comprehensive study guide*, 6th ed. American College of Emergency Physicians, McGraw-Hill Co; 2004: 1458.

Vassallo S, Hartstein M, Howard D, et al. Traumatic retrobulbar hemorrhage: Emergent decompression by lateral canthotomy and cantholysis. *J Emerg Med*. 2002;22(3):251–256.

68

Peritonsillar Abscess

Jenice Forde-Baker

Indications
- Clinical suspicion based on physical examination
  - Swollen and red peritonsillar region causing uvular shift
  - Fluctuant site
- Interim treatment for peritonsillar closed space infection until tonsillectomy

Contraindications
- Recurrent peritonsillar abscess (PTA)—needs tonsillectomy!
- Evidence of deep neck tissue extension
- Septicemia or toxic appearance
- Airway obstruction
- Severe trismus

Landmarks
- Superior lateral border of affected tonsil, or area of most fluctuance
- Aspirate superior pole of PTA first, then try middle pole, and then inferior pole of PTA

Technique
- **Patient Preparation**
  - Have a **cooperative** patient sitting upright in a chair with occipital support.
  - Consider IV narcotic analgesia or sedation.
  - Digital examination is key: Must feel abscess.
  - May use ultrasound to aid visualization of an abscess as well as its volume, location, and relationship to the carotid artery.
- **Needle Aspiration**
  - Anesthetize the area topically with benzocaine (Cetacaine) spray.
  - Use head lamp or other light source.
  - Apply tongue blade depressor for visualization.
  - Anesthetize locally with 1 to 2 mL of 1% lidocaine via 27-gauge needle.
  - Prepare 18-gauge needle with a 10-mL syringe attached.
  - Cut the distal 1 cm off of the needle cover and recap the needle, thereby preventing the needle from penetrating greater than 1 cm.
  - Insert 18-gauge needle at area of greatest fluctuance (usually the superior pole) and aspirate the pus.
  - If no pus is aspirated, insert needle in middle pole, and then in the inferior pole of the ipsilateral tonsil.
- **Incision and Drainage (I & D)**
  - If a large amount of pus is aspirated or continues to drain from aspiration site, an incision can be made.

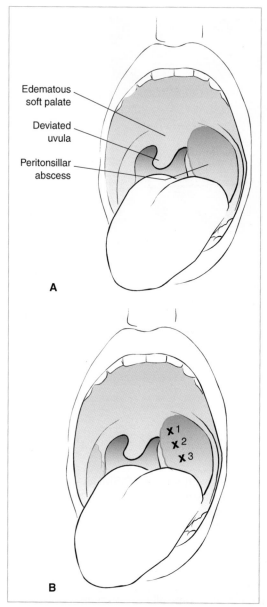

FIGURE 68.1: A: Peritonsillar abscess. The tonsil is displaced forward and inferomedial, the uvula is deviated toward the unaffected tonsil, and the soft palate is edematous and ruborous.
B: Recommended sites for three-point needle aspiration of a peritonsillar abscess. (From Saladino RA. Pharyngeal procedures. In: Henretig FM, King C, eds. *Textbook of pediatric emergency procedures.* Philadelphia: Williams & Wilkins; 1997:692, 696, with permission.)

- The area would already have been anesthetized from the aspiration.
- Obtain a no. 11 blade and tape the blade leaving only the distal 0.5 cm free, thereby preventing the scalpel from penetrating too deep.
- Incise the mucosa at the area of aspiration horizontally.
- Suction the area with a Frazier suction tip.
- Insert a Kelly clamp to break up loculations.

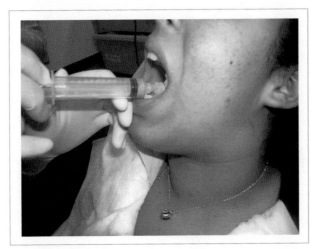

FIGURE 68.2: Needle aspiration.

- Have patient rinse and gargle with saline.
- Observe patient for at least 1 hour for complications.
- Postprocedure antibiotic treatment is with penicillin, clindamycin, or cephalosporin.
- All patients need 24-hour follow-up care with ENT physician.

Complications
- Airway obstruction
- Aspiration
- Carotid artery injury

Precautions
- **DO NOT** perform procedure on patient with severe **TRISMUS.**
- Always apply safeguards with needle cover and tape on the no. 11 blade to avoid aspirating/incising vascular structures.
- Remember to aspirate middle and lower poles if no aspirate is returned on first attempt.

Pearls
- Needle aspiration, I and D, and tonsillectomy all have excellent outcomes; no method has been demonstrated to be clearly superior.
- PTA is also known as "quinsy."
- Eighty percent of PTAs are felt on physical examination.
- During needle aspiration, orient needle in sagittal plane, not laterally, to avoid the carotid artery.
- Computed tomography (CT) scan is very useful for diagnostic purposes if the patient cannot open his or her mouth owing to trismus.
- Ultrasound guidance
  - Use a standard endocavitary 4 to 10 MHz probe (vaginal probe).
  - Look for dark fluid with swirls of white in the PTA.
  - Placing the probe on the normal contralateral side for comparison can be helpful.

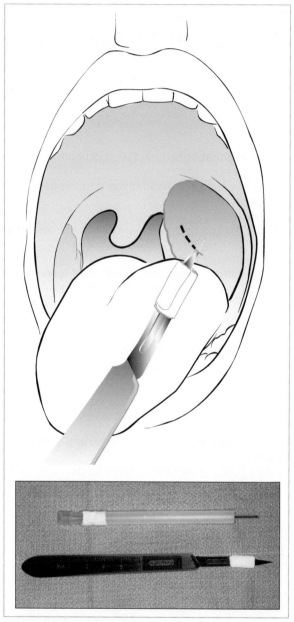

FIGURE 68.3: The depth of the needle and blade are controlled using a needle guard or an adhesive tape blade guard. (From Saladino RA. Pharyngeal procedures. In: Henretig FM, King C, eds. *Textbook of pediatric emergency procedures.* Philadelphia: Williams & Wilkins, 1997:695, with permission.)

Suggested Readings

Johnson RF, Stewart MG. The contemporary approach to diagnosis and management of peritonsillar abscess. *Curr Opin Otolaryngol Head Neck Surg.* 2005;13(3): 157–160.

69 Auricular Hematoma Drainage

Timothy C. Loftus and Joseph P. Underwood, III

Indications
- A subperichondrial hematoma that separates the perichondrium from the underlying auricular cartilage
  - Classically occurs as a result of a shearing force to the ear, but can also develop after blunt trauma.
  - Commonly seen in wrestlers.
  - The auricular cartilage derives its blood supply from the overlying perichondrium.
  - Early diagnosis and treatment is the key—necrosis begins within 24 hours.
  - In general, needle aspiration is sufficient. However, if a hematoma reaccumulates, incision and drainage may be indicated.

Contraindications
- There are no absolute contraindications.
- Anticoagulation is a relative contraindication. Consult with ENT specialist if there are any concerns.

Risks/Consent Issues
- Risk of infection is low. If clinical suspicion is high, an anti-staphylococcal antibiotic may be prescribed.
- Recurrent and untreated injuries allow new cartilage to develop, which leads to deformity of the auricle (cauliflower ear).

Landmarks
- The pinna is most commonly involved.
- The needle/scalpel is used in the area of greatest fluctuance.

Technique
- For needle aspiration, a 10-mL syringe and a 20-gauge needle are required.
  - Cleanse the outer ear with a topical antiseptic (e.g., povidone [Betadine] or chlorhexidine).
  - Local anesthesia is seldom required.
  - If local anesthesia is deemed necessary, avoid anesthetics containing epinephrine because of the risk of tissue necrosis.
  - Stabilize pinna with thumb and fingers.
  - Puncture area of greatest fluctuance with needle.
  - "Milk" hematoma with thumb and index finger until entire hematoma has been evacuated.
  - Maintain pressure on ear for 3 minutes after needle has been withdrawn.

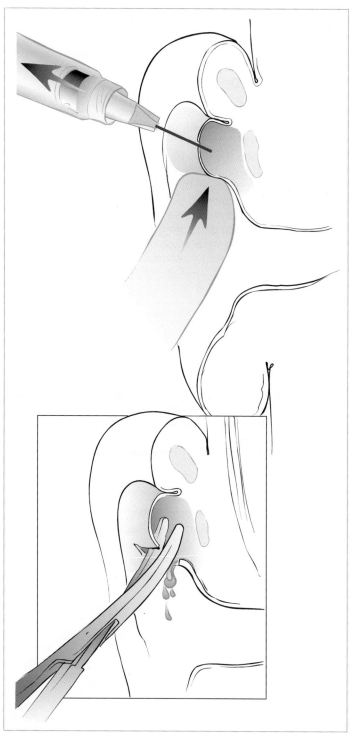

FIGURE 69.1: Evacuation of auricular hematoma. (From Pierce MC. External ear procedures. In: Henretig FM, King C, eds. *Textbook of pediatric emergency procedures*. Philadelphia: Williams & Wilkins; 1997:655, with permission.)

- Apply antibiotic ointment and a pressure dressing.
- Check ear again in 24 hours for reaccumulation of hematoma.
- Patient should be advised to avoid strenuous activity.
- Reaspiration may be required, whereas persistent reaccumulation warrants incision and drainage.
- For incision and drainage (I and D)
    - Cleanse the outer ear with a topical antiseptic (e.g., povidone [Betadine] or chlorhexidine).
    - Local anesthesia can be achieved with a small amount of 1% lidocaine (*without* epinephrine).
    - Using a no. 15 blade, incise the skin at the edge of the hematoma following the natural curvature of the pinna.
    - With the use of forceps, gently peel the skin and perichondrium off the hematoma and evacuate completely.
    - Irrigate the pocket with sterile normal saline.
    - Apply antibiotic ointment and a pressure dressing.
    - Reevaluate ear in 24 hours for recurrence of hematoma.
    - Patient should be advised to avoid strenuous activity.

Precautions
- Early diagnosis and treatment is the key.
- For severe or difficult cases, ENT specialist should be involved early on.

Pearls
- Needle aspiration may be attempted two to three times and is largely successful.
- If the hematoma persists, then I and D is indicated.
- If I and D is unsuccessful, then the patient should be promptly evaluated by ENT specialist.
- Drains are not necessary and may actually increase the risk of infection.

Suggested Readings
Pierce MC. External ear procedures. In: Henretig F King C, eds. *Textbook of pediatric emergency procedures*. Baltimore: Williams & Wilkens; 1997:654–655.

Section Editor: Jason A. Tracy

70

Intercostal Nerve Block

Jennifer V. Pope and Jason A. Tracy

Indications

- Used to provide analgesia for acute and chronic pain conditions affecting the thorax including the following:
  - Significant rib fractures causing hypoventilation, splinting respirations, or atelectasis
  - Chest wall/upper abdominal surgery: Thoracotomy, thoracostomy, gastrostomy tube placement
  - Neuralgia: Post-traumatic, post-herpetic (acute herpes simplex virus [HSV] infection), metastatic neoplasm of vertebral body

Contraindications

- Contralateral pneumothorax
  - Inadvertant creation of bilateral pneumothorax puts the patient at unnecessarily high health risk
- Relative contraindications
  - Routine rib fracture that is tolerating oral analgesia
  - Local infection
  - Lack of surgeon expertise
  - Serious hemostasis disorders, such as platelets <50,000 or international normalized ratio (INR) >1.0

Risk/Consent Issues

- Procedure can cause local pain. Local anesthesia will be given.
- Needle puncture can cause local bleeding, which is usually minimal. More significant bleeding can occur if the intercostal artery is punctured but care will be taken to avoid the artery.
- The needle could puncture the lung and cause a collapsed lung (pneumothorax). The risk is less than 1.5% and we have definitive treatment to reinflate the lung if the situation arises.
- Potential for introducing infection exists; however, this is extremely rare. Sterile technique will be utilized.

Landmarks

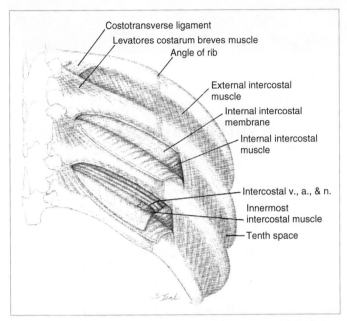

FIGURE 70.1: Exposure of the posterior part of intercostal spaces 8, 9, and 10. Note that the intercostal vein (*v.*), artery (*a.*), and nerve (*n.*) lie between the internal intercostal muscle and the innermost intercostal muscle layers. From the intervertebral foramen to the angle of the rib, the intercostal vessels and nerves are covered by the internal intercostal membrane. (Reprinted with permission from Blevins CE. Anatomy of the thorax. In: Shields TW, LoCicero J III, Ponn RB, et al. eds. *General thoracic surgery*, 6th ed. Vol. 1. Philadelphia: Lippincott Williams & Wilkins; 2005:11.)

- The intercostal nerves (ICNs) course in the subcostal groove parallel to the ribs. Within the subcostal groove, the ICNs lie inferior to the intercostal arteries (**v**ein, **a**rtery, **n**erve).
- Most ICN blocks are performed between the posterior and midaxillary line at a point proximal to the origin of the lateral cutaneous nerve. In adults, this correlates with 6 to 8 cm from the spinous process at the angle of the rib.

Technique
- **Collect Equipment**
  - Standard 25-gauge needle and 22-gauge 1.5-in. short-bevel needle
  - Sterile draping and sterile gloves
  - Povidone-iodine solution or chlorhexidine
- **Select Anesthetic of Choice**
  - For unclear reasons, the levels of local anesthetic in the blood are highest after ICN block as compared to any other block; therefore, the risk of systemic toxicity needs to be considered.
  - Bupivacaine 0.25% to 0.50% or lidocaine 1% to 2% with or without epinephrine can be used.
  - While bupivacaine has a longer duration of action, it can cause central nervous system (CNS) toxicity at smaller doses than lidocaine.

- Because of the increased systemic absorption, stay within the recommended dosing range (bupivacaine 3 mg/kg maximum, lidocaine 4.5 mg/kg and 7 mg/kg when used with epinephrine).

■ **Patient Preparation**

- The patient may be in a sitting position, prone, or lying with the unaffected side down. Ensure that the arms are forward in any position to pull the scapulae laterally to expose the posterior ribs.
- IV sedation with benzodiazepines, opioids, or ketamine may be needed and appreciated.
- Prepare the chest wall in a sterile manner with povidone-iodine solution or chlorhexidine.

■ **Skin Entry/Injection**

- Find the angle of the rib (costovertebral junction); in adults, this correlates with 6 to 8 cm from the spinous process (see Fig. 70.2). Anesthetize the skin surface by creating a wheal with 25-gauge needle and then switch to the 22-gauge needle.

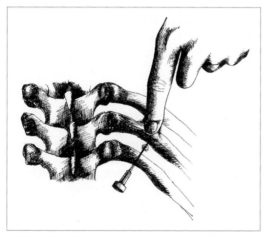

FIGURE 70.2: The intercostal nerve block. With the index finger of the left hand, palpate the rib to be injected and pull the skin overlying the rib cephalad. Insert the needle at a right angle to the skin and touch the rib. (Reused with permission from Simon RR, Brenner BE. *Emergency procedures and techniques*, 4th ed. Philadelphia: Lippincott Williams & Wilkins; 2002:143.)

- Use the index finger of the nondominant hand to retract the skin at the lower edge of the rib, cephalad and over the rib.
- With the syringe hand resting on the chest wall, advance the 22-gauge needle pointing cephalad at an 80-degree angle. The needle is advanced until it touches the lower border of the rib (less than 1 cm in depth).
- Inject local anesthetic to anesthetize the periosteum.
- With the nondominant hand, release the skin and hold the needle firmly while the syringe hand walks the needle caudally to just below the rib. Advance the needle 3 mm to reach the nerve in the intercostal space (see Fig. 70.3).
- With a negative aspirate, inject 3 to 5 mL of anesthetic.
- Repeat the above procedure on one to two ICNs above and below to cover overlapping innervation.

■ Postprocedure chest x-ray is recommended only if the patient develops symptoms of a pneumothorax including new cough, new pain, and/or shortness of breath.

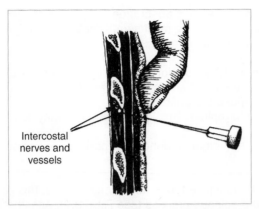

Intercostal
nerves and
vessels

FIGURE 70.3: The intercostal nerves lie beneath the rib margin, accompanied by the intercostal arteries. "Walk" the needle cautiously down the rib until it passes just beneath the inferior margin. Deposit the anesthetic solution here. Exercise caution not to go too deeply when passing the needle beneath the rib margin. (Reused with permission from Simon RR, Brenner BE. *Emergency procedures and techniques*, 4th ed. Philadelphia: Lippincott Williams & Wilkins; 2002:143.)

Complications
- Pneumothorax
  - In a large study of 100,000 ICN blocks performed by anesthesia residents, the rate of pneumothorax was 0.073%.
  - Another study of ICN blocks after rib fracture alone found the rate of PTX to be 1.4%.
- Systemic toxic reaction to the local anesthetic: Confusion, paresthesias, seizures
- Vasovagal reaction
- Abscess formation

Pearls
- The duration of action is approximately 12 hours and the effectiveness is operator dependent.
- Adequate sedation is important so the patient can tolerate the procedure.
- When compared with narcotics, ICN blocks have been shown to improve pulmonary function after rib fractures and chest surgery.
- ICN block may be a better alternative to narcotics for pain control in the elderly, as it will not impair their respiratory drive or their balance.
- Exercise greater caution in patients with chronic obstructive pulmonary disease (COPD).
  - Altered lung and pleural anatomy increase the risk of pneumothorax.
  - Pneumothorax may have more devastating outcome.

Suggested Readings
Kaplan JA, Miller EDE, Gallagher EG. Postoperative analgesia for throacotomy patients. *Anesth Analg*. 1975;54:773–777.

Moore DC. Intercostal nerve block for postoperative somatic pain following surgery of thorax and upper abdomen [Abstract only]. *Br J Anaesth*. 1975;47:284–286.

Moore DC. Intercostal nerve block. *Int Anesthesiol Clin*. 1998;36:29–34.

Orlinsky M, Dean E. Local and topical anesthesia and nerve blocks of the thorax and extremities. In: Roberts JR, Hedges JR. *Clinical procedures in emergency medicine*, 2nd ed. Philadelphia: WB Saunders; 1991.

Pardo M, Sonner JM. *The manual of anesthesia practice*. San Francisco: Pocketmedicine cominc; 2004.

Pedersen VM, Schulze S, Hoier-Madsen K, et al. Air-flow meter assessment of the effect of intercostal nerve block on respiratory function in rib fractures. *Acta Chir Scand*. 1983;149(2):119–120.

Shanti CM, Carlin AM, Tyburski JG. Incidence of pneumothorax from intercostal nerve block for analgesia in rib fractures. *J Trauma*. 2001;51: 536–539.

Watson DS, Panian S, Kendall V, et al. Pain control after thoracotomy: Bupivacaine versus lidocaine in continuous extrapleural intercostal nerve block. *Ann Thorac Surg*. 1999;67:825–829.

71

Dental Nerve Blocks

Julie A. Zeller and Peter B. Smulowitz

Indications

- Dental blocks are used to provide temporary analgesia for intraoral and dental pain related to the following:
    - Trauma requiring intraoral or facial laceration repair
    - Dental trauma resulting in fractured teeth
    - Infection (tooth abscess, root impaction, gum disease)
- Five most common types of blocks are described in Table 71.1

Contraindications

- **Absolute Contraindications**
    - Patient history of hypersensitivity/allergic reaction to local anesthetic agents
- **Relative Contraindications**
    - Coagulopathy patients
    - Infection at injection site
    - Uncooperative or obtunded patients

Risks/Consent Issues

- Dental blocks are intended for temporary pain relief and the procedure is not a substitute for prompt follow-up with a dentist
- Dental blocks are not 100% effective but should provide some immediate relief of pain in most cases
- Needle entry into the skin raises the possibility of introducing infection (sterile technique will be utilized)
- Needle puncture or accidental injury to vascular structures during the procedure can cause local bleeding
- Potential adverse reaction to the anesthetic
- Return of pain when the anesthetic wears off

Landmarks and Technique

- **Equipment and patient positioning:**
    - Adjust the examination chair to accommodate the patient's height.
    - Ensure there is adequate lighting to visualize oral landmarks.
    - Apply topical anesthetic, such as 20% benzocaine or 5% to 10% lidocaine ointment, before injection.
    - Assemble the necessary tools.
        - Sterile "thumb-control" Monoject aspirating dental syringe
        - A 1½ in. 25- to 27-gauge needle
        - Carpule cartridges containing anesthetic (either 2% lidocaine or 0.5% bupivacaine each with epinephrine 1:100,000 and 1:200,000 respectively)

TABLE 71.1: Types of dental blocks

Block	Area anesthetized	Comments
Supraperiosteal (local or apical)	Any individual maxillary tooth	▫ Straightforward, high success rate ▫ Not recommended for more than two adjacent teeth ▫ Works poorly on mandible because of bone density
Infraorbital (includes middle and anterior superior alveolar nerves)	▫ Maxillary teeth from midline through canine ▫ Buccal soft tissue of upper lip, lateral aspect of nose, lower eyelid	▫ Ideal for repairing upper lip lacerations ▫ Poor landmark identification could result in needle insertion into globe
Posterior superior alveolar	▫ Entire second and third maxillary molars ▫ First maxillary molar fully anesthetized in approximately 70% of patients	▫ Preferred block for pain in several maxillary molars ▫ Significant risk of hematoma, avoid overpenetration with needle; aspiration is crucial
Inferior alveolar	▫ All mandibular teeth to midline ▫ Anterior two-third of tongue (lingular branch) ▫ Floor of oral cavity ▫ Distribution of mental nerve	▫ Most widely used block, very effective when successful ▫ Failure rate high: 20%
Mental	▫ Mandibular teeth from midline to second premolar ▫ Buccal soft tissues from second premolar to midline, skin of lower lip and chin	▫ High success rate ▫ Ideal for repairing lower-lip and chin lacerations

> Cotton-tipped applicators for administering topical anesthetic and controlling bleeding
- Consider using lidocaine for laceration repairs and bupivacaine for dental blocks; 0.5% bupivacaine provides roughly 1 to 3 hours of dental pulp analgesia and 4 to 9 hours of soft tissue analgesia.
- Buffering with bicarbonate is not recommended for oral anesthesia.

Supraperiosteal Nerve Block
- Apply topical anesthetic to the apex of the mucobuccal fold adjacent to the affected tooth. The apex of the tooth is the target area and lies well above the patient's gum line.
- Lift the patient's upper lip and pull the tissue taut.
- Orient the needle and syringe parallel to the long axis of the tooth.
- Insert the needle into the target area with the bevel facing the bone.
- Advance and aspirate until the needle is a few millimeters beyond the apex of the tooth.
- If aspiration is negative then inject approximately 2 mL of anesthetic.

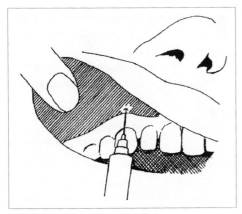

FIGURE 71.1: Supraperiosteal injection technique. (From Simon RR, Brenner BE. *Emergency procedures and techniques,* 4th ed. Philadelphia: Lippincott Williams & Wilkins; 2002:326, with permission.)

Infraorbital Nerve Block
See Chapter 72

Posterior Superior Alveolar Nerve Block
- Apply topical anesthetic to the apex of the mucobuccal fold above the second maxillary molar.
- Have the patient partially open the mouth and deviate the mandible toward the side of the pain to create more room.
- Using your index finger, retract the patient's cheek on the side being injected and pull the tissue taut.
- Insert the needle into the apex of the second maxillary molar, bevel facing bone.
- In one continuous movement, advance the needle through the soft tissue superiorly and medially (at a 45-degree angle to the plane of occlusion) and then posteriorly (at a 45-degree angle to the long axis of the second maxillary molar).

- The needle should penetrate approximately 15 mm in adults.
- Aspirate, then if blood is not aspirated, inject approximately 2 mL of anesthetic.

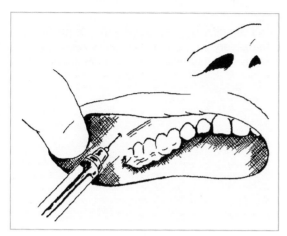

FIGURE 71.2: Posterior superior alveolar nerve injection technique. (From Simon RR, Brenner BE. *Emergency procedures and techniques*, 4th ed. Philadelphia: Lippincott Williams & Wilkins; 2002:326, with permission.)

Inferior Alveolar Nerve Block

- Stand opposite to the side being injected.
- Apply topical anesthetic on the mucosa at the site of the pterygomandibular triangle approximately 1 cm above the occlusal surface of the molars.
- Locate the anterior and posterior aspects of the mandibular ramus by placing the thumb of the nondominant hand intraorally and the index finger extraorally. The mandibular foramen is located between the index finger and thumb, slightly above the level of the mandibular molars and midway between the anterior and posterior borders of the ramus.

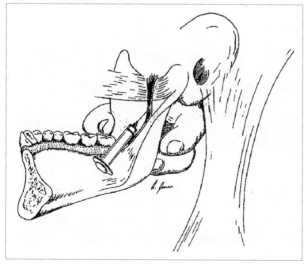

FIGURE 71.3: Inferior alveolar nerve injection. (From Simon RR, Brenner BE. *Emergency procedures and techniques*. 4th ed. Philadelphia: Lippincott Williams & Wilkins; 2002:327, with permission.)

- Orient the syringe so the barrel is in the opposite corner of the mouth, resting on the premolars.
- Aim toward your index finger and slowly penetrate the mucosa at the pterygomandibular triangle until you hit bone (approximately 2.5 cm).
- Failure to reach bone generally results from directing the needle too far posteriorly, toward the parotid gland. This risks temporary paralysis of the facial nerve.
- Once bone is contacted, withdraw slightly and aspirate. If no blood is aspirated, inject up to 2 mL of anesthetic.

Mental Nerve Block
See Chapter 72

Complications
- Nerve damage
- Localized hematoma
- Incomplete analgesia
- Infection
- Allergic reaction to anesthetic
- Intravascular injection
- Vasovagal syncope

Common Pitfalls
- Patient noncompliance secondary to pain if topical anesthesia before needle insertion is not used or anesthetic is injected too fast
- Incorrect identification of landmarks
- Failure to advance the needle to sufficient depth to reach apex of tooth
- Injecting directly into the foramen, which can cause nerve damage
- Injecting through an infected area, which can propagate the infection
- Changing the direction of the needle without first withdrawing, which can cause deep tissue damage and needle breakage

Pearls
- Take time to review the method, gather all necessary equipment, ensure adequate lighting, and identify landmarks before procedure.
- Always apply topical anesthetic to the mucosa before needle insertion.
- Provide verbal instruction to your patient throughout the procedure.
- Always insert the needle with the bevel toward bone.
- Always aspirate before injection of anesthetic.
- Inject slowly over at least 30 seconds in order to prevent additional pain from rapid tissue expansion.

Suggested Readings
Amsterdam JT, Kilgore KP. Regional anesthesia of the head and neck. In: Roberts JR, Hedges JR, eds. *Clinical procedures in emergency medicine*, 4th ed. Philadelphia: Elsevier Science; 2004:552–566.

Ferrera PC, Chandler R. Anesthesia in the emergency setting: Part II. Head and neck, eye and rib injuries. *Am Fam Physician*. 1994;50(3):569–573.

Henretig FM, King C. *Pediatric emergency procedures*. Baltimore: Williams & Wilkins; 1997.

Powell SL, Robertson L, Doty BJ. Dental nerve blocks: Toothache remedies for the acute-care setting. *Postgrad Med*. 2000;107(1):229–245.

Simon RR, Brenner BE. Common dental emergencies. In: *Emergency procedures and techniques*, 4th ed. Lippincott Williams & Wilkins; 2001:325–327.

Trott AT. *Wounds and lacerations: Emergency care and closure*, 2nd ed. St. Louis: Mosby; 1997.

72

Facial Nerve Blocks

Cathy Horwitz and Jason A. Tracy

Indications
- Used to provide anesthesia to the face and ears in order to facilitate the following:
    - Primary closure of facial lacerations
    - Incision and drainage
- Anesthetized distributions
    - Forehead (supraorbital and supratrochlear)
    - Infraorbital: Upper lip, cheek, lateral portion of the nose, and anterior maxillary teeth
    - Inferior alveolar: Lower jaw, lower lip, lower teeth to lower teeth, and anterior two-third of the tongue
    - Mental: Lower jaw, teeth, anterior tongue, and floor of the mouth
    - Auricular: External ear

Contraindications
- **Absolute Contraindications**
    - Patient history of hypersensitivity/allergic reaction to local anesthetic agents
- **Relative Contraindications**
    - Coagulopathy patients
    - Infection at injection site
    - Uncooperative or obtunded patients

Risks/Consent Issues
- Facial blocks are not 100% effective but should provide some immediate relief of pain in most cases.
- Needle entry into the skin raises the possibility of introducing infection (sterile technique will be utilized).
- Needle puncture or accidental injury to vascular structures during the procedure can cause local bleeding.
- Potential adverse reaction to the anesthetic
- Return of pain when the anesthetic wears off

Landmarks and Technique
- **Patient Preparation**
    - Consent for procedure
    - Supine position that allows ideal surgeon comfort
    - Adequate lighting to identify landmarks
- **Materials Preparation**
    - Use 25-gauge to 30-gauge needle
    - Prepare syringe filled with anesthetic of choice

- Local topical anesthetic cream (e.g., eutectic mixture of local anesthetics [EMLA], 20% benzocaine, or 5% to 10% lidocaine ointment) can be used before procedure to decrease the pain of needle insertion
- **Choice of Agent**
  - Lidocaine 1% to 2%
    - ▷ Onset of action: 4 to 10 minutes
    - ▷ Duration of action: 60 to 120 minutes
    - ▷ Maximum one time dose: 4.5 mg/kg
  - Bupivacaine 0.25%
    - ▷ Onset of action: 8 to 12 minutes
    - ▷ Duration of action: 240 to 480 minutes
  - Bicarbonate
    - ▷ Can be used in 1:10 dilution with above anesthetics to decrease the pain of infiltration
- **Sterile Technique**
  - Povidone-iodine solution or chlorhexidine on the skin (not mucosa!)
  - Sterile gloves

Forehead Nerve Block
- The supraorbital notch is located at the bisection of a vertical line through the pupil (when the eye is pointing forward) and a horizontal line at the superior edge of the orbit.
- Insert the needle just superior and medial to the supraorbital notch and inject 2 to 4 mL of anesthetic.
- Following anesthesia of the supraorbital nerve, anesthetize the supratrochlear nerve 0.5 to 1.0 cm medial to the supraorbital notch with an additional 2 to 4 mL of anesthetic.

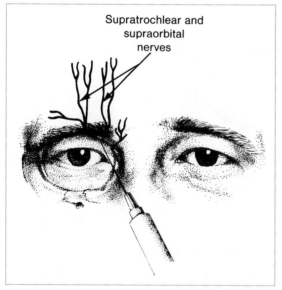

FIGURE 72.1: The supraorbital and supratrochlear nerves emerging through the notches at the upper border of the orbital ridge. (From Simon RR, Brenner BE. *Emergency procedures and techniques*, 4th ed. Philadelphia: Lippincott Williams & Wilkins; 2002:117, with permission.)

Infraorbital Nerve Block

▪ The infraorbital foramen is located just inferior to the bisection of a vertical line through the pupil (when the eye is pointing forward) and a horizontal line at the inferior edge of the orbit.

▪ Extraoral or intraoral approach can be used.

    ○ Extraoral

        ▷ Insert the needle 1 cm below the infraorbital foramen and inject 2 to 4 mL of anesthetic.

    ○ Intraoral

        ▷ Place one finger on the infraorbital foramen and retract the upper lip.

        ▷ Identify the first maxillary premolar, and insert the needle into the mucobuccal fold with the bevel facing the bone.

        ▷ Advance the needle toward the apex of the tooth or 1 cm below the infraorbital foramen.

        ▷ Take caution to avoid entering the orbit or the infraorbital foramen.

        ▷ If there is any paresthesia, retract the needle.

        ▷ Inject 2 to 4 mL of anesthetic.

Mental Nerve Block

▪ The mental foramen lies in the plane of the supraorbital and infraorbital foramina at the apex of the lower second premolar.

▪ Extraoral or intraoral approach can be used.

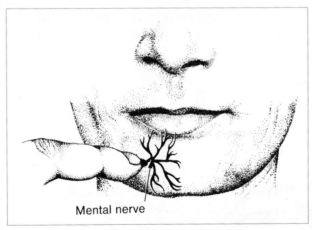

Mental nerve

FIGURE 72.2: The mental nerve supplies sensation to the skin and mucous membranes of the lower lip. (From Simon RR, Brenner BE. *Emergency procedures and techniques*. 4th ed. Philadelphia: Lippincott Williams & Wilkins; 2002:114, with permission.)

    ○ Extraoral

        ▷ Insert the needle 1 cm inferolateral to the foramen.

        ▷ Inject 2 to 4 mL of anesthetic.

    ○ Intraoral

        ▷ Retract the patient's lower lip.

        ▷ Locate the space between the premolar and molar teeth.

        ▷ At this site, insert the needle into the mucobuccal fold and advance toward the apex of the tooth and anterior to the mental nerve foramen.

        ▷ Aspirate. If no blood returns, inject 2 to 4 mL of anesthetic.

 ▷ Complete anesthesia should occur within 5 minutes of injection (lip usually starts to feel numb in 60 seconds).

Auricular Block

▪ First enter the skin superiorly and infiltrate along the superior/anterior aspect, and then infiltrate along the superior/posterior aspect of the ear.

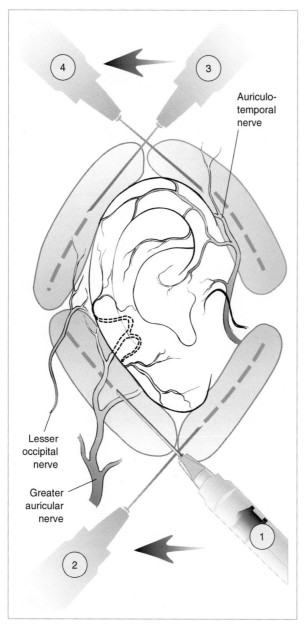

FIGURE 72.3: Regional auricular block. (From Kassutto Z, Helpin ML. Orofacial anesthesia techniques. In: Henretig FM, King C, eds. *Textbook of pediatric emergency procedures*. Philadelphia: Williams & Wilkins; 1997:719, with permission.)

- Next enter the skin inferior to the pinna and infiltrate along the inferior/anterior aspect and then along the inferior/posterior aspect.
- A total of 10 to 20 mL of anesthetic is injected in a diamond shape around the pinna.

Inferior Alveolar Nerve Block
See Chapter 71

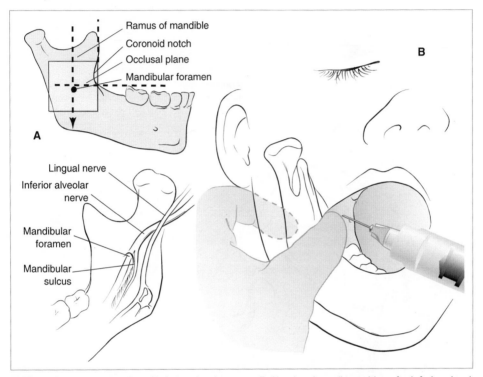

FIGURE 72.4: A: Localization of inferior alveolar nerve. **B:** Hand and needle positions for inferior alveolar nerve block. (From Kassutto Z, Helpin ML. Orofacial anesthesia techniques. In: Henretig FM, King C, eds. *Textbook of pediatric emergency procedures*. Philadelphia: Williams & Wilkins; 1997:719, with permission.)

Complications
- Nerve damage
- Localized hematoma
- Incomplete analgesia
- Infection
- Allergic reaction to anesthetic
- Intravascular injection
- Vasovagal syncope

Common Pitfalls
- Patient noncompliance secondary to pain if topical anesthesia before needle insertion is not used or anesthetic is injected too fast

- Incorrect identification of landmarks
- Failure to advance the needle to sufficient depth to reach apex of tooth
- Injecting directly into the foramen, which can cause nerve damage
- Injecting through an infected area, which can propagate the infection
- Changing the direction of the needle without first withdrawing, which can cause deep tissue damage and needle breakage

Pearls

- Take time to review the method, gather all necessary equipment, ensure adequate lighting, and identify landmarks before procedure.
- Always apply topical anesthetic to the mucosa before needle insertion.
- Provide verbal instruction to your patient throughout the procedure.
- Always insert the needle with the bevel toward bone.
- Always aspirate before injection of anesthetic.
- Inject slowly over at least 30 seconds in order to prevent additional pain from rapid tissue expansion.

Suggested Readings

Henretig FM, King C. *Pediatric emergency procedures*. Baltimore: Williams & Wilkins; 1997.

Hedges JR, Roberts JR. *Clinical procedures in emergency medicine*, 4th ed. Philadelphia: WB Saunders; 2004.

Simon RR, Brenner BE. *Emergency procedures and techniques*, 4th ed. Philadelphia: Lippincott Williams & Wilkins; 2002.

Tintinalli JE, Ruiz E, Krome RL. *Emergency medicine: A comprehensive study guide*, 4th ed. New York: McGraw-Hill; 1996.

Wolfson AB. *Harwood-Nuss' clinical practice of emergency medicine*. Philadelphia: Lippincott Williams & Wilkins; 2005.

Ankle and Foot Nerve Blocks
Matthew R. Babineau and Scott G. Weiner

Indications
- Used to provide regional anesthesia to the foot in order to facilitate the following:
  - Primary closure/exploration of foot wounds
  - Incision and drainage
  - Removal of foreign bodies
  - Operative intervention

Contraindications
- Very few; is a preferred technique because glabrous skin of the epidermis and fibrous septae in the dermis of the foot limit local diffusion of anesthetic
- Contraindications
  - Infection overlying injection sites
  - In cases of neurologic deficits, perform complete sensory examination before performing the block

Risks/Consent Issues
- Procedure can cause pain (local anesthesia will be given, several needle sticks are required)
- Needle puncture can cause local bleeding
- Whenever the skin is broken, there is potential for introducing infection (sterile technique will be utilized)
- Rare instances of persistent paresthesias, neuritis, or cardiotoxicity from anesthetic overdose or intravascular injection

Landmarks
There are five nerves which supply the entire surface of the foot (see Fig. 73.1)

Technique
- **Patient Preparation**
  - Consent for procedure
  - Supine position with knee in flexion and foot placed flat on the gurney or on a podiatric foot rest
- **Materials Preparation**
  - Use 25-gauge to 30-gauge needle
  - Prepare one to three 10-mL syringes filled with anesthetic of choice
  - Local topical anesthetic cream (e.g., eutectic mixture of local anesthetics [EMLA]) can be used before the procedure to decrease the pain of needle insertion

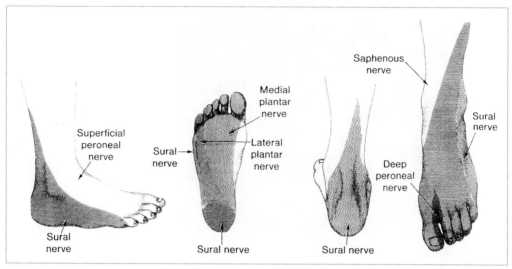

FIGURE 73.1: The sensory nerve supply to the foot. (From Simon RR, Brenner BE. *Emergency Procedures and Techniques.* 4th ed. Philadelphia: Lippincott Williams & Wilkins; 2002:136, with permission.)

- **Choice of Agent**
  - Lidocaine 1% to 2%
    - Onset of action: 4 to 10 minutes
    - Duration of action: 60 to 120 minutes
    - Maximum one-time dose: 4.5 mg/kg
  - Bupivacaine 0.25%
    - Onset of action: 8 to 12 minutes
    - Duration of action: 240 to 480 minutes
  - Bicarbonate
    - Can be used in 1:10 dilution with above anesthetics to decrease the pain of infiltration
- **Sterile Technique**
  - Povidone-iodine solution or chlorhexidine
  - Sterile draping
  - Sterile gloves

Posterior Tibial Nerve Block

- *Innervation*: Divides into medial and lateral plantar nerves to supply most of the plantar aspect of the foot.
- *Location*: Medial aspect of the ankle between medial malleolus and Achilles tendon.
- *Technique* (see Fig. 73.2)
  - Palpate posterior tibial artery posterior to medial malleolus.
  - Direct needle at 45-degree angle to mediolateral plane, posterior to artery.
  - At depth of artery (0.5 to 1 cm deep), wiggle needle to induce paresthesia.
  - If elicited, 3 to 5 mL of anesthetic are injected after aspiration.
  - Withdraw 1 mm, then infiltrate 5 to 7 mL of anesthetic while withdrawing 1 cm.

Sural Nerve Block

- *Innervation*: Lateral edge of foot, variable to fifth toe

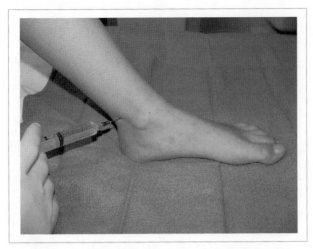

FIGURE 73.2: Approach for posterior tibial nerve block.

- *Location*: Lateral aspect of ankle between Achilles tendon and lateral malleolus
- *Technique* (see Fig. 73.3)

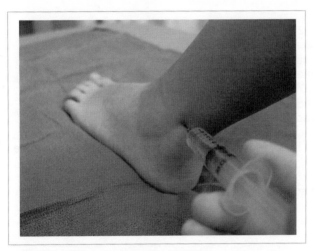

FIGURE 73.3: Approach for sural nerve block.

- Infiltrate 3 to 5 mL of local anesthetic in a band between Achilles tendon and lateral malleolus.

Deep Peroneal Nerve Block

- *Innervation*: Dorsal webspace between first and second toes
- *Location*: Anterior aspect of ankle, between extensor hallucis and anterior tibial tendons
- *Technique* (see Fig. 73.4)
  - Palpate tendons by having patient dorsiflex hallux and foot.
  - Raise subcutaneous wheal between the tendons.
  - Direct needle laterally at 30-degree angle under the extensor hallucis tendon until the tibia is met.
  - Withdraw needle 1 to 2 mm and infiltrate 1 mL of local anesthetic.

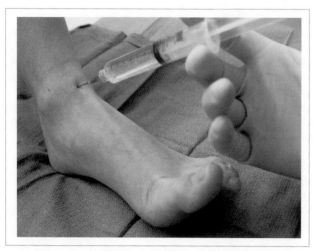

FIGURE 73.4: Approach for nerve block of deep peroneal nerve, superficial peroneal nerve, and saphenous nerve.

Superficial Peroneal Nerve Block
- *Innervation*: Dorsal aspect of foot, except webspace between first and second toes
- *Location*: Anterior aspect of ankle between extensor hallucis tendon and lateral malleolus
- *Technique*
  - Infiltrate 5 to 10 mL of local anesthetic subcutaneously in a band between extensor hallucis tendon and lateral malleolus. This can be done while withdrawing the needle from the deep peroneal nerve block.

Saphenous Nerve Block
- *Innervation*: Medial aspect of foot, variable to first toe
- *Location*: Anterior aspect of ankle between anterior tibial tendon and medial malleolus
- *Technique*
  - Infiltrate 3 to 5 mL of local anesthetic in a band between anterior tibial tendon and medial malleolus. This can be done while withdrawing the needle from the deep peroneal nerve block (Fig. 73.4).

Complications
- Infection (rare with sterile technique)
- Hematoma (minimize number of injections)
- Vessel puncture with subsequent cardiotoxicity (avoid greater saphenous vein at ankle; aspirate before injecting frequently)
- Nerve injury, neuritis (do not inject if patient complains of pain or high pressures, do not reinject deep nerves)

Common Pitfalls
- Failure to inform patient that technique does not always work on first attempt and may require reinjection
- Failure to respect maximum doses of anesthetic

Pearls

- Position the foot on a podiatric footrest, or with the knee in flexion and foot flat on a gurney, so all nerves can be accessed without repositioning patient or drapes.
- The superficial nerves (sural nerve, saphenous nerve, and superficial peroneal nerve) have extensive branches and anastomoses, so a generous subcutaneous infiltration will provide better anesthesia.
- For the deep nerve blocks (deep peroneal nerve and post tibial nerve) repeating the described procedures twice while "fanning" the needle 30 degrees medial and lateral will improve anesthesia.
- Alternatively, all five nerves can be blocked using three injections.
  - Block posterior tibial nerve as described.
  - Block sural nerve as described.
  - Block deep peroneal nerve as described; as the needle is withdrawn, fan medially and infiltrate to block the saphenous nerve, then fan laterally and infiltrate to block the superficial peroneal nerve.

74 Wrist Nerve Blocks

Jayson R. Pereira and Ryan P. Friedberg

Indications

- Used to provide anesthesia in distribution of median, ulnar, and/or radial nerves for the treatment of complex soft tissue or bony injuries of the hand
  - Irrigation of deep abrasions with embedded debris
  - Extensive or complex laceration repair
  - Burn injury pain control
  - Incision and drainage of abscess
  - Fracture/dislocation reduction
  - Traumatic amputation

Contraindications

- Overlying cellulitis at site of anticipated injection
- **Relative Contraindications**
  - Simple laceration or other injury that can be easily and adequately anesthetized with local infiltration or digital block

Risks/Consent Issues

- Procedure can cause pain
- Needle puncture can cause local bleeding
- Whenever the skin is broken, there is potential for introducing infection (sterile technique will be utilized)
- Risk of vascular or peripheral nerve injury is minimal, but present
- Allergic reaction to anesthetic solution may occur

Complications

- Hematoma formation and/or vascular injury
- Nerve injury
- Infection
- Allergic reaction

Ulnar Nerve Block

Landmarks

- Flexor carpi ulnaris tendon, pisiform bone, ulnar artery, proximal wrist crease (see Fig. 74.1)
- Ulnar nerve splits into dorsal and palmar branches approximately 5 cm proximal to the wrist crease

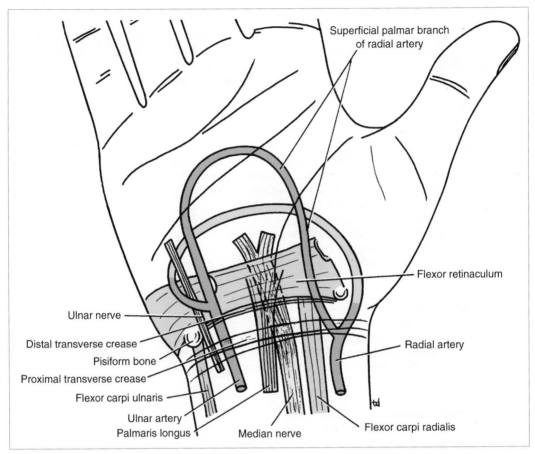

FIGURE 74.1: Surface anatomy of the wrist region. (From Snell RS. *Clinical anatomy*. 7th ed. Philadelphia: Lippincott Williams & Wilkins; 2004:534, with permission.)

■ Palmar branch runs between flexor carpi ulnaris tendon and the ulnar artery at the level of the proximal wrist crease

Technique
■ **Patient Preparation**
- Place the patient's affected hand comfortably on bedside procedure table with palmar surface up.
- Prepare wrist site in standard sterile manner (povidone-iodine solution or chlorhexidine).
- Have patient flex wrist against resistance to accentuate landmarks.
- Identify and mark flexor carpi ulnaris tendon from its insertion site at the pisiform bone to the ulnar nerve branch point (approximately 5 cm proximal to wrist crease).

■ **Injection**
- Approach the wrist medially and insert a small-bore (25-gauge) needle beneath the flexor carpi ulnaris tendon at the level of the proximal wrist crease (see Fig. 74.2)
  ▷ Inject approximately 2 mL of anesthetic solution (lidocaine/bupivacaine) beneath the tendon at its radial border.

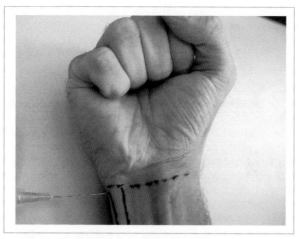

FIGURE 74.2: Injection site of an ulnar nerve block.

- ▷ Aspirate before injecting anesthetic to ensure that ulnar artery has not been inadvertently entered.
- ◦ To anesthetize the dorsal branch of the ulnar nerve use the same initial insertion site and technique. However, redirect needle 3 to 5 cm proximally toward the branch point.
  - ▷ Inject approximately 5 mL of anesthetic solution beneath the tendon at this branch point.

Common Pitfalls
- ▫ Inadequate anesthesia as a result of failure to redirect and inject at dorsal cutaneous branch point
- ▫ Depositing anesthetic solution too medially owing to fear of entering/injuring the ulnar artery

Pearls
- ▫ In patients in whom the proximal wrist crease cannot be easily identified the ulnar styloid can be used as an alternative landmark.
- ▫ If tendon is not identified initially have patient oppose thumb and fifth finger while flexing against resistance.
- ▫ If paresthesias are elicited at any point during advancement of the needle, stop and withdraw approximately 5 mm and inject the anesthetic.

Median Nerve Block

Landmarks
- ▫ Palmaris longus tendon, flexor carpi radialis tendon, proximal wrist crease (Fig. 74.1).
- ▫ Median nerve runs beneath palmaris longus tendon along its radial edge.
- ▫ For patients in whom the palmaris longus tendon is absent (approximately 15% of population) the median nerve can be found approximately 1 cm ulnar to flexor carpi radialis tendon.

- In contrast to the superficial position of the palmaris longus, the median nerve courses deep to the flexor retinaculum.

Technique
- **Patient Preparation**
  - Place the patient's affected hand comfortably on bedside procedure table with palmar surface up.
  - Prepare wrist site in standard sterile manner (povidone-iodine solution or chlorhexidine).
  - Have patient flex wrist against resistance to accentuate landmarks.
  - Identify and mark palmaris longus tendon and/or flexor carpi radialis tendon at the level of the proximal wrist crease.
- **Injection**
  - Approach the wrist from palmar side and insert a small-bore (25-gauge) needle through the proximal wrist crease at a right angle to the lateral border of the palmaris longus tendon (see Fig. 74.3).

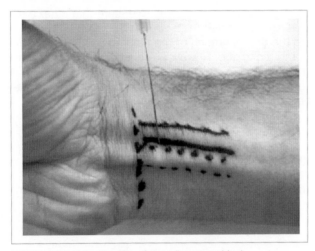

FIGURE 74.3: Injection site of a median nerve block.

  - Inject approximately 5 mL of anesthetic solution (lidocaine/bupivacaine) deep to the flexor retinaculum.
  - In patients without a palmaris longus, insert and inject 1 cm medial to flexor carpi radialis using the same approach and technique.

Common Pitfalls
- Injecting anesthetic superficial to flexor retinaculum which then blocks solution from contacting the nerve below.
- Mistaking the flexor carpi radialis tendon for the palmaris longus tendon in those patients in whom the palmaris longus is absent.

Pearls
- If tendons are not identified easily have patient oppose thumb and fifth finger while flexing against resistance.
- Feel for resistance as needle pierces the flexor retinaculum.

- To ensure that the injection is deep to the flexor retinaculum insert needle until bone is contacted, then withdraw 0.5 cm and deposit anesthetic solution.
- If paresthesias are elicited at any point during advancement of the needle, stop and withdraw approximately 5 mm and inject the anesthetic.

Radial Nerve Block

Landmarks
- Radial styloid, radial artery, proximal wrist crease, anatomic snuff box (see Fig. 74.4).

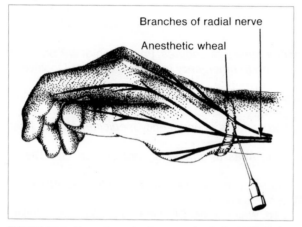

Branches of radial nerve

Anesthetic wheal

FIGURE 74.4: Deposit a subcutaneous wheal of anesthetic in a semicircle manner to block all branches of the radial nerve. (From Simon RR, Brenner BE. *Emergency procedures and techniques*, 4th ed. Philadelphia: Lippincott Williams & Wilkins; 2002:132, with permission.)

- Radial nerve follows the course of the radial artery breaking off into multiple deep and superficial branches before entering the hand.
- At the level of the proximal wrist crease all sensory branches of the radial nerve run superficially, providing an access point for complete anesthesia.

Technique
- **Patient Preparation**
  - Place the patient's affected hand comfortably on bedside procedure table with the ulnar surface down.
  - Prepare wrist site in standard sterile manner (povidone-iodine solution or chlorhexidine).
  - Identify and mark the radial artery at the level of the proximal wrist crease.
- **Injection**
  - Palpate for the radial styloid. Approach the wrist from palmar side and insert a small-bore (25-gauge) needle through the proximal wrist crease, immediately lateral to the radial artery.
    - Inject approximately 3 mL of anesthetic solution (lidocaine/bupivacaine) subcutaneously over the palmar aspect of the radial styloid.
  - Next ensure anesthesia of all the sensory branches. Using the same initial needle insertion point redirect the needle over the snuff box, and inject

approximately 5 mL of the anesthetic solution in a bandlike manner to the dorsal midline.

Common Pitfalls
- Failure to adequately block the dorsal sensory branches by stopping the bandlike injection short of the dorsal midline.

Pearls
- Avoid unnecessary patient discomfort when anesthetizing dorsal sensory branches; new needle insertions should be through areas of already anesthetized skin.

Suggested Readings
Dunmire S, Parris P. *Atlas of emergency procedures*. Philadelphia: WB Saunders; 1994.

Mitchell E, Medzon R. *Introduction to emergency medicine*. Boston: Lippincott Williams & Wilkins; 2005.

Mulroy M. *Regional anesthesia: An illustrated procedure guide*, 3rd ed. Virginia: Lippincott Williams & Wilkins; 2002.

Roberts J, Hedges J. *Clinical procedures in emergency medicine*, 4th ed. Philadelphia: WB Saunders; 2004.

Rosen P, Chan T, Vilke G, et al. *Atlas of emergency procedures*. San Diego: Mosby; 2001.

Simon RR, Brenner BE. *Emergency procedures and techniques*, 4th ed. Chicago: Lippincott Williams & Wilkins; 2002.

Snell R. *Clinical anatomy*, 7th ed. Washington, DC: Lippincott Williams & Wilkins; 2004.

Section Editor: Angela Tangredi

75   Intubation of the Pediatric Patient

Joshua S. Easter and Kevin M. Ban

Indications
- Inadequate oxygenation or ventilation
- Airway obstruction
- Loss of protective airway reflexes (e.g., depressed cough and gag reflex)
- Excess work of breathing
- Nonresponsive and apneic

Contraindications
- **Absolute Contraindications**
  - None for unstable patients
- **Relative Contraindications** (if possible, should involve anesthesia when these are present)
  - Epiglottitis; if stable, airway manipulation should be performed in the operating room (OR)
  - Significant facial or laryngeal edema with airway distortion
  - Significant airway distortion secondary to trauma

Risks/Consent Issues
- Airway trauma
- Aspiration of stomach contents
- Hypoxemia
- Pain
- Esophageal intubation
- Increase in blood pressure and intracranial pressure (ICP)

Landmarks
- Anatomical differences seen in children
  - Larger tongue
  - Larger and floppy epiglottis

- Narrow cricoid ring
- Larger occiput
- The glottic opening is more anterior in children due to a relatively high tracheal opening and can be seen at:
  - ▶ C1 in infancy
  - ▶ C3 to C4 at age 7
  - ▶ C4 to C5 in the adult

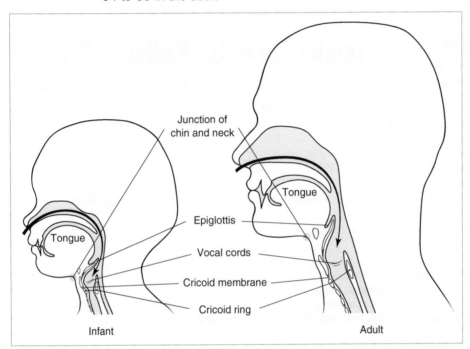

FIGURE 75.1: The anatomic differences particular to children are (a) higher, more anterior position of the glottic opening (note the relationship of the vocal cords to the chin/neck junction); (b) relatively larger tongue in the infant, which lies between the mouth and the glottic opening; (c) relatively larger and more floppy epiglottis in the child; (d) the cricoid ring is the narrowest portion of the pediatric airway versus the vocal cords in the adult; (e) position and size of the cricothyroid membrane in the infant; (f) sharper, more difficult angle for blind nasotracheal intubation; (g) larger relative size of the occiput in the infant.

Technique

The approach to the technique for rapid sequence intubation (RSI) can be summarized in seven discrete steps, each beginning with the letter P

- **Preparation:** Assemble the proper equipment
  - Cardiorespiratory monitor and pulse oximeter
  - Suction catheter
  - Bag valve mask (BVM) and oxygen source
  - Oral airway
    - ▶ Size based on Broselow tape or distance from the angle of the mouth to the ear tragus
  - Laryngoscope blade (see Table 75.1)
    - ▶ Straight/Miller blade is preferred to the curved blade for younger children to displace distensible anatomy and better visualize the anterior glottic opening size based on Broselow tape

TABLE 75.1: Pediatric laryngoscope blade sizes

Age/weight	Size (type)
2.5 kg	0 (straight)
0–3 mo	1.0 (straight)
3 mo–3 yr	1.5 (straight)
3–12 yr	2.0 (straight or curved)[a]
12–18 yr	3.0 (straight or curved)

[a]A curved blade may be used for older children, but a straight blade is generally preferred.
From King C, Stayer SA. Emergent endotracheal intubation. In: Henretig FM, King C, eds. *Textbook of pediatric emergency procedures*. Philadelphia: Williams & Wilkins, 1997:185, with permission.

- Endotracheal tube size based on Broselow tape or calculated as follows (see Table 75.2):
  - ▸ Calculated: (age in years + 16)/4
  - ▸ Uncuffed tube is preferable in children younger than 8 years
  - ▸ Have two extra endotracheal tubes that are a size larger and smaller than the estimated size
  - ▸ Place stylet to provide rigidity

TABLE 75.2: Pediatric endotracheal tube sizes

Weight/age	Internal diameter (mm)[a]	Tube marking at lips (cm)
Under 1,500 g	2.5 uncuffed	wt in kg 6.0 cm
1,500–5,000 g	3.0 uncuffed	wt in kg 6.0 cm
5,000 g–6 mo	3.5 uncuffed	12.0–13.0
6–18 mo	3.5–4.0 uncuffed	13.0–14.0
18 mo–3 yr	4.0–4.5 uncuffed	13.5–14.5
3–5 yr	4.5 uncuffed	14.5–15.5
5–6 yr	5.0 uncuffed	15.5–17.0
6–8 yr	5.5–6.0 uncuffed	17.0–19.0
8–10 yr	5.5–6.0 cuffed	19.0–20.0
10–12 yr	6.0–6.5 cuffed	20.0–21.0
12–14 yr	6.5–7.0 cuffed	21.0–22.0
14–16 yr	7.0–7.5 cuffed	22.0–23.0

[a]Two additional endotracheal tubes (one-half size larger and smaller) should also be readily available in case the initial estimation proves incorrect.
From King C, Stayer SA. Emergent endotracheal intubation. In: Henretig FM, King C, eds. *Textbook of pediatric emergency procedures*. Philadelphia: Williams & Wilkins, 1997:185, with permission.

- End tidal CO_2 monitor
  - In children weighing<15 kg, must use pediatric monitor
- Have airway alternatives available (e.g., laryngeal mask airway [LMA], needle cricothyrotomy equipment)

Preoxygenation
- Theoretically, deliver 100% oxygen for 3 minutes; nonrebreather mask delivers approximately 70%
- If child is breathing, use well fitting mask with 100% O_2 (nonrebreather mask with O_2 flow of 10 to 15 L/minute is preferred)
  - Pediatric basal O_2 consumption is twice adult values; children tend to desaturate more quickly than adults because of limited oxygen reserve
- If child is not breathing, use BVM ventilation
  - Tilt the head back and use three fingers under the angle of the mandible to lift up the jaw
  - Place remaining fingers on mask to form ''C'' lock
  - If two people are available, one person maintains mask seal while the other compresses the bag
  - Use the rhythm ''squeeze, release, release'' to allow enough time for exhalation
  - Apply cricoid pressure if the patient is unconscious
  - Insert an oral airway in the unconscious pediatric patient in whom it is difficult to ventilate

Pretreatment: This refers to the administration of medications to attenuate the potential adverse side effect of intubation (see Table 75.3)
- **Atropine:** 0.01 to 0.02 mg/kg; minimum dose of 0.1 mg (to prevent paradoxical bradycardia)
  - Reduces vagal stimulation and oral secretions
  - Use for all children younger than 1 year
  - Use in all children who are receiving ketamine or succinylcholine
- **Lidocaine:** 1 to 2 mg/kg
  - Use in case of suspected increased ICP (e.g., head injury)
  - Use in asthmatics
- **Vecuronium:** 0.01 mg/kg
  - Inhibits the muscle fasciculations caused by succinylcholine
  - Use in case of suspected increased ICP (e.g., head injury)
- **Fentanyl:** 1 to 3 μg/kg
  - For analgesia
  - Use in case of suspected increased ICP (e.g., head injury)

Protection and Positioning
- Pull up on child's chin to create sniffing position to relieve airway flexion due to relatively large occiput
  - Infants often require a towel behind their shoulders to elevate their torso
  - When in proper position, external auditory canal should be anterior to the shoulders
- Maintain C-spine immobilization when concerned about a potential cervical spine injury

Paralysis and Induction
- Induction agents
  - **Etomidate:** 0.2 to 0.4 mg/kg IV
    - Onset is at 30 to 40 seconds, duration is 5 to 8 minutes
  - **Ketamine:** 1 to 2 mg/kg IV, 4 mg/kg IM
    - Also provides analgesia

TABLE 75.3: Pretreatment drugs

Drugs	Dose	Special considerations
Drugs for rapid sequence intubation		
Atropine	0.01–0.02 mg/kg	Minimum dose 0.1 mg Use in infants <1 year of age Use with ketamine to reduce salivation
Lidocaine	1–2 mg/kg	Use with increased ICP
Vecuronium	0.01 mg/kg	Use with succinylcholine to reduce fasciculations
Fentanyl	1–3 μg/kg	
Sedation drugs One of the following		
Etomidate	0.2–0.4 mg/kg	Onset at 1 min, lasts 3–12 min
Ketamine	1–2 mg/kg IV 4 mg/kg IM	Onset at 1–2 min, lasts 10–30 min; use atropine to reduce salivation; may increase ICP
Propofol	1–2 mg/kg	Onset at 30–60 sec, lasts 10–15 min; may decrease BP
Thiopental	3–5 mg/kg	Onset at 10–20 sec, lasts 10–30 min; may decrease BP
Paralysis drugs One of the following		
Succinylcholine	1–2 mg/kg	Onset at 30–45 sec, lasts 3–12 min; contraindication with high ICP, rhabdomyolysis, high K^+, renal failure
Rocuronium	0.6–1.2 mg/kg	Onset at 30–90 sec, lasts 30–90 min
Vecuronium	0.1 mg/kg	Onset at 90–120 sec, lasts 25–120 min

ICP, intracranial pressure; BP, blood pressure.

- Avoid in children with suspected increased ICP or intraocular pressure (IOP)
- Helpful for patients with status asthmaticus
- Onset is at 1 to 2 minutes, duration is 30 to 60 minutes
  - **Propofol:** 2 mg/kg IV
  - **Thiopental:** 3 to 5 mg/kg IV
    - For head injury patients who are normotensive
- Paralysis agents: Confirm paralysis with absence of spontaneous movements, respiratory effort blink reflex, and by jaw relaxation
  - **Succinylcholine:** 1 to 2 mg/kg
    - Avoid when suspect rhabdomyolysis or hyperkalemia
    - Onset is at 30 to 60 seconds, duration is 3 to 5 minutes
  - **Rocuronium:** 0.6 to 1.2 mg/kg
    - Onset is at 60 seconds, duration is 30 to 60 minutes
  - **Vecuronium:** 0.1 mg/kg
    - Onset is at 90 seconds, duration is 30 to 60 minutes
- **Placement of Tube and Proof of Placement**
  - Blade insertion
    - Place laryngoscope blade in left hand and insert into right side of mouth
    - Once the tip of the blade is at the base of the tongue sweep the tongue to the left with the blade

- ▷ If using a straight blade, the tip of the blade should be used to lift the epiglottis
- ▷ If using a curve blade, insert the tip into the vallecula then pull upward in the direction of the long axis of the laryngoscope handle
- ▷ Use suction if necessary to clear the airway

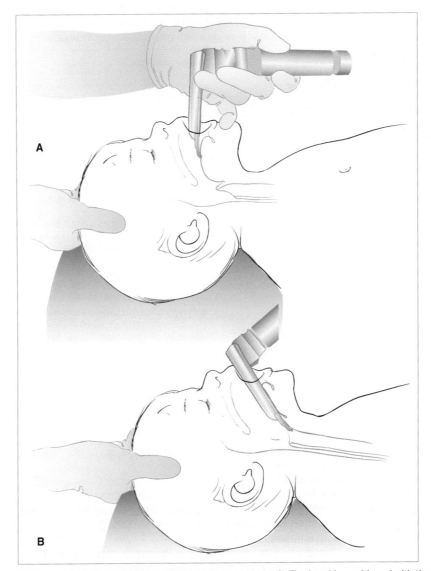

FIGURE 75.2: Direct laryngoscopy using a straight blade. **A:** The head is positioned with the right hand and the mouth is opened using the fifth finger of the left hand (if necessary). **B:** The tip of the blade is used to directly retract the epiglottis, revealing the vocal cords and glottic opening. (From King C, Stayer SA. Emergent endotracheal intubation. In: Henretig FM, King C, eds. *Textbook of pediatric emergency procedures*. Philadelphia: Williams & Wilkins, 1997:199, with permission.)

- Endotracheal tube (ETT) insertion
  - ▷ Keep the vocal cords visualized at all times and insert the tube through the glottic opening

  ▷ Place the tube's black glottic marker at the level of the vocal cords
  ▷ Remove the laryngoscope and stylet from the tube
  ▷ Maintain control of the ETT with your hand until properly secured
- Proof of tube placement
  ▷ Look for symmetric chest rise and condensation of the tube
  ▷ Listen for bilateral breath sounds over the chest and absence of breath sounds over the stomach
  ▷ Use end tidal CO_2 detector—yellow color change indicates proper placement
- Secure the tracheal tube with tape
- **Postintubation Management**
  - Place a nasogastric (NG) or orogastric (OG) tube to decompress the stomach
  - Obtain a post intubation chest x-ray
  - Administer sedation to keep patient comfortable

Complications
- Incorrect tube placement: Esophageal airway or mainstem intubation
- Aspiration
- Broken teeth, excessive bleeding secondary to mucosal damage
- Pneumothorax and pneumomediastinum
- Cardiac dysrhythmia
- Complications or side effects due to pharmacologic therapy, including hypotension

Common Pitfalls
- Failure to appreciate anatomic differences of children compared to adults
- Failure to confirm IV access and patency
- Not allowing onset of action of sedation and paralysis medications before attempting intubation
- Failure to maintain visualization of cords when passing the endotracheal tube
- Using the laryngoscope as a lever

Pearls
- Children have smaller airways and are therefore more prone to obstruction.
- Children's tongues occupy relatively more space in the oropharynx than in adults and therefore oral airways are extremely helpful in preventing airway obstruction.
- Crying increases a child's work of breathing by 32 times. Therefore, keep a conscious child in a comfortable position in the company of family.
- If a child will not tolerate a nonrebreather mask, consider a face tent or oxygen hood.
- Children have higher oxygen consumption rates than adults and decreased residual capacities, leading them to desaturate faster. As a result each attempt at intubation should not last longer than 30 seconds.
- Use the Broselow tape to identify the proper equipment size. Excellent technique cannot overcome incorrectly sized equipment.
- Succinylcholine's advantage of short duration of action is not as useful in children because they typically do not recover spontaneous ventilation after being sedated. Therefore, other paralytics such as rocuronium are also appropriate.
- During passage of the endotracheal tube, insert the tube into the right corner of the mouth to avoid obscuring the view of the vocal cords.

- Children require smaller tidal volumes and higher rates than adults for ventilation.
- NG tube placement is crucial in children because BVM may cause substantial gastric insufflation impairing ventilation.
- The tonsils and adenoids are larger in children, rendering blind nasotracheal intubation dangerous in children younger than 10 years.
- Even with severe obstruction, BVM ventilation with two-person technique and a tight fitting mask is usually adequate to oxygenate for a short period. It is often preferable to provide oxygen via needle cricothyrotomy while mobilizing the OR for definitive airway management.
- Needle cricothyrotomy should be used only if a child cannot be intubated or ventilated, and there is an obstruction proximal to the glottic opening. Often in children, the cricothyroid membrane cannot be palpated and so the catheter should just be placed anywhere in the proximal trachea.
- If a child has epiglottitis and is stable, do not manipulate the airway in the emergency department (ED). If unstable and BVM ventilation is unsuccessful, attempt intubation with a tube 1 mm smaller than estimated, and if this is unsuccessful perform a needle cricothyrotomy.
- If a child has croup, needle cricothyrotomy may not help because the airway obstruction is distal to the glottic opening.

Suggested Readings
Walls RM. *Manual of emergency airway management*. Philadelphia: Lippincott Williams & Wilkins; 2000; 105–118, 143–152.

76 Sedation and Analgesia for the Pediatric Patient

Veda Maany, Oscar Rago, and Angela M. Tangredi

Indications

- To provide anxiolysis, analgesia, sedation, and motor control during unpleasant diagnostic or therapeutic procedures. Decisions regarding appropriate sedation practices depend on:
  - Type of procedure or treatment
  - Age and medical condition of the patient
  - Skill and experience of practitioner
  - Available staff
  - Policies and procedures of the institution

Contraindications

- No absolute contraindications to analgesia other than significant allergies
  - Pain control is an essential component of good emergency care.
  - Choice of agent depends on level of pain, speed of action, medical condition, and age of patient.
- **Relative Contraindications**
  - Presence of acute or chronic conditions which make the patient ASA class III or higher (anesthesiology should be involved in the care of these patients; general anesthesia in the operating room [OR] may be indicated)
  - Inadequate personnel available
    - ▷ Except for mild anxiolysis (oral benzodiazepines) or analgesia without sedation, person administering sedation cannot be the same person performing the procedure
    - ▷ At a minimum, two physicians (one to manage sedation, one to perform procedure) and a nurse must be available for the duration of the sedation

Risk/Consent Issues

- Inadvertent deep sedation or general anesthesia
- Hypoxia/hypoventilation
- Nausea and vomiting
- Medication reactions
  - Fentanyl: Respiratory depression, rigid chest (more likely with rapid delivery)
  - Morphine: Histamine release
  - Benzodiazepines, barbiturates: Paradoxical reaction of restlessness or agitation
  - Ketamine: Laryngospasm, emergence reactions

Classification

- In general, moderate sedation is the goal for emergency department procedural sedation. However, one must be aware of the possibility of the patient passing into a state of deep sedation and be able to manage this occurrence. Advanced airway management skills are required for anyone performing procedural sedation.

- **Minimal/mild sedation:** Impaired cognitive function and coordination but unaffected ventilatory and cardiovascular functions; able to respond to verbal commands
- **Moderate sedation:** Blunted anxiety/pain responses but intact airway reflex; normal cardiovascular function; patient should respond to verbal commands (possibly with addition of light tactile stimulation).
- **Dissociative sedation:** Profound analgesia and amnesia with retention of airway reflexes, spontaneous respirations and cardiovascular function
  ▶ State induced by ketamine
- **Deep sedation:** Difficult to arouse; can respond purposefully to repeated or painful stimulation; partial or complete loss of airway reflexes is possible; cardiovascular function usually intact

TABLE 76.1: American Society of Anesthesiologists physical status classification

ASA Class	Examples
I: Healthy patient	Unremarkable past medical history
II: Mild systemic disease—no functional limitation	Mild asthma without active wheezing, well controlled diabetes, VSD without failure
III: Severe systemic disease with functional limitation	Active wheezing, poorly controlled diabetes or seizure disorder, history of CHF
IV: Severe systemic disease that is a constant threat to life	Advanced degree of cardiac, pulmonary, renal, or endocrine insufficiency
V: Moribund patient who is not expected to survive without procedure	Septic shock, severe trauma

VSD, ventricular septal defect; CHF, congestive heart failure.

Presedation Considerations

All patients should have a presedation assessment, which includes the following:

- Consider type and severity of underlying medical conditions; consult anesthesiology for patients of ASA class III and higher (see Table 76.1).
- Consider current medications and allergies especially regarding previous adverse experiences with analgesia/anesthesia.
- Inspect airway for abnormalities or limited neck mobility that may impair rescue airway intervention (short neck, obesity, large tonsils/tongue, small mandible).
- Determine time and nature of last meal: Fasting recommendations for elective procedures are 2 to 3 hours for liquids and 4 to 8 hours for solids; in an emergency situation, these guidelines are often not realistic; document the time of last intake and the need for emergent treatment.
- Perform a general physical examination, concentrating on cardiac and lung auscultation, presence of active upper respiratory infection (URI), and baseline neurologic state.
- Assemble all equipment you may need for sedation and potential complications:
  - Suction
  - Oxygen delivery system (face mask or nasal cannula of appropriate size)

- Airway equipment
- Monitors (pulse oximeter, cardiorespiratory, blood pressure, capnography)
- Medications, including recovery drugs

Technique

- Choice of agent depends on the following:
  - Age of patient
  - Goal of your intervention (see Table 76.2)

TABLE 76.2: Goal of intervention

Goal	Recommended medication or intervention
Motion control	Sedative or dissociative
Anxiolysis	Guided imagery/distraction, nitrous, sedative or dissociative
Sedation	Sedative or dissociative
Analgesia alone	Acetaminophen, ibuprofen, opioid
Amnesia	Opioids, dissociative, sedative

- Type of procedure (see Table 76.3)

TABLE 76.3: Type of procedure

Type of procedure	Specific examples	Recommended medication or intervention
Nonpainful	Diagnostic imaging	Pentobarbital (PO, PR, IM, IV) Midazolam (PO, PR, IV) Propofol (IV)
Minimally painful	Minor trauma Instrumentation Peripheral access	Nitrous oxide Topical/local anesthesia (LET/EMLA) Midazolam (PO, PR, IV) Sucrose (PO—infants only)
Painful	Fracture reduction Central access	Ketamine (IM, IV) Fentanyl + midazolam (IV) Propofol ± fentanyl (IV) Regional anesthesia/hematoma block

EMLA, eutectic mixture of local anesthetic; LET, lidocaine epinephrine tetracaine.

- Duration of procedure
- Titrate dose to desired effect or to predetermined maximum (see Table 76.4)
- Continue monitoring through recovery period
- See Table 76.5 for information on selected agents.

Common Pitfalls

- Premature cessation of monitoring vital signs after the procedure is done despite the fact that the patient is still sedated
- Failing to provide adequate sedation
- Misconception that infants cannot feel or remember pain because they cannot talk

TABLE 76.4: Doses of selected analgesics

Medication	Dose	Comments
Sucrose	0.5–1 mL PO, then dip pacifier in solution	Newborn to 3–6 months
Acetaminophen (PO, PR)	10–15 mg/kg	
Ibuprofen (PO)	5–10 mg/kg	Do not use if <6 months of age
Ketorolac	0.5–1 mg/kg, (maximum 30 mg)	
Morphine	0.1 mg/kg/dose; repeat q5–10 min until desired effect	Monitor respiratory status

TABLE 76.5: List of selected agents

Sedative-hypnotic	Dose	Onset	Duration	Comments
Midazolam	IV: Initially 0.1 mg/kg; titrate to maximum 0.5 mg/kg	2–3 min	20–60 min	1.5–5 times stronger than diazepam Dose in small increments Wait 2 min in between doses
	IM: 0.1–0.15 mg/kg	10–20 min	60–120 min	
	PO: 0.5–1 mg/kg; maximum 20 mg	15–30 min	60–90 min	Use IV formulation added to flavored syrup
	IN, PR: 0.3 mg/kg	IN: 60 min PR: 10–30 min	IN: 60 min PR: 60–90 min	Intranasal route is uncomfortable
Pentobarbital	IV: 1–6 mg/kg, adjust increments of 2 mg/kg IM: 2–6 mg/kg to a maximum of 100 mg	1 min		
	PO or PR age<4 y: 6 mg/kg to maximum: 100 mg	10–15 min	60–120 min	
	PO or PR age>4 y: 3 mg/kg to maximum: 100 mg	15–60 min	60–240 min	
Etomidate	IV: 0.1–0.3 mg/kg/dose	30–60 sec	3–5 min	May cause emesis, myoclonus
Methohexitol	PR: 25 mg/kg; maximum 500 mg	10–15 min	60 min	
Thiopental	PR: 10–25 mg/kg	10–15 min	60–120 min	
Analgesic	**Dose**	**Onset**	**Duration**	**Comments**
Fentanyl	IV: 1 μg/kg/dose; may repeat every 2–3 min; titrate to desired effect	2–3 min	30–60 min	Exhibits little hypnosis Rare histamine release May cause respiratory depression May cause chest wall rigidity (more likely with higher doses, rapid rate)

TABLE 76.5: (Continued)

Dissociative agent	Dose	Onset	Duration	Comments
Ketamine	IV: 1–2 mg/kg; repeat dose 0.5 mg/kg; maximum 500 mg or 5 mg/kg, whichever is less	1–5 min	10–150 min	Administer IV: over 1–2 min Note: Prior to ketamine, give atropine 0.01 mg/kg or glycopyrrolate, 0.005 mg/kg
	IM: 4 mg/kg of ketamine mixed with atropine in the same syringe	5–15 min		May cause hallucinations up to 48 hr
				Patients may not perform skilled or hazardous tasks for 48 hr
				Contraindicated in patients with URI with significant nasal discharge or for procedures which stimulate posterior pharynx
				May cause increased intracranial or intraocular pressure

Inhalation agent	Dose	Onset	Duration	Comments
Nitrous oxide	30%–70% concentration; continuous flow or demand valve	<5 min	<5 min after discontinuation	Up to 80% nonresponders Do not use in combination with other drugs

Reversal agents	Dose	Onset	Duration	Comments
Naloxone	IV, IM, SQ: 0.1 mg/kg to maximum of 2 mg; may repeat every 2 min	IV: 2 min	IV: 20–40 min	DO NOT use routinely
		IM, SQ: 10–15 min	IM, SQ: 60–90 min	May cause hypertension and pulmonary edema Use cautiously in opiate dependence
Flumazenil	IV: 0.01–0.03 mg/kg; maximum 0.2 mg	1–2 min	30–60 min	Contraindicated in patients on benzodiazepine for seizures Administer IV over 15 sec

URI, upper respiratory infection.

Pearls

- Patients should be discharged with specific sedation-related discharge instructions.
  - Close supervision for at least 24 hours
  - Light diet for 24 hours
  - Return to the emergency department (ED) for lethargy, persistent vomiting, or any unusual behavior

- Use of age-appropriate nonpharmacologic techniques can decrease the dose of medication needed, or eliminate it entirely.
  - Quiet room with dimmed lighting
  - Stereo headphones, movies, or toys
  - Storytelling, guided imagery, or singing
- Always use the parents to calm the child as they can play a major role in reducing the child's stress.
- Warn parents about the nystagmus and trancelike cataleptic state resulting from ketamine administration.
- Be prepared for the possibility of disinhibitory effects of benzodiazepines.
- Avoid painful IM injections whenever possible.
- Reversal agents are reserved for emergencies since the half-life of the reversal agent may be shorter than the sedative and the patient may become sedated again at home.
- Do not use sedation without analgesia for painful procedures.
- Chloral hydrate and the ''lytic cocktail'' or ''DPT'' (combination of meperidine, promethazine, and chlorpromazine) are not recommended due to unpredictable depth of sedation and prolonged effect.

77   Ear Foreign Body Removal

Elad Bicer and Kathleen G. Reichard

Indications

- Removal of foreign matter lodged within the external auditory canal
  - Organic matter (beans, flowers)
  - Inorganic matter (plastic, metal, pebbles, etc.)
  - Live/dead insects

Contraindications

- Irrigation technique is contraindicated in the following instances:
  - Patients with suspected or known tympanic membrane (TM) perforation or tympanostomy tubes
  - Patients with organic foreign bodies because the water may make the object swell and make further attempts at removal more difficult

Technique

- **Patient Preparation**
  - Place patient in a supine position.
  - Restrain patient and immobilize the head using an assistant, if necessary.
    - ▶ Consider sedation for patients unable to cooperate with the procedure and those difficult to restrain
  - In patients presenting with live insects in the auditory canal, instill 1 to 2 mL of mineral oil or 2% lidocaine directly into the canal through a 5-mL syringe in an attempt to kill the insect.
    - ▶ Death generally occurs in less than 1 minute
- **Irrigation**
  - Before the procedure, perform pneumatic otoscopy in patients with suspected TM perforation to document an intact TM.
    - ▶ Pull the pinna superiorly, posteriorly, and laterally in order to straighten the external auditory canal and allow for a more complete visualization of the foreign matter and TM.
  - Attach a 20-mL syringe to a 16- or 18-gauge IV catheter or a 2-in. section of butterfly needle tubing (cut off the needle assembly).
  - Use water at body temperature to avoid vestibular stimulation.
  - Insert the catheter or tubing 1 to 1.5 cm into the canal, aimed superiorly and posteriorly, and irrigate with mild to moderate pressure on the syringe.
- **Instrumentation**
  - Use only when able to visualize the object.
    - ▶ Use a speculum to visualize the object while attempting removal.
  - Various instruments can be used, including alligator forceps, curettes, right-angle hooks, or bayonet forceps.
    - ▶ Alligator and bayonet forceps are useful to remove insects or other irregular objects, as well as compressible objects (such as paper), which

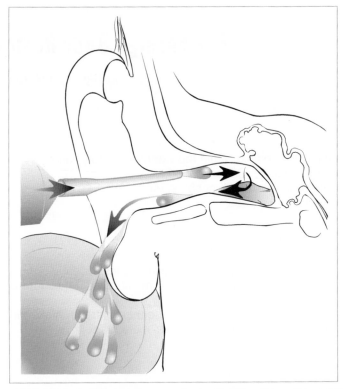

FIGURE 77.1: Syringing cerumen or a foreign body from the auditory canal with an intravenous catheter attached to a 20-mL syringe. The irrigating stream is directed at the posterior, superior wall of the canal. (From Fuerst RS. Removal of cerumen impaction. In: Henretig FM, King C, eds. *Textbook of pediatric emergency procedures*. Philadelphia: Williams & Wilkins; 1997:643, with permission.)

can be "grabbed." Occasionally, separation of the foreign body may occur, necessitating further attempts.

▶ Curettes and right-angle forceps are useful when the hooked end can be passed beyond the foreign body. At that point, rotate the instrument and allow it to drag the object as you pull.

■ **Suction Catheter**
- May work for round objects that are difficult to grasp.
- Inflexible devices such as a Frazier suction device work better than flexible suction catheters. If a flexible catheter is used, choose one with no side holes, or cut the distal portion with the side holes off and be sure to smooth the cut edges.
- Attach a suction catheter device to wall suction and gently advance the catheter tip until it abuts the foreign object. Apply suction and slowly remove the catheter with the foreign body attached.
- Warn patient about noise.

■ **Cyanoacrylate (Superglue)**
- Used for removal of round, dry objects that are difficult to grasp.
- Apply a small amount of glue to the wood end of a cotton-tip applicator, place against the object, allow to dry, then slowly remove the applicator with the foreign body attached.
- Use with caution in uncooperative patients to avoid applying instilling glue into the canal.

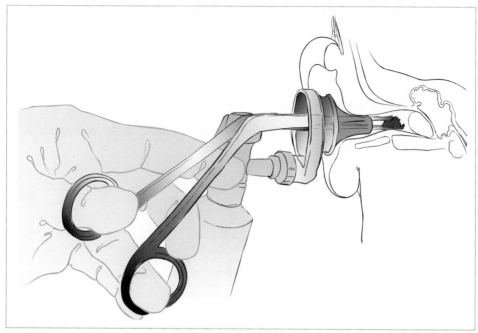

FIGURE 77.2: Cerumen or a foreign body is removed from the auditory canal under direct visualization with an alligator forceps and an operating head otoscope. (From Fuerst RS. Removal of cerumen impaction. In: Henretig FM, King C, eds. *Textbook of pediatric emergency procedures*. Philadelphia: Williams & Wilkins; 1997:644, with permission.)

Complications
- Pain, bleeding, infection due to irritation or manipulation of external auditory canal
- Nausea, vomiting, vertigo due to irrigation of external canal
- Iatrogenic TM perforation
- Ossicle disruption

Common Pitfalls
- Inadequate immobilization of the patient
- Failure to consult the ENT specialist early for anticipated difficult extractions
- Failure to document TM examination following the procedure

Pearls
- Instrumentation should be attempted only when direct visualization of the foreign body is adequate and the patient is cooperative or can be adequately restrained or sedated.
- Batteries lodged in the external canal should be removed expeditiously as they may cause corrosion into the middle ear.
- Patient should be referred to ENT specialist for outpatient treatment in following instances:
  - Unable to adequately sedate an uncooperative patient
  - Foreign body is abutting the TM
  - Unable to remove the object after multiple attempts

- Local anesthetic drops and/or anti-inflammatory drops can be prescribed (for nonorganic matter) until the follow-up appointment.
- Consider prescribing topical antibiotic/corticosteroid after extraction.

Suggested Readings

Simon RR, Brenner BE. *Emergency procedures and techniques*, 4th ed. Philadelphia: Lippincott Williams & Wilkins; 2002.

Roberts JR, Hedges JR. *Clinical procedures in emergency medicine*, 4th ed. Philadelphia: WB Saunders; 2004.

78 Nasal Foreign Body Removal

Keeli A. Hanzelka and Kathleen G. Reichard

Indications
- Presence of foreign material within the nostril

Contraindications
- If the foreign body entered the nose traumatically and there is concern it has penetrated the cranial cavity
- If there is danger of obstructing the airway

Technique
- **Patient Preparation**
    - An uncooperative child should be properly immobilized or sedated.
        - An option is to papoose the child in a blanket in the supine position with the arms at the sides and an assistant holding the head still.
    - Using a syringe as a dropper, instill either lidocaine and phenylephrine or lidocaine with epinephrine in the nostril to optimize the visual field and provide anesthesia, decongestion, and hemostasis.
    - Dosing for nasal phenylephrine
        - Six months to 2 years: 1 to 2 drops per nostril of a 0.1255 solution
        - Two to 6 years: 2 to 4 drops per nostril of a 0.1255 solution
        - Older than 6 years: 2 to 3 drops per nostril of a 0.1255 solution
    - Make sure you have a good light source and suction.
    - Consider anxiolysis or sedation in the uncooperative child, especially in those who require more urgent removal of the foreign body, as in the case of button batteries.

Methods of removal

Manual removal
Suction catheter
Positive pressure
Foley catheter
Cyanoacrylate glue
Nasal wash

- **Manual Removal**
    - A directly visualized object can be removed with alligator forceps or a curette with or without the assistance of a nasal speculum.
    - Alligator forceps are best used for easily grasped, solid or compressible (e.g., paper) objects in the anterior nostril.
    - A round and smooth object may be removed with an angled wire loop/curette or right-angle hook. It is inserted along the nasal floor or septum until it is

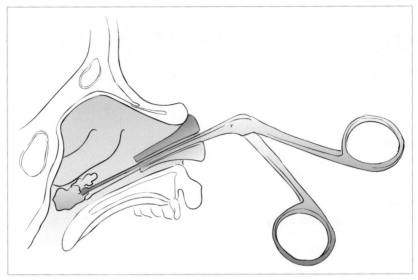

FIGURE 78.1: Removal of an intranasal foreign body using forceps. (From Issacman DJ, Post JC. Nasal foreign body removal. In: Henretig FM, King C, eds. Textbook of Pediatric Emergency Procedures. Philadelphia: Williams & Wilkins, 1997: 684, with permission.)

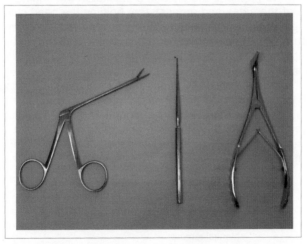

FIGURE 78.2: From left to right—alligator clips, right-angle hook, nasal speculum.

    behind the object and rotated so that the angled end is caught behind the object; the object can then be pulled out.
- If no wire loop is available a makeshift one can be constructed with a paperclip (see Fig. 78.3).

■ **Suction Catheter**
- Using a small suction catheter connected to wall suction, gently put the suction catheter up to the visible side of the object.
  ▷ Be careful not push the object further back.
- When the object becomes attached to the end of the suction catheter, slowly withdraw both the catheter and foreign body.
- Rigid suction catheters usually work better than flexible catheters.

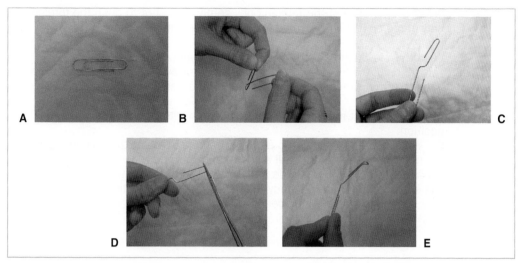

FIGURE 78.3: Pull the paperclip apart as shown and use forceps to bend the end to a right angle.

- The presence of side holes will prevent a vacuum from occurring at the tip. Choose a catheter without side holes, or trim the catheter tip to remove the side holes, leaving only an end opening.
  - Trim any sharp edges from the cut end to prevent trauma.
- **Positive Pressure**
  - The parent or the physician can do this technique. The parent may assist with this procedure and therefore reduce the child's anxiety.
  - Instruct the parent to gently occlude the nostril without the foreign body with finger pressure.
  - Give one quick puff of air into the child's mouth.
    - To put the child at ease, the parent can say she/he is going to give the child a big kiss.
  - The puff of air should push the foreign body out of the nostril.
  - Alternatively, the physician can provide positive pressure using an Ambu bag:
    - Place the Ambu bag over the child's mouth leaving the nose free from the mask; gently occlude the unobstructed nostril.
    - Give one quick squeeze on the Ambu bag; the resultant positive pressure to the obstructed nostril should push the foreign body out.
  - This technique is best for large objects that occlude the entire passage and would be difficult to slide an instrument past or grasp onto.
- **Foley Catheter**
  - Use a no. 4 to no. 8 Fogarty vascular catheter or a 5 or 6 French balloon Foley catheter.
  - Lubricate the balloon end of the catheter with lidocaine jelly or Surgilube and slide the catheter past and behind the object.
  - Inflate with 2 to 3 mL of air and pull the Foley catheter forward to force the foreign body out.
  - This technique is best used for a visualized, partially obstructing foreign body.
- **Cyanoacrylate Glue**
  - On the wooden end of a cotton swab, or the cut end of a hollow plastic swab apply a dot of cyanoacrylate glue.
    - Use a very small amount so it will not drip.
  - Insert the tip into the nostril, making sure not to touch the nasal mucosa.

- Press the tip against the foreign body gently so as not to push the foreign body more posterior, and hold for 30 to 60 seconds to allow for it to dry.
- Withdraw slowly the swab with attached foreign body.
- This technique should be used with caution, or avoided, in an uncooperative patient to avoid the risk of getting glue on the nasal mucosa.

Nasal Wash

- Place the patient in an upright sitting position with the neck in a neutral position.
- Put 7 mL of sterile saline into a bulb syringe, and insert the bulb syringe into the nonobstructed nostril until a good seal is created.
- In one quick squeeze push the sterile saline into the nostril.
- The saline and the foreign body will be expressed out of the opposite nostril.
- This technique should likely be reserved for an older cooperative child because of risk of saline aspiration.

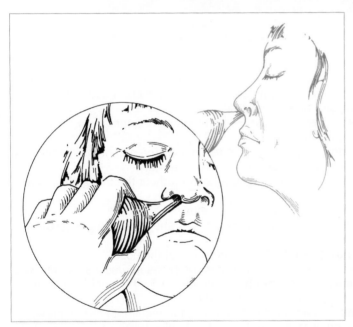

FIGURE 78.4: Nasal wash technique.

Complications

- **General**
  - Epistaxis
  - Nasal infection
  - Aspiration of foreign body
  - Partial removal of foreign body
  - Mucosal damage
  - Cribriform plate damage
- **Procedure Specific**
  - *Nasal wash:* Reflux of saline into the eustachian tubes or aspiration of saline
  - *Positive pressure:* Barotrauma to the tympanic membrane

Common Pitfalls
- Inadequate immobilization—even in a cooperative patient proper immobilization is important because they will tend to flinch when instruments are in the nostrils, putting them at risk for trauma.
- Not recognizing that unilateral purulent discharge or epistaxis could be due to a foreign body.

Pearls
- Sedation is an option if immobilization alone is not adequate.
- Health care workers should adhere to universal precautions and therefore wear a face-shield mask.
- If the foreign body is a button battery it should be removed without delay as it can cause ulceration of nasal mucosa and even perforation in a short amount of time.
- Talk the child through the procedure and involve the parents, if possible, to reduce anxiety.
- Patient should be referred to ENT specialist for outpatient treatment in following instances:
  - Unable to adequately sedate an uncooperative patient
  - Unable to remove the object after multiple attempts

Suggested Readings
Backlin SA. Positive pressure technique for nasal foreign body removal in children. *Ann Emerg Med*. 1995;25(4):534–535.

Kadish HA, Corneli HM. Removal of nasal foreign bodies in the pediatric population. *Am J Emerg Med*. 1997;15(1):54–56.

Lichenstein R. Giudice EL: Nasal wash technique for nasal foreign body removal. *Pediatr Emerg Care*. 2000;16(1):59–60.

Reichman EF, Simon RR. *Emergency medicine procedures*. New York: McGraw-Hill; 2004:1286–1290.

Simon RR, Brenner BE. *Emergency procedures and techniques*. 4th ed. Philadelphia: Lippincott Williams & Wilkins; 2002.

Umbilical Vein Catheterization

Ann Vorhaben and Ramona S. Sunderwith

Indications
- To provide rapid vascular access in neonates up to 2 weeks of age for resuscitation in which all other access attempts have failed
- To provide rapid administration of IV fluids, medications, and blood

Contraindications
- ### Absolute Contraindications
  - None for the unstable newborn with respiratory failure or cardiovascular compromise
- ### Relative Contraindications
  - Successful peripheral or central venous access
  - Umbilical vein catheter (UVC) placement in newborns with omphalocele, gastroschisis, omphalitis, peritonitis, or necrotizing enterocolitis as circulation is often compromised in these situations
  - Cellulitis or impetigo of the abdominal skin

Landmarks
- The umbilicus consists of one large, thin walled vein in between two smaller, thick walled arteries.

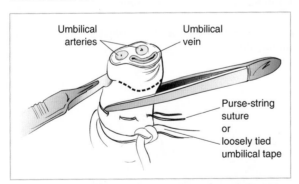

FIGURE 79.1: Introduction of the umbilical vein catheter. (From Lipton JD, Schafermeyer RW. Umbilical vessel catheterization. In: Henretig FM, King C, eds. *Textbook of pediatric emergency procedures.* Philadelphia: Williams & Wilkins, 1997:519, with permission.)

- After cord transection, the arteries physiologically constrict making it sometimes more difficult to distinguish between artery and vein.

Equipment
- Personal protective equipment (face mask, eye protection, gown, sterile gloves)
- Cardiac monitor with pulse oximetry

- Antiseptic prep solution, sterile drapes, gauze pads, antibiotic ointment
- External heat source
- No. 11 or 15 blade surgical scalpel
- Small hemostat
- Umbilical tape or silk suture (3-0 or 4-0) on straight or curved needle
- Size 5 French umbilical catheter
- A 10-mL syringe
- Three-way stopcock
- Bag of saline solution

Technique
- **Patient Preparation**
  - Use universal precautions
  - Place newborn in the supine and frog-leg position on a radiant warmer bed. (Place soft limb restraints only if necessary.)
  - Continuously monitor vital signs and oxygen saturation.
  - Using sterile technique: Prep the umbilicus and entire abdomen with antiseptic solution.
  - Place sterile drapes, leaving the prepped umbilicus exposed.
  - Consider placement of nasogastric tube (NGT) to prevent aspiration of gastric contents.
- **Equipment Preparation**
  - Connect umbilical catheter to one port of three-way stopcock, syringe to second port, and tubing to bag of saline solution to third port.
  - Flush catheter with saline solution
- **Procedural Technique**
  - Using umbilical tape or silk suture, loosely tie a purse string at the base of the umbilicus.
  - Cut the umbilical cord with a scalpel 1 to 2 cm from abdominal wall.
  - Expose the umbilical vessels by attaching two clamps/hemostats to the stump, thereby everting the edges.
  - Identify the centrally located thin walled vein and dilate its lumen with forceps. Remove any visible clot with forceps.
  - Holding the umbilical catheter near its distal end, advance the catheter tip until blood returns freely.
  - Secure the catheter in place by tightening the purse-string suture or the umbilical tape.
  - Tape the catheter in place.

Complications
- Infection
- Thrombosis
- Perforation
- Portal vein thrombosis

Common Pitfalls
- Mistaking artery for vein
- Obstruction during advancement of catheter
- Advancing catheter too far and infusing fluids directly into liver

Pearls
- A UVC may be placed up to 7 to 14 days after birth.
- To overcome obstruction during catheter advancement, gently pull the umbilicus toward the head of the neonate or apply continuous gentle pressure.
- If an attempt at relieving obstruction fails, consider umbilical arterial catheterization as an alternative.
- The UVC is a temporary line—it should be withdrawn as soon as possible after resuscitation (after alternate access is obtained) to prevent complications.
- Consider antibiotic prophylaxis for all neonates with UVCs.

Suggested Readings

Fleisher G, Ludwig S, Henretig F. *Textbook of pediatric emergency medicine*, 5th ed. Lippincott Williams & Wilkins; 2006:1874–1877.

Henretig F, King C. *Textbook of pediatric emergency procedures*. Williams & Wilkins; 1997:517–523.

Simon RR, Brenner BE. *Emergency procedures and techniques*, 3rd ed. Williams & Wilkins; 1994:419–425.

80 Nursemaid's Elbow (Radial Head Subluxation)

Adrian Martinez and Emilola Ogunbameru

Definition
- Radial head subluxation is also known as "nursemaid's elbow" or "pulled elbow."
- A common injury in children between the ages of 2 and 5 years.
  - In children there is little structural support between the radius and humerus.
  - Sudden traction on the hand or forearm pulls the annular ligament that attaches the radius to the humerus over the radial head.

Indications
- Clinical suspicion of a nursemaid's elbow.
  - Refusal to use affected arm
  - Typical posture (see Fig. 80.1)
  - Often (but not always) a history of a pull on the child's extended arm

Contraindications
- Swelling or bony deformity

Landmarks
- Child has affected arm held close to the body with the elbow slightly flexed and forearm pronated. The child is usually in no distress unless the arm is moved.

Technique
- **Patient Preparation:** Have caretaker/parent hold child in her/his lap, restraining the unaffected arm
- **Supination/Flexion Method**
  - Grasp the elbow with the thumb over the region of the radial head.
  - Place the other hand on the wrist and gently apply traction before supination.
  - Supinate the forearm fully and then flex the elbow, all in one motion.
  - A sudden release of resistance accompanied by a palpable click signifies reduction but may not be present always.
- **Hyperpronation Method**
  - Examiner grasps the child's upper arm, with the elbow flexed.
  - With the other hand, the examiner rapidly hyperpronates the arm at the wrist.
  - A sudden release of resistance accompanied by a palpable click signifies reduction but may not be present always.
- **Post Procedure**
  - Reevaluate child in 10 to 15 minutes to note use of arm.
    - The child will generally regain use of the arm quickly.

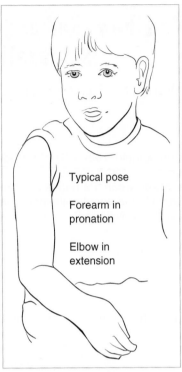

Typical pose

Forearm in
pronation

Elbow in
extension

FIGURE 80.1: Typical posture for child with radial head subluxation. (From Young GM. Reduction of common joint dislocations and subluxations. In: Henretig FM, King C, eds. *Textbook of pediatric emergency procedures*. Philadelphia: Williams & Wilkins; 1997: 1078, with permission.)

- If the child has not regained use of arm by 10 to 15 minutes and no click was detected during procedure, the procedure should be repeated.
- Radiography should be performed if the child has not regained use of arm after a reasonable time and no click was detected.

Complications
- Pain
- Unsuccessful reduction

Pearls
- Both methods of reduction have equal efficacy and are both well tolerated.
- Reduction is generally performed without premedication.
  - If subluxation has been present for hours, oral anxiolysis can be used to overcome the child's anxiety.
- Explain to caretaker that reduction will likely cause discomfort but this is transient.
- If reduction has been achieved clinically and maintained, analgesics and follow-up visits are unnecessary.
- Need for a splint or sling after reduction is very rare.
- Explain to parents that there is risk of repeat subluxation; they should use caution when holding child by the hand and avoid twisting movements of arm (i.e., when putting on a t-shirt).

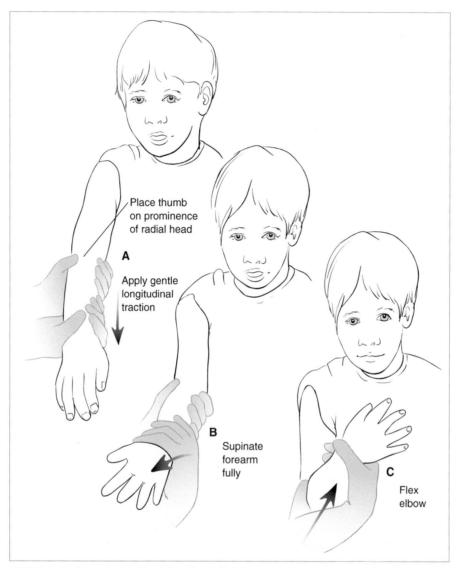

Place thumb on prominence of radial head

A

Apply gentle longitudinal traction

B

Supinate forearm fully

C

Flex elbow

FIGURE 80.2: Procedure for reduction of radial head subluxation. (From Young GM. Reduction of common joint dislocations and subluxations. In: Henretig FM, King C, eds. *Textbook of pediatric emergency procedures*. Philadelphia: Williams & Wilkins; 1997: 1078, with permission.)

Suggested Readings

Henretig FM, King C. *Textbook of pediatric emergency procedures*. Philadelphia: Lippincott Williams & WilkIns; 1997:1075–1079.

Simon RR, Brenner BE. *Emergency procedures and techniques*, 4th ed. Philadelphia: Lippincott Williams & Wilkins; 2002;281–282.

Roberts JR, Hedges JR. *Clinical procedures in emergency medicine*, 4th ed. WB Saunders; 2004; 967–969.

Section Editor: David C. Riley

81 Bedside Gallbladder Ultrasonography: Limited, Goal-Directed

Kaushal Shah

Indications

- Yes or no:
    - Are gallstones present?
    - Is the gallbladder (GB) wall >3 mm?
    - Is a sonographic Murphy sign present?
- Clinical suspicion of cholecystitis or biliary colic
    - Right upper quadrant (RUQ) pain, epigastric pain, abdominal pain, right flank pain
    - Right shoulder pain
    - Nausea/vomiting
    - Sepsis without source

Contraindications

- None: No contrast or radiation involved

Risks/Consent Issues

- The only theoretical risk is allergy to the ultrasonography gel

Landmarks

- Initially place ultrasound probe in RUQ of abdomen where you suspect the GB to be located

Technique

- Using a standard 3.5 to 5.0 MHz probe, scan the RUQ of the abdomen in the longitudinal plane under the costal margin using the liver as an acoustic window (see Fig. 81.1)
- If the GB is not readily identified, try the following techniques:
    - Ask the patient to take slow deep breaths because the GB moves significantly with respiration
    - Change the position of the patient to the left lateral decubitus position
    - Place the probe in the intercostal space to avoid bowel gas and rib shadows

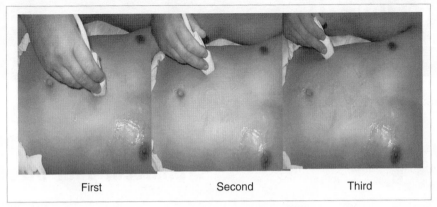

First   Second   Third

FIGURE 81.1: Biliary ultrasonography: Costal margin sweep; first to locate the gallbladder (GB).

■ Once the GB is identified, confirm the structure is in fact the GB by identifying associated structures
   • Echogenic gallstones in the lumen casting echolucent shadows (see Fig. 81.2)

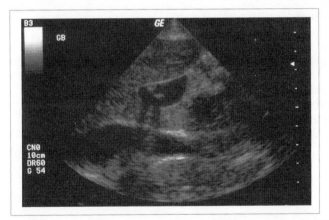

FIGURE 81.2: Echogenic gallstones casting acoustic shadows. (Courtesy of Kaushal Shah, MD.)

   • Main lobar fissure of the liver points toward the GB neck and also connects the portal vein
   • Common bile duct (CBD) usually runs between the GB and the portal vein (see Fig. 81.3)
   • Identify signs of cholecystitis (see Table 81.1)

TABLE 81.1: Sonographic signs of cholecystitis

▷ Presence of gallstones
▷ Sonographic Murphy sign: tenderness with probe pressure directly on the sonographically identified GB
▷ GB wall thickness >3 mm
▷ Pericholecystic fluid
▷ Common bile duct >6 mm (more consistent with choledocholithiasis)

GB, gallbladder.

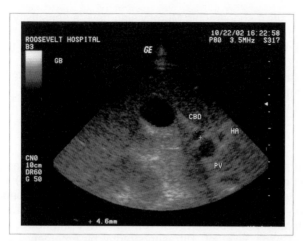

FIGURE 81.3: "Mickey Mouse" sign is comprised of the common bile duct (*CBD*), portal vein (*PV*), and hepatic artery (*HA*). (Courtesy of Kaushal Shah, MD.)

Common Pitfalls

- Limited, goal-directed ultrasonography is within the capacity of the emergency physician (EP). The EP is not expected to identify subtle abnormalities in the hepatobiliary system.
- Always visualize the GB in various planes (e.g., longitudinal and transverse) in order to see the entire extent of the GB.
- GB wall thickening is a nonspecific finding because it can occur with other disease states, such as congestive heart failure (CHF), liver disease, and renal disease.

Pearls

- Figure 81.4 shows the recommended clinical approach to bedside ultrasonography of the GB.

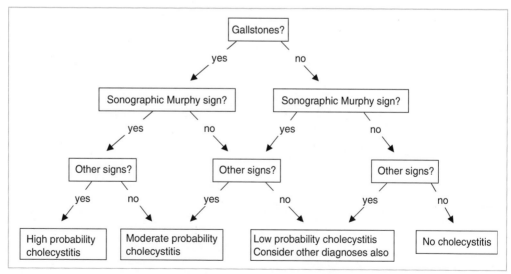

FIGURE 81.4: Algorithmic approach to bedside ultrasound of the gallbladder.

■ Gallstones and a positive sonographic Murphy sign have a sensitivity >90% in the hands of EP in multiple studies.

■ "Halo" sign occurs when echolucent pericholecystic fluid surrounds the entire GB owing to inflammation; it is a very specific sign for cholecystitis.

■ "WES sign" is present when the GB is contracted around a gallstone; ultrasonography demonstrates only the anterior GB **W**all, the **E**chogenicity of the stone, and a **S**hadow.

Suggested Readings

Blaivas M, Harwood RA, Lambert MJ. Decreasing length of stay with emergency ultrasound examination of the gallbladder. *Acad Emerg Med*. 1999;6(10):1020–1023.

Kendall JL, Shimp RJ. Performance and interpretation of focused right upper quadrant ultrasound by emergency physicians. *J Emerg Med*. 2001;21(1):7–13.

Ma OJ, Mateer JR. *Emergency ultrasound*. New York: McGraw-Hill; 2003.

Rosen CL, Brown DF, Chang Y, et al. Ultrasonography by emergency physicians in patients with suspected cholecystitis. *Am J Emerg Med*. 2001;19(1):32–36.

Shah K, Wolfe R. Hepatobiliary ultrasound. *Emerg Med Clin North Am*. 2004;22(3): 661–673.

Bedside Echocardiography: Limited, Goal-Directed

Robert Favelukes and Nelsson Becerra

Indications
- Yes or no: Is the heart beating and is there fluid around the heart?
- Cardiac arrest
  - To distinguish asystole versus ventricular fibrillation
- Clinical suspicion of pericardial effusion
  - Pleuritic and positional chest pain, tachycardia, friction rub, distant heart sounds
- Hypotension of unclear etiology
  - To diagnose/rule out cardiac tamponade
- Acute chest pain
  - Diagnosing myocardial ischemia
  - Assessing right ventricle (RV) dysfunction in cases of pulmonary embolus (PE)

Contraindications
- None: No contrast or radiation involved

Risk/Consent Issues
- None: The only theoretical risk is allergy to ultrasonography gel

Standard Views
- **Subcostal Four Chambers:** Right atrium (RA), right ventricle (RV), left atrium (LA), left ventricle (LV) (see Fig. 82.1)

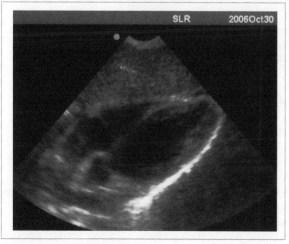

FIGURE 82.1: Subcostal four chamber: Right atrium (RA), right ventricle (RV), left atrium (LA), left ventricle (LV).

■ **Parasternal Long Axis** (see Fig. 82.2)

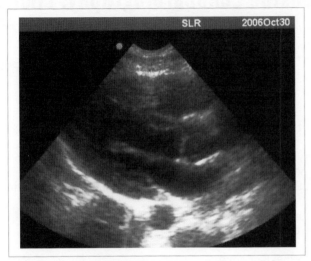

FIGURE 82.2: Parasternal long axis.

■ **Parasternal Short Axis:** Pulmonary artery (PA) (see Fig. 82.3)

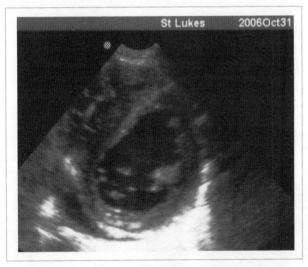

FIGURE 82.3: Parasternal short axis: Pulmonary artery (PA).

■ **Apical Four Chambers** (see Fig. 82.4)

Landmarks and Technique
■ Use a standard 2.0 to 5.0 MHz microconvex or phased array probe to scan at least two of the four views of the heart.
■ **Subcostal Four Chambers**
● Place probe in subxyphoid position of abdomen, facing toward patient's heart with probe marker located to left of patient.

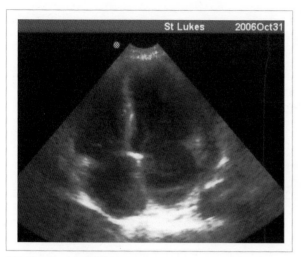

FIGURE 82.4: Apical four chamber.

- If the heart is not adequately viewed, move the probe to the patient's right using the liver as an acoustic window. Asking the patient to take a deep breath will push the heart inferior toward the probe (see Fig. 82.5).

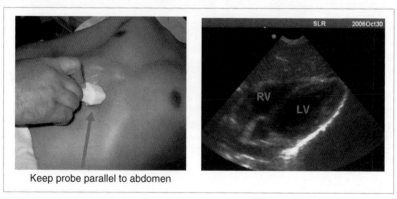

Keep probe parallel to abdomen

FIGURE 82.5: Subcostal four chamber view.

- **Parasternal Long Axis**
  - Place probe in third/fourth intercostal space just left of the sternum directed toward the patient's heart, with probe marker directed toward the patient's left elbow.
  - Moving the probe to the left and then up and down along the anterior posterior axis may help obtain a better view.
  - The pericardium always connects to the descending aorta, and fluid above the pericardium is pericardial fluid and fluid below the pericardium is pleural fluid. (See Fig. 82.6)
- **Parasternal Short Axis**
  - Place probe in same location as the parasternal long axis view, but rotate the probe marker toward the patient's right hip (see Fig. 82.7).
- **Apical Four Chamber**
  - Place probe at apex of heart which is usually along the nipple line at the left fifth intercostal space at the point of maximal impulse (PMI), with the probe marker directed toward the right elbow, at 8 o'clock position (see Fig. 82.8).

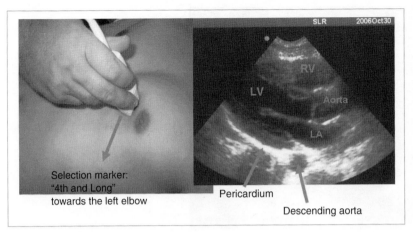

FIGURE 82.6: Parasternal long axis view.

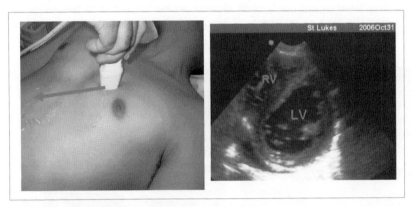

FIGURE 82.7: Parasternal short axis view.

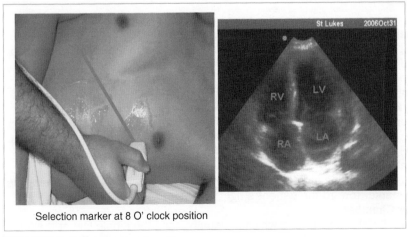

FIGURE 82.8: Apical four chamber view.

Sonographic Signs to Identify in Emergency Bedside Echocardiography
- Ventricular fibrillation
  - Fine fibrillatory movements of the left ventricle
- Pericardial effusion
  - Anechoic fluid (dark) collection between the parietal and visceral pericardium
- Cardiac tamponade
  - Pericardial fluid collection with the following:
    - ▸ Right atrial collapse during systole
    - ▸ Right ventricular collapse during diastole ("scalloping") (see Fig. 82.9)

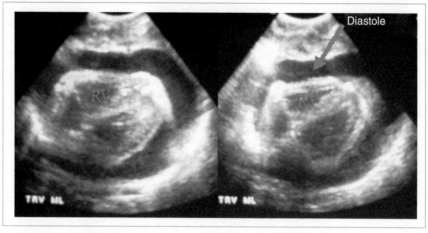

FIGURE 82.9: Cardiac tamponade: Diastolic collapse of the right ventricle.

- Myocardial ischemia
  - Abnormal wall motion and abnormal ventricular emptying or relaxation
    - ▸ Hypokinesis (reduced wall thickening and motion)
    - ▸ Akinesis (absent wall thickening and motion)
    - ▸ Dyskinesia (paradoxical motion of wall; outward movement of wall during systole)
  - Increased left ventricular size
  - Reduction of left ventricular ejection fraction
- Right ventricular dysfunction in cases of PE
  - Right ventricular dilatation: RV end diastolic diameter greater than LV end diastolic diameter
  - Right ventricular hypokinesis

Common Pitfalls
- Mistaking the motion caused by positive pressure ventilation for cardiac motion. In a code, briefly stop ventilations during bedside echocardiography
- Failure to note diastolic collapse of right ventricle suggestive of cardiac tamponade when a pericardial effusion is present.
- Failure to note evidence of loculation when pericardial fluid is noted.
- Confusion of right and left heart chambers owing to improper transducer orientation.
- Overdiagnosing pericardial effusion: Mistaking an anterior pericardial fat pad or pleural effusion for a true pericardial effusion.

Pearls

- Limited, goal-directed echocardiography is within the capacity of the emergency physician. The emergency physician is not expected to identify subtle abnormalities.
- Always visualize the heart in more than two views.
- Patients with subcutaneous emphysema, pneumopericardium, and large anterior–posterior girth can be difficult to image.
- Fluid will appear anechoic; however, a blood clot may be echogenic initially with an anechoic stripe at the borders. Viewing other windows may assist in finding fluid in other areas of the pericardium.
- Echocardiography has not proven sufficient for accurate diagnosis of PE by itself. It may help expedite diagnosis, but failure of diagnosis by echocardiography should not rule out PE.
- Identification of regional wall motion abnormalities is a sensitive predictor of Q-wave myocardial infarction (MI). The limitations lie in non–Q-wave MIs where patients may have normal wall motion.
- New regional wall motion abnormalities cannot be differentiated from old abnormalities.
- Methods of enhancing image acquisition include the following:
  - Keep the complete ultrasound probe in contact with the chest wall and angle, rotate, and tilt the ultrasound probe as necessary.
  - Use an adequate amount of gel during bedside echocardiography.
  - Try alternative cardiac echocardiography views.
  - Turn the patient in the left lateral decubitus position to bring the heart up closer to the anterior chest wall.

Suggested Readings

Ma OJ, Mateer JR. *Emergency ultrasound*. New York: McGraw-Hill; 2003.

Mandavia DP, Hoffner RJ, Mahaney K, et al. Bedside echocardiography be emergency physicians. *Ann Emerg Med*. 1991;38(4):377–382.

Plummer D, Brunette D, Asinger R, et al. Emergency department echocardiography improves outcome in penetrating cardiac injury. *Ann Emerg Med*. 1992;21(6):709–712.

83 Bedside FAST: Focused Assessment with Sonography for Trauma

Andreana Kwon and David C. Riley

Indications
- Yes or no: Is there intra-abdominal fluid or fluid around the heart?
- Assessment of blunt thoracoabdominal trauma with significant mechanism of injury
- Assessment of penetrating torso trauma if operative management is not immediately indicated

Contraindications
- The (FAST) examination should never delay a patient's transport to the operating room (OR) when operative management is clearly indicated.

Risks/Consent Issues
- The only theoretical risk is allergy to the ultrasonography gel.

Advantages
- Noninvasive and no sedation is required.
- Can be performed at the bedside while resuscitative efforts are simultaneously being performed.
- Can be performed at the bedside on patients too unstable for the computed tomography (CT) imaging suite.
- Can be repeated serially along with changes in symptoms or hemodynamic stability.

Landmarks
- Subcostal
  - Probe placed in the subxiphoid region pointed toward the heart, detects fluid in pericardial sac.
- Hepatorenal
  - Probe placed in the right midaxillary line between the 8th and 11th ribs, detects fluid in the hepatorenal space (Morison pouch).
- Splenorenal
  - Probe placed in the left posterior axillary line between the 8th and 11th ribs, detects fluid in the splenorenal recess.
- Suprapubic
  - Probe placed 2 cm superior to the symphysis pubis, detects fluid in the retrovesical or retrouterine space.

Technique
- The standard four FAST views: **Subcostal, hepatorenal-Morison pouch, splenorenal, and suprapubic**

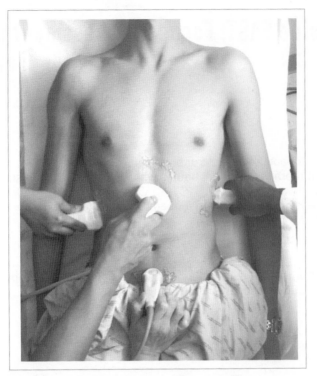

FIGURE 83.1: The four views of the FAST examination.

Subcostal View

- With the probe in the transverse plane, place it in the subxiphoid area and aim towards the patient's left shoulder to see a four-chambered view of the heart.
- Sweep the probe anteriorly and posteriorly to view the entire pericardium.
- Unclotted blood will appear as an anechoic black "stripe" within the hyperechoic pericardial sac.

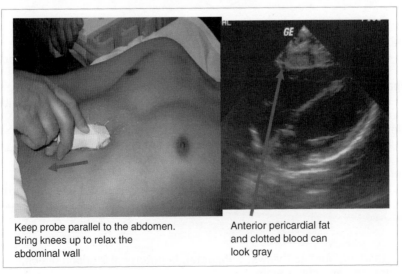

Keep probe parallel to the abdomen. Bring knees up to relax the abdominal wall

Anterior pericardial fat and clotted blood can look gray

FIGURE 83.2: Subcostal view.

Hepatorenal-Morison Pouch View
- With the indicator pointed toward the patient's right axilla, place probe in the midaxillary line between 8th and 11th ribs.
- Hold the probe in a longitudinal or an oblique plane to aid visualization through rib spaces.
- Unclotted blood or fluid will appear as an anechoic black "stripe" in the space between the liver and right kidney.

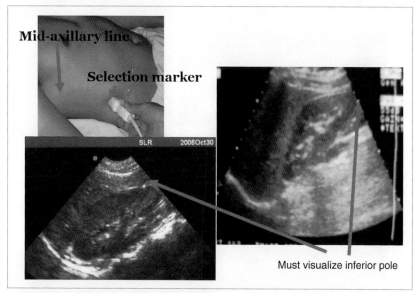

FIGURE 83.3: Hepatorenal-Morison pouch view.

Splenorenal View
- With the indicator pointed toward the patient's left axilla, place the probe in the left posterior axillary line between the 8th and 11th ribs, also at an oblique plane.
- Turn the probe longitudinally to enhance your view.
- Unclotted blood or fluid will appear as an anechoic black "stripe" in the space between the spleen and left kidney.

Suprapubic View
- This view is facilitated by a full bladder.
- With the indicator pointing toward the patient's head, place the probe 2 cm superior to the symphysis pubis along the midline.
- Aim the probe caudally into the pelvis.
- Rotate the probe 90 degrees counterclockwise for transverse images.
- Look for anechoic blood adjacent to the bladder and anterior peritoneum.

Common Pitfalls
- Sensitivity of the examination may be dependent on several factors including the experience of the sonographer, position of patient, equipment used, and the number of serial examinations performed.
- Examination may be obscured by obese body habitus, subcutaneous air, pregnancy, pre-existing peritoneal fluid, or increased bowel gas.
- Inferior pole of both kidneys must be visualized to avoid missing early fluid/blood accumulation.

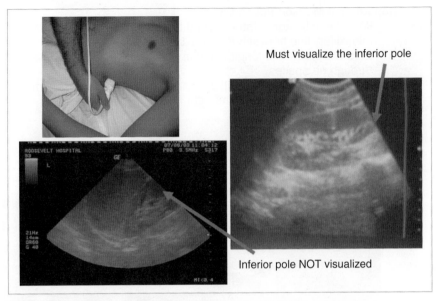

FIGURE 83.4: Splenorenal view.

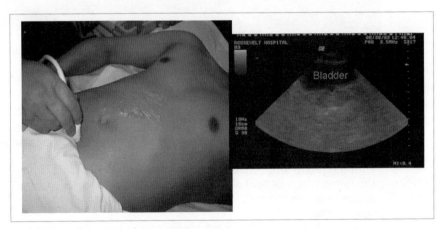

FIGURE 83.5: Suprapubic view.

- The FAST examination should *not* be used for the following:
  - Detecting contained solid organ injuries
  - Detecting bowel injuries
  - Detection of blood in the retroperitoneum or pelvis

Pearls

- Placing the patient in Trendelenburg position makes the examination of the right upper quadrant (RUQ) and left upper quadrant (LUQ) more sensitive.
- Remember that fresh unclotted blood will appear anechoic, but fibrin formation during the clotting process can produce variable echoes.
- The sensitivity of the examination will be increased with increasing volume of fluid in the peritoneum.

Suggested Readings

Kimura A, Otsuka T. Emergency center ultrasonography in the evaluation of hemoperi-
toneum: A prospective study. *J Trauma*. 1991;31:20–23.

Ma OJ, Mateer JR. *Emergency ultrasound*. New York: McGraw-Hill; 2003.

Ma OJ, Mateer JR, Ogata M, et al. Prospective analysis of a rapid trauma ultrasound
examination performed by emergency physicians. *J Trauma*. 1995;38:879–885.

84 Bedside Obstetric/Gynecologic Ultrasonography: Limited, Goal-Directed

Daniel Munoz and Manny A. Colon

Indications

- Yes or no: Is an intrauterine pregnancy (IUP) (defined as yolk sac or fetal parts) present and is the endomyometrial mantle >8 mm?
- Abdominal or pelvic pain
- Suspected ectopic pregnancy or risk factors for ectopic pregnancy
- Vaginal bleeding
- Unexplained syncope, or hypotension
- Pelvic mass

Contraindications

- Absolute: None
- Relative (transvaginal approach): Recent major pelvic surgery

Risks/Consent Issues

- All patients undergoing a pelvic ultrasonography need to give verbal or written consent for the procedure, except in extremis situations.
- There are no documented harmful effects on the fetus or the mother due to ultrasound exposure.

Landmarks

- Transabdominal
  - Place probe on anterior abdominal wall, at the level of the symphysis pubis.
  - For advanced gestations, place the probe more proximally.
- Transvaginal
  - Insert the probe into the vaginal canal.
- The uterus is midline, posterior to the bladder and anterior to the rectum.
- The right and left ovaries are lateral to the uterus and anteromedial to the right and left iliac vessels.

Technique

- Transabdominal
  - Have the patient lie supine.
  - The bladder should be full in order to have an adequate acoustic window.
  - Use a standard curved 3.5 to 5.0 MHz probe to scan the lower abdomen.
- Transvaginal
  - Place patient in supine position with her legs and hips flexed or on a pelvic examination table with stirrups.
  - The bladder should be empty to avoid displacement of structures.
  - Insert a standard endocavitary 4 to 10 MHz probe into the vagina.

- For both
  - Identify the uterus in the longitudinal plane and scan it entirely. The uterus will appear pear-shaped; the widest part is the fundus, the narrowest is the cervix (see Figs. 84.1A and 84.2).

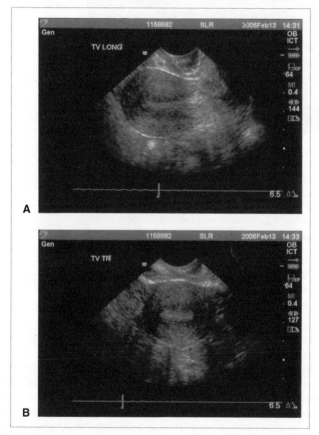

FIGURE 84.1: Transvaginal views of the uterus. **A:** Sagittal view. **B:** Transverse view.

  - Rotate the probe 90 degrees and identify the uterus in the transverse plane.
  - Scan from the fundus to the cervix. The uterus will appear round in shape (see Figs. 84.1B and 84.2).
  - Note the presence or absence of an IUP or free fluid in the anterior and posterior cul-de-sac.
  - If an IUP is present, look for and document the presence of a yolk sac, fetal parts, and/or fetal heart rate (using M-mode).
  - After scanning the uterus, scan each of the adnexa in both transverse and longitudinal planes.
  - Identify each of the ovaries.
  - Note the presence or absence of an ectopic pregnancy and look for other findings suggestive of an ectopic pregnancy (see Table 84.1).

Common Pitfalls

- Inform all pregnant patients that limited, goal-directed obstetric ultrasonography performed by emergency physicians (EPs) is not used to detect fetal anomalies or

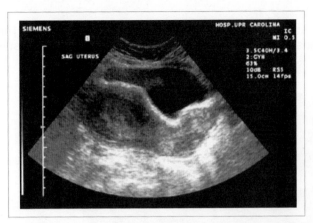

FIGURE 84.2: Transabdominal view of the uterus with a possible intrauterine pregnancy.

TABLE 84.1: Sonographic findings in ectopic pregnancy

Definite ectopic
▷ Extrauterine gestational sac, yolk sac, embryo, or fetus

Probable ectopic

▷ Free fluid in the pelvis
▷ Complex adnexal mass
▷ Tubal ring
▷ Intraperitoneal free fluid (Morison pouch)

to assess fetal health. This is out of the scope of emergency medicine and should be evaluated with a formal examination.

▪ Although the presence of an IUP (defined as yolk sac or fetal tissue, not gestational sac) virtually rules out the possibility of an ectopic pregnancy, some patients can present with an IUP and a concurrent ectopic pregnancy (heterotopic pregnancy). Suspect this diagnosis in patients on fertility treatment.

▪ Early cornual or interstitial ectopic pregnancies can be indistinguishable from a normal IUP. An early clue to unruptured cornual ectopic pregnancy is a thinning of the endomyometrium around the gestational sac (specifically, an endomyometrial mantle <8 mm).

▪ Set strict sonographic criteria for diagnosing an IUP. In the setting of a positive beta human chorionic gonadotropin (b-hCG), do not assume that an empty uterus or a small intrauterine sac (pseudo-gestational sac) is an early gestation. They can both be ectopic pregnancies.

Pearls

▪ Perform the obstetric-gynecologic ultrasonography simultaneously with every pelvic examination. You can find out if a patient has an ectopic pregnancy, an IUP, or other pathology hours before any laboratory or radiology result comes back.

▪ Do not use history of recent last menstrual period, sterilization, tubal ligation, or history of sexual inactivity to screen out patients for a limited, goal-directed bedside ultrasonography. Any sexually active female of reproductive age must be assumed to be pregnant.

▪ A quantitative b-hCG level below 1,000 mIU/mL does not rule out an ectopic pregnancy. An empty uterus with levels above 1,000 mIU/mL can be indicative of an early gestation or even an ectopic pregnancy. Correct interpretation of b-hCG levels must be done together with clinical and sonographic findings (Fig. 84.3 shows the suggested approach).

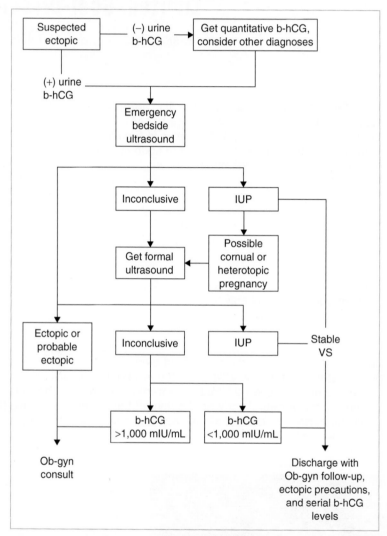

FIGURE 84.3: Emergency obstetric ultrasonography algorithm. b-hCG, beta human chorionic gonadotropin; IUP, intrauterine pregnancy; VS, vital signs.

Suggested Readings

Burgher SW, Tandy TK, Dawdy MR. Transvaginal ultrasonography by emergency physicians decreases patient time in the emergency department. *Acad Emerg Med.* 1998;5(8):802–807.

85

Bedside Aortic Ultrasonography: Limited, Goal-Directed

Jessica Paisley and Lekha Ajit Shah

Indications
- Yes or no: Is the aorta >3.0 cm and are the iliac arteries >1.5 cm?
- Clinical suspicion of abdominal aortic aneurysm (AAA)
  - Unexplained abdominal, back, or flank pain in the older patient
  - Unexplained hypotension (in the setting of abdominal pain)
  - Syncope in the setting of abdominal pain
  - Pulsatile abdominal mass

Contraindications
- None: No contrast or radiation involved

Risk/Consent Issues
- None: Only theoretical risk is allergy to gel

Landmarks
- The proximal aorta is located in the subxiphoid area.
- The aorta bifurcates into the iliac vessels at the level of the umbilicus.
- On the *ultrasound display* (see Fig. 85.1), the transverse proximal aorta is located above (anterior to) the vertebral body, to the right of the inferior vena cava (IVC) (anatomically the aorta is to the left of the IVC), and below (posterior to) the superior mesenteric artery.

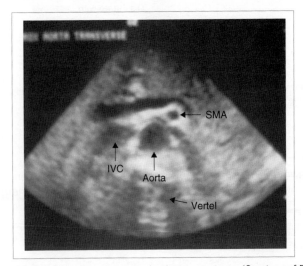

FIGURE 85.1: Transverse proximal aorta anatomy. (Courtesy of David Riley, MD.)

Technique

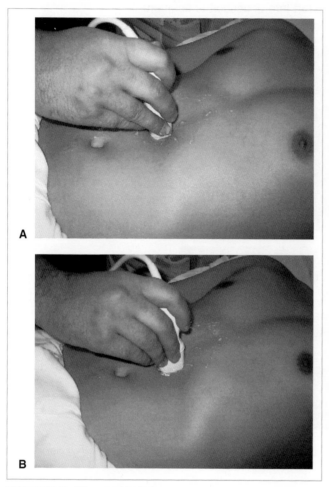

FIGURE 85.2: Ultrasound technique.

- Apply ultrasound gel on the patient's abdomen, from the xiphoid process to just distal to the umbilicus.
- Using a standard 3.5 to 5.0 MHz probe with the selection marker to the patient's right, identify the proximal aorta in the epigastric area.
- Once the aorta is identified, scan the entire length of the vessel to the iliac bifurcation at the umbilicus.
- Measure vessel diameter from outer wall to outer wall.
- Vessel measurement in the following views permits adequate screening for AAA:
  - Transverse proximal aorta
  - Transverse middle aorta
  - Transverse distal aorta
  - Transverse view iliac vessels at the bifurcation
  - Longitudinal aorta
- If the aorta is not readily identified, try the following techniques:
  - Apply gentle downward pressure with the probe to displace bowel gas.
  - Increase the depth of penetration on the ultrasound display.

- Reimaging after several minutes may permit improved visualization as intestinal peristalsis displaces bowel.
- Place the patient in the left lateral decubitus position.

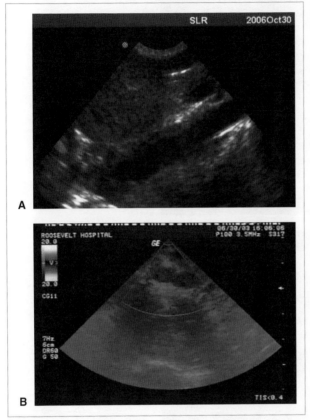

FIGURE 85.3: **A:** Longitudinal aorta. **B:** Transverse image of the common iliac bifurcation. (Images courtesy of David Riley, MD.)

Sonographic signs of abdominal aortic aneurysm

- Aortic diameter measuring 3 cm or greater
- Iliac vessel measuring 1.5 cm or greater

Complications
- Delay in definitive surgical treatment in order to perform study. Computed tomographic (CT) evaluation typically poses a greater time delay.

Common Pitfalls
- Large body habitus and small amounts of air, commonly from overlying bowel gas, may prevent adequate visualization. Increasing pressure or repositioning may overcome this obstacle.

- Failure to visualize the entire extent of the abdominal aorta and iliac bifurcation.
- Incorrect identification of the IVC as the aorta; the aorta lies to the left of the IVC. The aorta is pulsatile, thick-walled, and noncompressible, in contrast to the nonpulsatile, thin-walled, compressible IVC.
- Underestimation of aortic diameter as a result of measuring inner wall to inner wall; note that the extramural clot may occupy a significant portion of the lumen (see Fig. 85.4).

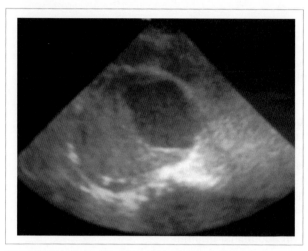

FIGURE 85.4: Large thrombus within the aortic lumen.

Pearls

- Always consider the diagnosis of AAA in the older patient with abdominal, back, or flank pain, especially in the setting of hypotension.
- Renal colic is the leading misdiagnosis for AAA. Exercise caution in attributing hematuria, flank pain, or hydronephrosis to nephrolithiasis in elderly patients.
- Young intravenous drug abuse patients can have mycotic AAAs.
- Free fluid in the abdomen may be absent because AAAs commonly rupture into the retroperitoneum. Ultrasound is a poor imaging modality for this area.
- Smaller aneurysms rupture less frequently than larger aneurysms; 22% of aneurysms >5 cm in diameter will rupture within 2 years.

Suggested Readings

Nevitt MP, Ballard DJ, Hallet JW Jr. Prognosis of abdominal aortic aneurysms. *N Engl J Med*. 1989;321:1009–1014.

Phalen MP, Emerman CL. Focused aortic ultrasound to evaluate the prevalence of abdominal aortic aneurysm in ED patients with high-risk symptoms. *Am J Emerg Med*. 2006;24(2):227–229.

Tayal VS, Tayal CD, Gibbs MA. Prospective study of accuracy and outcome of emergency ultrasound for abdominal aortic aneurysm over two years. *Acad Emerg Med*. 2003;10:867–871.

Indications

- Yes or no: Is there hydronephrosis suggestive of ureteral obstruction?
- Clinical suspicion of nephrolithiasis or ureteral colic
  - Abdominal or flank pain
  - Hematuria
  - Groin pain
- Other indications include the following:
  - Acute urinary retention
  - Known or suspected acute renal failure
    - Laboratory evidence of renal failure
    - Oliguria or anuria
    - Painless hematuria or proteinuria
  - Suspected renal abscess
    - Infected urine with fever and abdominal or flank pain
  - Suspected or known abdominal trauma

Contraindications

- None: No contrast or radiation involved

Risks/Consent Issues

- The only theoretical risk is allergy to the ultrasonography gel

Landmarks

- The right kidney is usually located inferior and posterior to the liver and can be located by placing the probe in the right upper quadrant (RUQ) and scanning laterally to the right flank.
- The left kidney is located inferior to the spleen and is most easily located by placing the probe over the left flank at the posterior axillary line (probe hand will likely need to be against the bed).
- The bladder should be imaged with the transducer placed suprapubically.

Technique

- A 3.5-MHz probe is commonly suitable for most adults although a 5.0-MHz probe can be used in patients with a thinner body habitus and in children.
- **The Right Kidney**
  - With the patient supine, start at the midaxillary line at the level of the lower ribs holding the probe in the longitudinal axis or slightly oblique and scan laterally until the sagittal view of the hepatorenal space (Morison pouch) and the right kidney are visible.

- Rotate the probe 90 degrees to obtain a transverse image of the kidney. Once in the transverse plane, move the probe superiorly and inferiorly to locate the renal hilum and visualize the full extent of the parenchyma.

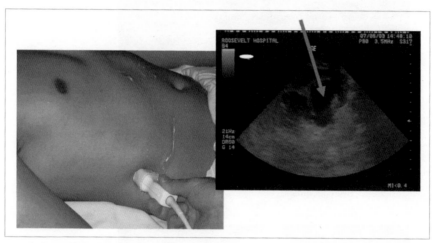

FIGURE 86.1: Renal ultrasonography.

- **The Left Kidney**
  - The left kidney is most easily located by placing the probe hand against the bed while scanning the left flank at the posterior axillary line at the level of the lower ribs.
  - The probe should be rotated 90 degrees to obtain a transverse view of the left kidney.
- **The Bladder**
  - The bladder is best imaged when it is moderately filled at the time of examination.
  - Place the probe suprapubically in the transverse plane. Angle the probe toward the patient's feet. Color Doppler techniques can be used over the trigone area to verify the presence of ureteral flow jets indicating urine flow into the bladder.
  - Once a transverse image of the bladder is obtained, rotate the probe 90 degrees to obtain a sagittal view.

Sonographic Signs of Obstructive Uropathy
- Hydronephrosis: Large, echofree areas seen within the echogenic renal sinus (see Fig. 86.2)
- Hydroureter: Echofree tubular structure arising from the renal sinus
- Stones: Ureteral stones are rarely visualized. These will appear as echogenic structures with posterior acoustic shadowing (see Fig. 86.3).
- Absence of ureteral flow jets

Other Common and Emergent Abnormalities
- Renal abscesses: Typically solitary, round hypoechoic masses
- Renal masses: May be isoechoic, hypoechoic, or hyperechoic in their appearance
- Renal cysts: Anechoic, smooth surface, round or oval, typically eccentrically placed

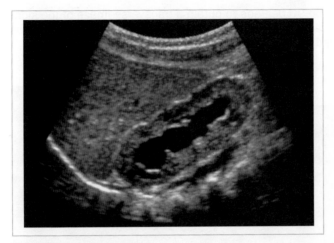

FIGURE 86.2: Hydronephrosis.

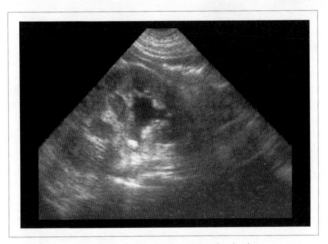

FIGURE 86.3: Echogenic stone casting acoustic shadow.

Common Pitfalls

- Limited, goal-directed ultrasonography of the kidneys looking for hydronephrosis as evidence of ureteral obstruction is within the scope of the emergency physician. The emergency physician is not expected to identify subtle abnormalities in the kidneys, ureters, or bladder.
- Always visualize the kidney and bladder in two planes (e.g., sagittal and transverse).
- Hydronephrosis is a nonspecific finding because it can occur with other states, such as abdominal aortic aneurysm, pregnancy, or intra-abdominal masses compressing the ureters and urinary outlet obstruction (see Fig. 86.4).
- Presence of hydronephrosis may be masked by dehydration.
- Prominent renal pyramids and renal cysts can mimic hydronephrosis.
- The afferent and efferent vessels of the kidney can sometimes be mistaken for a dilated ureter, and color Doppler can help differentiate mild hydronephrosis from blood vessels.

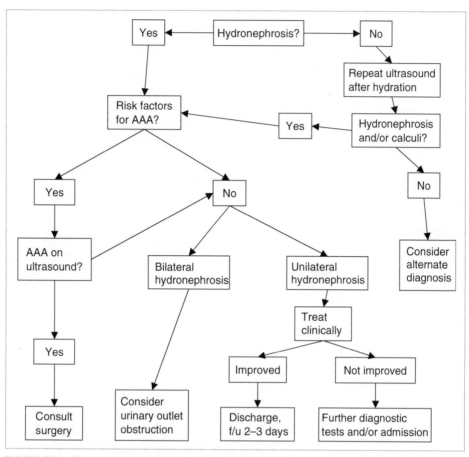

FIGURE 86.4: Hydronephrosis algorithm. AAA, abdominal aortic aneurysm.

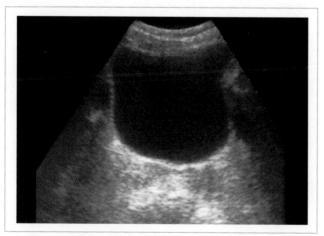

FIGURE 86.5: Bladder filled with urine.

Pearls

- When looking to detect clinically relevant abnormalities due to nephro/urolithiasis, (e.g., unilateral hydronephrosis and/or urolithiasis in patients with an obstructing calculus) the sensitivity of ultrasonography is 92%.
- Always scan both kidneys. If hydronephrosis is seen bilaterally, suspect a urinary outlet obstruction, particularly if there is a distended bladder (see Fig. 86.5) and oliguria.
- False-negative scans are encountered in markedly dehydrated patients.
- In the absence of trauma, a perinephric fluid collection may represent calyceal rupture and extravasation of urine resulting from high-grade obstruction.
- Always scan the aorta to rule out an abdominal aortic aneurysm (AAA) in the patient with flank/abdominal pain with risk factors of AAA.

Suggested Readings

Ma OJ, Mateer JR. *Emergency ultrasound*. New York: McGraw-Hill; 2003.

Brown DF, Rosen CL, Wolfe RE. Renal ultrasonography. *Emerg Med Clin North Am.* 1997;15(4):877–893.

Index

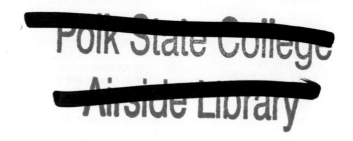